# Polytrauma Rehabilitation

*Editors*

BLESSEN C. EAPEN
DAVID X. CIFU

# PHYSICAL MEDICINE AND REHABILITATION CLINICS OF NORTH AMERICA

www.pmr.theclinics.com

*Consulting Editor*
SANTOS F. MARTINEZ

February 2019 • Volume 30 • Number 1

**ELSEVIER**

1600 John F. Kennedy Boulevard • Suite 1800 • Philadelphia, Pennsylvania, 19103-2899

http://www.theclinics.com

**PHYSICAL MEDICINE AND REHABILITATION CLINICS OF NORTH AMERICA** Volume 30, Number 1
February 2019 ISSN 1047-9651, ISBN 978-0-323-65517-0

Editor: Lauren Boyle
Developmental Editor: Meredith Madeira

*Reprints.* For copies of 100 or more of articles in this publication, please contact the Commercial Reprints Department, Elsevier Inc., 360 Park Avenue South, New York, NY 10010-1710. Tel.: 212-633-3874; Fax: 212-633-3820; E-mail: reprints@elsevier.com.

*Physical Medicine and Rehabilitation Clinics of North America* (ISSN 1047-9651) is published quarterly by Elsevier Inc., 360 Park Avenue South, New York, NY 10010-1710. Months of issue are February, May, August, and November. Business and Editorial Offices: 1600 John F. Kennedy Blvd., Suite 1800, Philadelphia, PA 19103-2899. Customer Service Office: 3251 Riverport Lane, Maryland Heights, MO 63043. Periodicals postage paid at New York, NY and additional mailing offices. Subscription price per year is $304.00 (US individuals), $600.00 (US institutions), $100.00 (US students), $366.00 (Canadian individuals), $790.00 (Canadian institutions), $210.00 (Canadian students), $429.00 (foreign individuals), $790.00 (foreign institutions), and $210.00 (foreign students). Foreign air speed delivery is included in all *Clinics* subscription prices. All prices are subject to change without notice. **POSTMASTER:** Send address changes to *Physical Medicine and Rehabilitation Clinics of North America*, Customer Service Office: Elsevier Health Sciences Division, Subscription Customer Service, 3251 Riverport Lane, Maryland Heights, MO 63043. **Customer Service: 1-800-654-2452 (US). From outside of the United States, call 314-447-8871. Fax: 314-447-8029. E-mail: JournalsCustomer Service-usa@elsevier.com (for print support); JournalsOnlineSupport-usa@elsevier.com (for online support).**

*Physical Medicine and Rehabilitation Clinics of North America* is indexed in *Excerpta Medica, MEDLINE/ PubMed (Index Medicus), Cinahl, and Cumulative Index to Nursing and Allied Health Literature.*

# Contributors

## CONSULTING EDITOR

**SANTOS F. MARTINEZ, MD, MS**
Diplomate of the American Academy of Physical Medicine and Rehabilitation,
Certificate of Added Qualification Sports Medicine, Assistant Professor, Department
of Orthopaedics, Campbell Clinic Orthopaedics, University of Tennessee, Memphis,
Tennessee

## EDITORS

**BLESSEN C. EAPEN, MD**
Chief, Department of Physical Medicine and Rehabilitation, VA Greater Los Angeles Health
Care System, Los Angeles, California

**DAVID X. CIFU, MD**
Department of Physical Medicine and Rehabilitation, Virginia Commonwealth University,
U.S. Department of Veterans Affairs, VA/DoD Chronic Effects of NeuroTrauma
Consortium, Richmond, Virginia

## AUTHORS

**JOSEPH F. ALDERETE, MD**
Center for the Intrepid, Department of Orthopaedic Surgery, Brooke Army Medical Center,
JBSA Fort Sam Houston, San Antonio, Texas

**MEREDITH ANDERSON, DO**
Department of Physical Medicine and Rehabilitation, Tufts Medical Center, Boston,
Massachusetts

**MICHAEL ARMSTRONG, MD**
Service Chief, Assistant Professor, Department of Physical Medicine and Rehabilitation,
Minneapolis VA Health Care System, University of Minnesota, Minneapolis, Minnesota

**LAUREN AVELLONE, PhD, BCBA**
Research Associate, Rehabilitation Research and Training Center, Virginia
Commonwealth University, Richmond, Virginia

**OGO AZUH, MD**
Department of Physical Medicine and Rehabilitation, Tufts Medical Center, Boston,
Massachusetts

**KATHLEEN M. BAIN, PhD**
Neuropsychology Fellow, Polytrauma Transitional Rehabilitation Program (PTRP),
South Texas Veterans Health Care System (STVHCS), San Antonio, Texas

**SHANNON L. BARNICOTT, MS, OTR**
Center for the Intrepid, Department of Rehabilitation Medicine, Brooke Army Medical
Center, JBSA Fort Sam Houston, San Antonio, Texas

**SHARON BARTON, MS, CRC, CRP**
Vocational Rehabilitation Counselor, Service Member Transitional Advanced
Rehabilitation (STAR) Program, Hunter Holmes McGuire VA Medical Center, Richmond,
Virginia

**SAURABHA BHATNAGAR, MD**
Associate Director Physical Medicine and Rehabilitation Residency, Department of
Physical Medicine and Rehabilitation, Harvard Medical School, Massachusetts General
Hospital, Spaulding Rehabilitation Hospital, Boston, Massachusetts

**AMY O. BOWLES, MD**
Chief, Brain Injury Rehabilitation Service, Deputy Chief, Department of Rehabilitation
Medicine, Brooke Army Medical Center, JBSA, Fort Sam Houston, San Antonio, Texas;
Associate Professor of Physical Medicine and Rehabilitation, Uniformed Services
University of the Health Sciences, Bethesda, Maryland

**JILL M. CANCIO, OTD, OTR/L, CHT**
Center for the Intrepid, Department of Rehabilitation Medicine, Brooke Army Medical
Center, Extremity Trauma and Amputation Center of Excellence, JBSA Fort Sam
Houston, San Antonio, Texas

**JULIE CHAMPAGNE, MD**
Medical Director, Polytrauma Transitional Rehabilitation, Minneapolis VA Health Care
System, Minneapolis, Minnesota

**WALTER LEE CHILDERS, PhD, CP**
Center for the Intrepid, Department of Rehabilitation Medicine, Brooke Army Medical
Center, Extremity Trauma and Amputation Center of Excellence, JBSA Fort Sam
Houston, San Antonio, Texas

**MICHAEL CHU, DO**
Department of Physical Medicine and Rehabilitation, Tufts Medical Center, Boston,
Massachusetts

**SAMUEL T. CLANTON, MD, PhD**
Traumatic Brain Injury/Polytrauma Fellow, Hunter Holmes McGuire VA Medical Center,
Virginia Commonwealth University, Richmond, Virginia

**MICAELA CORNIS-POP, PhD**
National Polytrauma Program Manager, Rehabilitation and Prosthetic Services, McGuire
VA Medical Center, Associate Professor, Physical Medicine and Rehabilitation, Virginia
Commonwealth University School of Medicine, Richmond, Virginia

**EDAN CRITCHFIELD, PsyD, ABPP-CN**
Neuropsychologist, Polytrauma Transitional Rehabilitation Program (PTRP), South Texas
Veterans Health Care System (STVHCS), San Antonio, Texas

**LESLI CULVER, LCSW**
Telerehabilitation Enterprise-Wide Initiative Director, Department of Physical Medicine
and Rehabilitation, James A. Haley Veterans' Hospital, Tampa, Florida

**SALLY H. DANG, OD**
Optometry Service, VA Long Beach Healthcare System, Long Beach, California

**WILLIAM SCOTT DEWEY, PT**
Chief, Rehabilitation Services, Army Burn Center, U.S. Army Institute of Surgical
Research, JBSA Fort Sam Houston, Texas

**BLESSEN C. EAPEN, MD**
Chief, Department of Physical Medicine and Rehabilitation, VA Greater Los Angeles
Health Care System, Los Angeles, California

**INBAL ESHEL, MA, CCC-SLP**
Senior Principal Scientist, General Dynamics Health Solutions (GDHS), Contractor
Employee Supporting the Defense & Veterans Brain Injury Center, Clinical Affairs Division,
Silver Spring, Maryland

**SANDRA M. FOX, OD**
Surgical Service, Ophthalmology, Polytrauma Rehabilitation Center, South Texas
Veterans Health Care System (STVHCS), San Antonio, Texas

**PAWAN GALHOTRA, PT**
Polytrauma Director, Polytrauma Rehabilitation Center, Palo Alto Health Care System,
Palo Alto, California

**CHRISTOPHER J. GILLIS, OTR**
Occupational Therapist, Polytrauma Transitional Rehabilitation Program (PTRP), South
Texas Veterans Health Care System (STVHCS), San Antonio, Texas

**DAVID GLAZER, MD**
Medical Director, Polytrauma Rehabilitation Center, Hunter Holmes McGuire VA Medical
Center, Richmond, Virginia

**LANCE L. GOETZ, MD**
Spinal Cord Injury and Disorders Service, Hunter Holmes McGuire VA Medical Center,
Department of Physical Medicine and Rehabilitation, Virginia Commonwealth University,
Richmond, Virginia

**BRANDON J. GOFF, DO**
Center for the Intrepid, Department of Rehabilitation Medicine, Brooke Army Medical
Center, JBSA Fort Sam Houston, San Antonio, Texas

**MARIA TERESA GOMEZ-LANSIDEL, QTR, ABLS**
Occupational Therapist, Polytrauma Transitional Rehabilitation Program (PTRP), South
Texas Veterans Health Care System (STVHCS), San Antonio, Texas

**PRAVEEN GOOTAM, MD**
James A. Haley Veterans Hospital, Department of Psychiatry and Behavioral
Neurosciences, University of South Florida Medical School, Tampa, Florida

**CRYSTAL GOUDEAU, PT, DPT**
Physical Therapist, Polytrauma Transitional Rehabilitation Program (PTRP), South Texas
Veterans Health Care System (STVHCS), San Antonio, Texas

**MARY HIMMLER, MD**
Medical Director, Polytrauma Rehabilitation Center (4K), Minneapolis VA Health Care
System, Minneapolis, Minnesota

**SIDNEY R. HINDS II, MD, FAAN, COL, MC, USA**
Assistant Professor, Department of Neurology and Radiology, Uniformed Services
University of the Health Sciences, Bethesda, Maryland; Blast Injury Research Program
Coordinating Office (PCO), United States Army Medical Research and Materiel Command
(USAMRMC), Fort Detrick, Frederick, Maryland

**ANDREA J. IKEDA, MS, CP**
Center for the Intrepid, Department of Rehabilitation Medicine, Brooke Army Medical Center, Extremity Trauma and Amputation Center of Excellence, JBSA Fort Sam Houston, San Antonio, Texas

**BOOKER T. KING, MD, FACS**
COL, Medical Corps US Army, Co-Director, Army Burn Center, U.S. Army Institute of Surgical Research, JBSA, Fort Sam Houston, Texas

**PAUL KOONS, MS, OMS, CLVT, CBIS**
Blind Rehabilitation Service, Major Charles Robert Soltes, Jr. O.D. Blind Rehabilitation Center (BRC), Tibor Rubin VA Medical Center, Long Beach, California

**TRACY KRETZMER, PhD**
James A. Haley Veterans Hospital, Department of Psychology, University of South Florida Medical School, Tampa, Florida

**DANIEL KUO, DO**
Department of Physical Medicine and Rehabilitation, Tufts Medical Center, Boston, Massachusetts

**TIMOTHY LAVIS, MD**
Spinal Cord Injury and Disorders Service, Hunter Holmes McGuire VA Medical Center, Department of Physical Medicine and Rehabilitation, Virginia Commonwealth University, Richmond, Virginia

**KENNETH K. LEE, MD**
Chief, Spinal Cord Injury Division, Clement J Zablolcki Veterans Affairs Medical Center, Associate Professor, Department of Physical Medicine and Rehabilitation, Medical College of Wisconsin, Milwaukee, Wisconsin; Medical Director, National Veterans Wheelchair Games, U.S. Department of Veterans Affairs, Washington, DC

**TAMARA L. MCKENZIE-HARTMAN, PsyD**
James A. Haley Veterans Hospital, Tampa, Florida; Defense and Veterans Brain Injury Center (DVBIC), Silver Spring, Maryland

**BRYAN P. MERRITT, MD**
Assistant Professor, James A. Haley Veterans Hospital, Department of Neurology, University of South Florida Medical School, Tampa, Florida

**DIANE SCHRETZMAN MORTIMER, MD, MSN**
Assistant Professor, Department of Physical Medicine and Rehabilitation, University of Minnesota, Medical Director, Polytrauma Network Site, Minneapolis VA Health Care System, Minneapolis, Minnesota

**MELISSA OLIVER, MS, OTR/L**
Occupational Therapist, Assistive Technology Program Coordinator, McGuire VA Medical Center, Richmond, Virginia

**FREDERICK PECHARKA, MA, CRC, LPC-S**
Specialty Vocational Programs Manager, Supervisory Vocational Rehabilitation Counselor, Louis Stokes Cleveland VA Medical Center, Cleveland, Ohio

**MICHELLE PETERSON, DPT**
Emerging Consciousness Program Coordinator, Lead Physical Therapist, Polytrauma Rehabilitation Center (4K), Minneapolis VA Health Care System, Minneapolis, Minnesota

**LINDA M. PICON, MCD, CCC-SLP**
Senior Consultant for TBI, Rehabilitation and Prosthetic Services, Veterans Health Administration, Washington, DC

**CINDY POORMAN, MSPT**
National Telerehabilitation Program Manager, Physical Medicine and Rehabilitation, U.S. Department of Veterans Affairs, Washington, DC

**MELISSA R. RAY, MS, CCC-SLP**
Speech Language Pathologist, Brain Injury Rehabilitation Service, Brooke Army Medical Center, JBSA Fort Sam Houston, Texas

**KAVITHA P. REDDY, MD**
Whole Health System Clinical Director, Primary Care, VA St. Louis Health Care System, Assistant Clinical Professor, Emergency Medicine, Washington University School of Medicine, St Louis, Missouri

**WILLIAM A. ROBBINS, MD**
Medical Director, Polytrauma Transitional Rehabilitation Program (PTRP), Servicemember Transitional Advanced Rehabilitation (STAR) Program, Hunter Holmes McGuire VA Medical Center, Richmond, Virginia

**JOEL SCHOLTEN, MD**
Director, Physical Medicine and Rehabilitation, U.S. Department of Veterans Affairs, Washington, DC

**KATTI SORBORO, MEd, CRC, PHR**
Special Emphasis Program Manager - Disability, Vocational Rehabilitation Counselor, Louis Stokes Cleveland VA Medical Center, Cleveland, Ohio

**REBECCA N. TAPIA, MD**
Medical Director, Polytrauma Network Site, South Texas Veterans Health Care System, San Antonio, Texas, Adjunct Assistant Professor, Department of Rehabilitation Medicine, UT Health San Antonio, San Antonio, Texas

**MICHAEL J. UIHLEIN, MD**
Associate Medical Director, Emergency Medicine, Director, Adaptive Sports Medicine Clinic, Clement J. Zablocki Veterans Affairs Medical Center, Assistant Professor, Department of Emergency Medicine, Medical College of Wisconsin, Milwaukee, Wisconsin; Team Physician, Men's U.S. National Sled Hockey Team, USA Hockey, Colorado Springs, Colorado

**JOSEPH B. WEBSTER, MD**
Associate Professor, Department of Physical Medicine and Rehabilitation, Virginia Commonwealth University School of Medicine, Staff Physician, Physical Medicine and Rehabilitation, Hunter Holmes McGuire VA Medical Center, Richmond, Virginia

**PAUL WEHMAN, PhD**
Professor of Physical Medicine and Rehabilitation, Chairman, Division of Rehabilitation Research, Director of VCU-RRTC, Virginia Commonwealth University School of Medicine, Richmond, Virginia

**ALAN W. YOUNG, DO, FAAPMR**
Chief, Complementary and Integrative Medicine Service, Department of Pain Management, Brooke Army Medical Center, JBSA Fort Sam Houston, Texas; Clinical Assistant Professor, Rehabilitation Medicine, UT Health San Antonio, San Antonio, Texas

**CYNTHIA YOUNG, MS, CRC**
Vocational Rehabilitation Counselor, Service Member Transitional Advanced
Rehabilitation (STAR) Program, Hunter Holmes McGuire VA Medical Center, Richmond,
Virginia

# Contents

The Department of Veterans Affairs Polytrauma Transitional Rehabilitation
Program was established to extend the rehabilitation of veterans and
active duty service members past the acute phase and reintegrate them
into the community. Effective community reintegration is best achieved
with a diverse interdisciplinary team that treats patients' physical, cognitive, and psychological deficits in a collaborative approach. Barriers,
such as lack of accurate awareness of functional limitations and premorbid
psychosocial stressors, can limit the recovery process. Recovery from polytrauma injuries is often a lifelong process, with the goal of maximizing
functional independence and quality of life.

Spinal cord injury results in multiple secondary comorbidities, which vary
based on injury severity and other characteristics. Persons with spinal
cord injury are at lifelong risk for many complications, most of which are
at least partially preventable with proper medical care. The Veterans Health
Administration Spinal Cord Injury and Disorders (SCI&D) System of Care offers these evaluations to all persons in their registries. Annual evaluations
are performed at any of the 24 SCI&D Veterans Administration Centers
nationwide. This allows veterans to receive the care from an interdisciplinary team that specializes in the care of veterans with spinal cord injury.

The hand and arm are exceptionally dexterous, exquisitely sensitive, and
proficient in performing tasks and functions. Given the invaluable functions
of the upper extremity in daily life, replacement of a missing limb through
prosthetic substitution is challenging. Prosthetic and rehabilitation needs
of injured Service members from recent military conflicts have brought upper extremity amputation to the forefront, which has led to an increase in
attention and resource allocation. This article provides an overview of the
care of the upper extremity amputee including surgical considerations,
prosthetic design and fitting, and preprosthetic and post-prosthetic rehabilitation considerations.

Traumatic amputation can result from injuries sustained both within and
outside the military setting. Individuals with trauma-related amputations
have unique needs and require specialized management with an interdisciplinary team approach and care coordination across the continuum of

care to facilitate optimal outcomes. Management considerations include issues with the amputation itself, issues related to injury of other body parts, and the management of longer-term secondary conditions. Some of these issues are more prevalent and of greater severity in the early recovery period, whereas others develop later and have the potential for progressive worsening over time.

individuals who have experienced a TBI/concussion should be screened for vision symptoms and visual dysfunction. A TBI-specific eye examination is necessary to identify the visual sequelae of TBI and address any vision/ocular issues that may be contributing to other post-TBI complaints. A vision rehabilitation plan that includes vision therapy can improve visual dysfunction secondary to TBI. Combining office-based and home-based vision therapy training will maximize visual potential and functional results.

# PHYSICAL MEDICINE AND REHABILITATION CLINICS OF NORTH AMERICA

**FORTHCOMING ISSUES**

*May 2019*
Technological Advances in Rehabilitation
Joel Stein and Leroy R. Lindsay, *Editors*

*August 2019*
Medical Impairment and Disability
Evaluation, and Associated Medicolegal
Issues
Robert D. Rondinelli and
Marjorie Eskay-Auerbach, *Editors*

*November 2019*
Rehabilitation in Developing Countries
Joseph Jacob, *Editor*

**RECENT ISSUES**

*November 2018*
Value-Added Electrodiagnostics
Karen Barr and Ileana M. Howard, *Editors*

*August 2018*
Muscle Over-activity in Upper Motor
Neuron Syndrome: Assessment and
Problem Solving for Complex Cases
Miriam Segal, *Editor*

*May 2018*
Para and Adapted Sports Medicine
Yetsa A. Tuakli-Wosornu and
Wayne Derman, *Editors*

---

**SERIES OF RELATED INTEREST**

*Orthopedic Clinics*
*Clinics in Sports Medicine*

---

**VISIT THE CLINICS ONLINE!**
Access your subscription at:
www.theclinics.com

# Foreword
# A Heritage to Remember

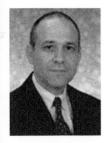

Santos F. Martinez, MD
*Consulting Editor*

In a world where medical specialties become ever more compartmentalized, we are reminded that the Physiatrist is trained with special qualities serving as a hub and catalyst for a team of gifted interdisciplinary practitioners. This culture of teamwork for achieving optimal functional outcome is imbedded in the Physiatrist's DNA and becomes particularly evident in caring for these warriors. From the tragedies and casualties of armed conflict emerged a specialty dedicated to reestablish one's dignity and functional return to society. This issue of the *Physical Medicine and Rehabilitation Clinics of North America* is very special and addresses difficult topics that have not previously been compiled in such a useful format.

Dr Eapen and Dr Cifu have completed a noble feat and have humbly given a gift to us all. The repercussions and benefits to future veterans, their families, and rehabilitation specialists will undoubtedly be impacted from this work. We owe them gratitude for reminding us all of the cost of freedom and for providing a guide for taking care of our fallen comrades.

Santos F. Martinez, MD
American Academy of Physical Medicine
and Rehabilitation
Campbell Clinic Orthopaedics
Department of Orthopaedics
University of Tennessee
Memphis, TN 38104, USA

*E-mail address:*
smartinez@campbellclinic.com

Phys Med Rehabil Clin N Am 30 (2019) xv
https://doi.org/10.1016/j.pmr.2018.10.002
1047-9651/19/© 2018 Published by Elsevier Inc.

pmr.theclinics.com

# Preface

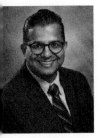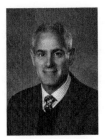

Blessen C. Eapen, MD    David X. Cifu, MD
*Editors*

It is a great privilege to have developed this issue of the *Physical Medicine and Rehabilitation Clinics of North America* dedicated to upholding Abraham Lincoln's declaration during his second Inaugural Address, *"To care for him who shall have borne the battle and for his widow, and his orphan,"* by focusing on the specialized rehabilitation needs of Polytrauma Rehabilitation in the Military and Veteran Populations. Polytrauma, defined as "two or more injuries, one of which may be life threatening, sustained in the same incident that affect multiple body parts or organ systems and result in physical, cognitive, psychological, or psychosocial impairments and functional disabilities," occurred in nearly 500,000 American service members during the Afghanistan and Iraqi Wars, and these complex injuries spurred yet another surge in the field of Physical Medicine and Rehabilitation (PM&R) ranging from the "signature injury" of traumatic brain injury, to the life-changing major physical injuries of burns, amputation, spinal cord injury, to the challenging physical and psychosocial insults of posttraumatic stress disorder, depression, and chronic pain. No other field but PM&R (including all team members) is so ideally suited to provide for the full range of acute and long-term needs of individuals who have sustained these polytrauma injuries and insults, during war time, and yet the degree of specialized training, knowledge, and experience required to apply all of the key aspects of PM&R care may be lacking in many practitioners. Thus, it was with considerable deliberation that we have assembled the foremost experts in the field of polytrauma rehabilitation medicine to construct this special issue.

The twin goals of this special issue on Polytrauma Rehabilitation in the Military and Veteran Populations are to provide readers with both a detailed overview of the current state of ever-expanding science supporting the diagnoses and management of the complex injuries and insults of war time, while at the same time providing a practical overview of the clinical advances in the field of PM&R that can be applied to this polytrauma population. In order to provide the often overlooked historical context of combat-related care, we also describe the legacy of the close collaboration between the Department of Defense (established around 1776) and the Department of Veterans Affairs (established around 1865) in caring for these complex patient populations. Finally,

Phys Med Rehabil Clin N Am 30 (2019) xvii–xviii
https://doi.org/10.1016/j.pmr.2018.10.001
1047-9651/19/© 2018 Published by Elsevier Inc.

pmr.theclinics.com

we have also made sure to provide reviews of the vast array of cutting-edge and innovative new rehabilitation treatment options that are being used and are being researched on these unique populations ranging from coma care to community reintegration.

We are thankful to all of our contributing authors for their hard work and dedication to both this special issue and the individuals that they care for. We would like to dedicate this issue not only to all of America's Heroes who are struggling daily to preserve all of our freedoms but also to those brave individuals who have sacrificed "the full measure" and given their lives in the protection of our great nation. This compilation is a small step in saluting all public servants, and we are hopeful that it can further the impact of PM&R providers in enhancing recoveries and supporting a return to wellness.

Blessen C. Eapen, MD
Department of Physical Medicine and Rehabilitation
VA Greater Los Angeles Health Care System
11301 Wilshire Boulevard
Los Angeles, CA 90073, USA

David X. Cifu, MD
Department of Physical Medicine and Rehabilitation
Virginia Commonwealth University
US Department of Veterans Affairs
VA/DoD Chronic Effects of
NeuroTrauma Consortium
1223 East Marshall Street
PO Box 980677
Richmond, VA 23284-0667, USA

E-mail addresses:
blessen.eapen2@va.gov (B.C. Eapen)
david.cifu@vcuhealth.org (D.X. Cifu)

# Rehabilitation in the Department of Veterans Affairs Polytrauma System of Care

## Historical Perspectives

Micaela Cornis-Pop, PhD[a,b,*], Sidney R. Hinds II, MD[c,d], Linda M. Picon, MCD, CCC-SLP[e], Rebecca N. Tapia, MD[f,g]

## KEYWORDS

- Screening • Evaluation • Plan of care • Practice guideline • Follow-up
- Longitudinal research

## KEY POINTS

- The Department of Veterans Affairs Polytrauma System of Care is a nationwide system of specialized rehabilitation programs.
- More than 1.1 million veterans were screened for a deployment-related traumatic brain injury.
- The Department of Veterans Affairs/Department of Defense Clinical Practice Guidelines for mild traumatic brain injury inform the provision of rehabilitation services and care.
- Department of Veterans Affairs and Department of Defense researchers collaborate in the study of the long-term effects of traumatic brain injury.

## INTRODUCTION

Although Operation Iraqi Freedom and Operation Enduring Freedom brought "invisible wounds of wars" into the households of around the country, organizations and systems of care were created before 9/11 to address the concerns of traumatic brain

Disclosure Statement: The authors have nothing to disclose.
[a] Rehabilitation and Prosthetic Services, McGuire VA Medical Center, 1201 Broad Rock Boulevard, Richmond, VA 23249, USA; [b] Physical Medicine and Rehabilitation, Virginia Commonwealth University-Medical College of Virginia, Richmond, VA, USA; [c] United States Army Medical Research and Material Command, 810 Schrieder Street, Fort Detrick, MD 21702-5012, USA; [d] Department of Neurology and Radiology, Uniformed Services University of the Health Sciences, Bethesda, MD, USA; [e] Rehabilitation and Prosthetic Services, Veterans Health Administration, 810 Vermont Avenue, Washington, DC 20420, USA; [f] Polytrauma Network Site, South Texas Veterans Health Care System, 7400 Merton Minter Blvd San Antonio, TX 78229; [g] Department of Rehabilitation Medicine, UT Health-San Antonio, San Antonio, TX, USA
* Corresponding author.
E-mail address: micaela.cornispop@va.gov

injury (TBI). In 1992, the Defense and Veterans Brain Injury Center (DVBIC) was created from what was formerly the Vietnam Veterans Head Injury Program.[1] DVBIC has always been an organization that has emphasized the strong foundation and belief of clinical care, research, and education. In fact, the introduction of the clear majority of professional articles written on military TBI quote the work of DVBIC when reporting the TBI worldwide numbers of service members and veterans.[2] From the beginning, DVBIC has been a partnership between the Department of Veterans Affairs (VA) and the Department of Defense (DoD). The importance of this fact is 2-fold: 4 VA facilities became DVBIC network sites in 1992 and these sites would later become hubs for the VA Polytrauma System of Care (PSC).[3,4] The success of this collaboration was instrumental in the 2005 VA mandate that would establish the PSC. The mandate was necessary to address the needs of those with TBI, but more specifically address the need for those who suffer polytrauma, which included TBI.[5] The purpose of this article is to inform the reader of the historical aspects of the PSC, understand the solutions that were implemented in addressing the continuum of care needs for service members and veterans, and provide an understanding of ongoing research efforts that will inform future solutions to strategically identified future care needs.

## EVOLUTION OF THE POLYTRAUMA SYSTEM OF CARE

Times of war have led to significant developments in armed combat and technology throughout history. Warfare also has provided the stimulus for major advancements in medical care and rehabilitation.[6] The Vietnam War, the Persian Gulf War, and more recently the wars in Afghanistan and Iraq served as catalysts for change in TBI rehabilitation. They effected change in medical and rehabilitation care for military-related TBI and activated the development of programs and services for TBI and polytrauma within DoD and VA.

A major expansion of knowledge about TBI in the military, particularly penetrating TBI, came from the landmark Vietnam Veterans Head Injury Study, which collected retrospective data on more than 1000 Vietnam Veterans who sustained a TBI between 1967 and 1970.[7] The Vietnam Veterans Study created the first TBI longitudinal patient registry, collecting data for more than 14 years and providing the most comprehensive insights to date into the medical, physical, neuropsychological, and social-behavioral characteristics of patients after military-related TBI. This study provided the foundational research for clinical care and rehabilitation of TBI in the military for years to come.

The VA has a long and distinguished history of providing rehabilitation services for veterans beginning with developing prosthetic devices for veterans with amputations returning from World War II. After the Vietnam War, the range of rehabilitation services increased to include "training for employment and independence in daily living."[8] During this time, rehabilitation for TBI was typically included with care for other neurogenic disorders.

Specialized TBI rehabilitation in VA can be traced back to congressional legislation that authorized the creation of the Defense and Veterans Head Injury Program in 1992. This program was the first that coordinated the care for TBI patients between 3 military facilities (the Walter Reed Army Medical Center, the Wilford Hall Medical Center, and the Naval Medical Center San Diego) and 4 VA TBI Lead Centers located at the medical centers in Minneapolis, Palo Alto, Richmond, and Tampa. This partnership led to a Memorandum of Agreement between the VA and the DoD to provide expert TBI rehabilitation care for service members at the 4 VA TBI Lead Centers. The centers offered comprehensive TBI rehabilitation care in dedicated inpatient bed units using interdisciplinary teams of rehabilitation providers and medical experts available for consultation at these tertiary care hospitals. VA specialists had the opportunity to participate in collaborative research projects that provided the impetus for the TBI clinical and research advancements that began with the wars in Afghanistan and Iraq.

Renamed the DVBIC in 2001, the DoD–VA collaboration for TBI care and research celebrated its 25th anniversary in 2017. This partnership enabled the development of leading clinical, research, and educational resources for service members and veterans with military-related TBI, their families, and their care providers. The first large-scale, randomized, controlled trial of cognitive rehabilitation for military-related TBI,[9] and the VA TBI Screening and Evaluation program described herein, are two of the remarkable collaborative accomplishments of this robust relationship.

Notably, DVBIC provided the foundation for the development of the VA PSC in 2005 beginning with the designation of the TBI Lead Centers as Polytrauma Rehabilitation Centers (PRCs). This pivotal partnership changed TBI care for service members and veterans by coordinating and advancing TBI research, education, policy, and clinical management. It created early opportunities that continue to this day to coordinate investigations, and develop provider tools and training, and educational products for patients, caregivers, and families.

## POLYTRAUMA SYSTEM OF CARE TODAY

Since its inception in 2005 with a focus on inpatient rehabilitation for the severely wounded, the VA PSC has evolved into a nationwide, integrated network of 124 rehabilitation programs dedicated to the care of veterans and service members with deployment- and non–deployment-related TBI and polytrauma.[10] Through this program, the VA continues to advance the diagnosis, evaluation, treatment, and understanding of TBI in a variety of ways, including establishing standardized diagnostic and assessment protocols, developing and implementing best clinical practices for care, collaborating with strategic partners, educating and training in TBI-related care and rehabilitation, and conducting, interpreting, and translating research findings into improved patient care and caregiver support. The PSC has grown, improved, and maintained its readiness through a coordinated program of education, training, and research (including integration with the DoD, academic partners, and private industry), and is continually working to socialize its services in ways that make it accessible to all veterans.

With its 4-tiered organizational setup, the PSC is designed to ensure access to a continuum of rehabilitation services, case management, family education and support, psychosocial services, and community reintegration assistance based on the needs of the veteran and proximity to the community where they live (**Fig. 1**).

### Polytrauma Rehabilitation Center

The PSC has 5 PRCs located at the medical centers in Minneapolis, Palo Alto, Richmond, San Antonio, and Tampa. The PRCs serve as regional referral centers for comprehensive acute inpatient rehabilitation. A dedicated staff of rehabilitation professionals and consultants is available to address complex and severe TBI and associated polytrauma. The PRCs function as resources for consultations and care coordination in their regions. Their staff participates in the development of clinical guidance and best practices, and integration of research activity and findings into the care system through education and knowledge translation. The PRCs are accredited by the Commission on Accreditation of Rehabilitation Facilities using Brain Injury Program standards.

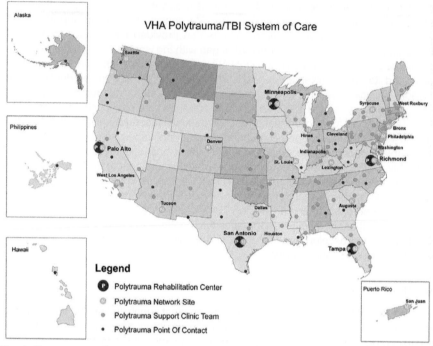

**Fig. 1.** Department of Veterans Affairs Polytrauma/traumatic brain injury system of care. (*From* https://www.polytrauma.va.gov/system-of-care/index.asp. Accessed October 10, 2018; with permission.)

## Polytrauma Network Site

The PSC operates 23 Polytrauma Network Sites (PNSs) distributed, 1 or 2, in each Veterans Integrated Service Network. Rehabilitation care at the PNSs focuses on outpatient services, but inpatient bed units are also available to address postacute and chronic complications. PNSs maintain a full complement of rehabilitation professionals on staff to address TBI- and polytrauma-related symptoms and functional deficits. PNS staff provide clinical and administrative oversight of the PSC programs within their Veterans Integrated Service Network, including care coordination, managing referrals, and consultations and advising on the collection and reporting of access and outcome data. The inpatient rehabilitation bed units at the PNSs maintain Commission on Accreditation of Rehabilitation Facilities accreditation for a Comprehensive Integrated Inpatient Rehabilitation Program.

## Polytrauma Support Clinic Team

PSC oversees 91 polytrauma support clinic teams distributed across VA medical centers and facilities. The polytrauma support clinic teams provide and coordinate outpatient interdisciplinary rehabilitation care for veterans and service members typically focused on the catchment area of their medical facility. Polytrauma support clinic teams also conduct comprehensive evaluations of patients with positive TBI screens, and develop and implement rehabilitation and community reintegration plans of care.

## Polytrauma Point of Contact

PSC has 34 polytrauma points of contact that deliver a more limited range of rehabilitation services, including evaluations for TBI and polytrauma related problems and treatments delivered by individual rehabilitation providers. Whenever necessary, the polytrauma point of contact works with the PNS in their Veterans Integrated Service Network for consultations and direct services using telehealth solutions.

## POLYTRAUMA SYSTEM OF CARE IN NUMBERS

- There were 3944 veterans and service members with severe TBI and polytrauma treated at the PRCs from 2003 to 2017.
- There were 165 veterans and service members with disorders of consciousness treated at the PRCs from 2010 to 2017.
- More than 1000 veterans enrolled in the VA PRC TBI Model Systems project to track long-term outcomes.
- There were 86,877 veterans with TBI who health care services in the VA in 2017.
- There were 8431 Individualized Rehabilitation and Community Reintegration (IRCR) Care Plans completed in 2017.
- More than 1.1 million post 9/11 veterans screened for possible TBI from 2007 to 2017.
- There was a $284.1 million VA investment in TBI care for veterans in 2017.
- There was $34 million in VA direct funding for 151 projects in TBI research in 2017.

## SCREENING AND EVALUATION OF TRAUMATIC BRAIN INJURY

In April 2007, the VA initiated a nationwide, evidence-supported screening program to identify veterans with deployment-related exposure to potentially concussive events. Veterans with positive screening results are offered a uniform assessment procedure, available in-person or virtually, to evaluate and diagnose TBI-related symptoms and to guide management interventions using a nationally developed Clinical Practice Guideline (see the Clinical Practice Recommendations section, elsewhere in this article).

Mandatory screening for deployment-related TBI includes 4 sets of questions related to the initial mechanism of injury, symptoms synchronous with the injury event, and their persistence or resolution up to the current week. TBI screening is based on a measure developed by the DVBIC that had limited field testing.[11] The goal of the VA's TBI screen is to identify veterans with symptoms related to a history of mild TBI who would otherwise not be identified or receive appropriate rehabilitation care.

Based on extensive research, the VA-TBI Screening Tool has revealed good sensitivity and acceptable specificity allowing VA to identify symptomatic veterans and develop appropriate plans of care.[12] Of the more than 1.1 million veterans who have been screened for deployment related TBI between 2007 and 2017, approximately 20% had positive screens and were referred for further evaluation.

TBI specialists conducted approximately 154,350 Comprehensive TBI Evaluations between 2007 and 2017 to establish a diagnosis and make treatment recommendations. The TBI diagnosis was confirmed in 93,916 cases (61%) and veterans were referred for services, as appropriate. Similar actions were taken if the diagnosis was not confirmed but the veterans needed services to address health care concerns.

The Comprehensive TBI Evaluation is a structured clinical interview that includes a detailed history related to the initial injury exposure, immediate symptoms after the injury, completion of the Neurobehavioral Symptom Inventory,[13] confirmation of the TBI diagnosis, and development of a care plan. Treatment varies by the type and severity of the initial injury and subsequent residual symptoms, and is delivered within the context of an individualized care plan that integrates veteran's rehabilitation goals with services from an interdisciplinary team of rehabilitation specialists.

## INDIVIDUALIZED REHABILITATION AND COMMUNITY REINTEGRATION CARE PLAN

Given the multiple comorbidities often associated with TBI, the hallmark of TBI rehabilitation in PSC is interdisciplinary care. In outpatient settings, however, the management of services can be particularly challenging owing to the need to coordinate schedules and priorities across patients, clinicians, and locations. Effective communication among all parties involved becomes essential for the delivery of integrated care. To support this requirement, the PSC implemented a templated electronic IRCR Care Plan that serves to ensure that goals are communicated and coordinated, interventions are prioritized to focus on maximum functional improvement, and treatment efforts are not duplicated or in conflict.[14]

IRCR care plans are used to document interdisciplinary rehabilitation care and case management delivered across all PSC programs. The care plan follows from the comprehensive interdisciplinary assessment and addresses the following elements:

a. Rehabilitation goals that reflect the veteran's rehabilitation priorities and target maximizing independence and community reintegration,
b. Specific rehabilitation treatments and other services necessary to achieve the rehabilitation goals, including the type, frequency, estimated duration, and location of such treatments and services,
c. Plan reviews conducted on schedule and ad hoc to gauge the effectiveness of the plan and to apply modifications, as necessary, and
d. Access to all appropriate rehabilitative components of the PSC continuum and including community reintegration options and services.

A spectrum of treatment options based on the VA/DoD Clinical Practice Guidelines (CPGs) and other nationally developed best practice recommendations are available to veterans with TBI in all PSC programs. These services can take many forms, including but not limited to health care services, individual and group therapy, education and counseling, vocational and employment services, social and independent living skills, healthy living recommendations, and telerehabilitation. Services provided are based on the individual veteran's clinical preferences and needs. Not all veterans require the entire continuum of services. Veterans must be able to move among the levels of the continuum as is clinically appropriate, with minimal disruption in treatment, and in a manner that facilitates positive treatment outcomes.

In the past year, the VA developed the capacity to examine the IRCR care plans longitudinally to ensure that veterans with chronic problems related to TBI and polytrauma receive proactive, coordinated services.

### Long-Term Management of Traumatic Brain Injury/Polytrauma-Related Disabilities

In the last decade, the medical community has increasingly recognized the long-term neurologic effects of TBI. The concept of brain injury as a chronic condition was originally introduced by Masel and DeWitt,[15] who emphasized the importance of managing the symptoms of brain injury beyond the acute setting to address ongoing needs including prevention of medical complications and providing services geared toward community reintegration. Following along these lines, participants at the 2013 Galveston Brain Injury Conference developed a set of recommendations toward the implementation of a Chronic Care Model in Brain Injury, including the importance of clinical guidelines and surveillance technologies, improved specialist–primary care provider communication, and risk-stratified self-management support and case management.[16]

As a system of care, PSC was the first adopter of the TBI chronic care model focusing initially on the care of veterans with moderate to severe TBI and later including patients with mild injuries and complex comorbidities who have difficulties with community reintegration and those who experience functional decline over time. The PSC provides long-term rehabilitation management services to sustain and prevent loss of functional gains and to contribute to maximizing the veteran's independence and quality of life. The long-term management of rehabilitation needs for veterans with TBI and polytrauma is coordinated through their primary care clinicians and supported by teams of rehabilitation specialists with veteran-centric training and experience.

In designing a disease management approach to chronic brain injury, the PSC took the following steps.

a. Developing a framework for identifying veterans at risk for functional and participation decline using *International Classification of Diseases,* 10th edition, codes, longitudinal review of the IRCR care plans and score on the Mayo Portland Participation Index indicative of community reintegration difficulties. Programs are encouraged to use clinical judgment to develop their own lists of candidates for follow-up services.

b. Creating an automated report system that tracks IRCR care plans and Mayo Portland Participation Index results across episodes of care.

c. Establishing joint educational encounters and resource sharing opportunities with primary care and mental health providers to establish frameworks for referrals and consultations.

d. Fast growing use of telehealth technologies including in-home telehealth to connect veterans with TBI specialists and allow effective monitoring of rehabilitation needs.

**Table 1** describes the guidance disseminated across the PSC regarding the conduct of follow-up rehabilitation care.

## COLLABORATIONS WITH STRATEGIC PARTNERS

The VA maintains ongoing collaboration with the DoD, DVBIC, the Centers for Disease Control and Prevention, and National Institutes of Health, specifically focusing on ways to (1) improve TBI identification, (2) enhance standardized TBI reporting, (3) diagnose severity of TBI, and (4) improve treatment of TBI. The VA maintains ongoing collaboration with the National Institute on Disability and Rehabilitation Research Traumatic Brain Injury Model Systems Program to enable VA to perform multicenter research protocols in collaboration with academic centers of excellence in TBI.[17] Along with the 16 academic Traumatic Brain Injury Model Systems centers, the VA PRCs are now full voting members of the core Traumatic Brain Injury Model Systems program.

## CLINICAL PRACTICE GUIDELINES

The VA and DoD have worked closely over the last decade to standardize care to reduce unintended variations in clinical practice and services that could negatively impact outcomes after TBI. They also work closely with academic partners and industry to evaluate, classify, and deliver care that meets the highest level of evidence

**Table 1**
**Stratification for Acquired Brain Injury follow-up care**

| | Description | Management | Follow-up |
|---|---|---|---|
| ABI1 | Totally dependent, 24-h caregiving, including disorders of consciousness | Management centered around avoidance of adverse events (skin breakdown, aspiration, infections), supporting caregivers, life-planning, respite, nutrition, bowel/bladder, spasticity, and secretions | Annual and as needed Clinic visit Family conference IRCR review |
| ABI2 | High-need, 24-h caregiving, alert and able to communicate but dependent for most care, lacks capacity | Management centered around avoidance of adverse events, supporting caregivers, life planning, respite, and nutrition | Annual and as needed Clinic visit Family conference IRCR review |
| ABI3 | Ambulatory, largely independent for self-care (bathing, showering, toileting), alert and conversational but lacks capacity for medical decisions and requires 24-h supervision | Management centered around behavioral modification, setting boundaries, family dynamics, and respite | Annual and as needed Clinic visit Family conference IRCR review |
| ABI4 | Independent for self-care, does not require supervision but may receive help from others, reintegration is below expected level of function and may have active rehabilitation goals, retains capacity but may involve POA | Determining limitations or barriers to reintegration, symptom-based approach, Neuropsychological testing, behavioral modification, mental health, and family support | Annual and as needed More frequent with active rehabilitation goals IRCR review |
| ABI5 | Independent for self-care, but still struggling with sequelae such as neurogenic bowel, headaches, decision making, and higher level life skills; retains capacity | Supporting current level of reintegration, addressing individual symptoms, and ongoing psychological or family support | Annual and as needed Clinic visit IRCR review |
| ABI6 | Fully reintegrated, no ongoing needs related to traumatic brain injury | Educating patient about resources available, addressing individual symptoms, discussion of indications to return for care | As needed |

*Abbreviations:* IRCR, Individualized Rehabilitation and Community Reintegration; POA, power of attorney.

available. Their combined clinical, education, and research missions as well as collaboration with other federal and external partners provides the synergistic platform for the identification of knowledge gaps, study development, translation of findings, and dissemination and implementation of best practices.

The VA/DoD CPG are based on an intensive search and review of the highest level of evidence available at the time of publication.[18] Cpgs are not intended to define a standard of care or prevent a provider from using clinical judgment and patient-centered options. Rather, they provide practitioners with a comprehensive look at the state of the science and offer evidence-based management guidance.

The VA and DoD initially published the CPG for the management of concussion/mild TBI in 2009 and updated it in 2016. It covers the management of postacute (>7 days after onset) and chronic (any length of time >30 days) symptomatic mild TBI. The mild TBI CPG is not applicable to the acute concussion period, that is, less than 7 days after onset. Experts involved in the development of the mild TBI CPG took into consideration the strength of the evidence, but also balancing positive outcomes with potential harms of treatment, equity of resource availability, the intended population and settings of care, and the potential for variations in provider and patient values and preferences.

The mild TBI CPG is formatted into 23 best practice recommendations covering symptoms commonly reported by those with a history of mild TBI stratified into physical symptoms (eg, headache, dizziness and balance disruptions, sensory abnormalities, sleep disturbances), cognitive symptoms (eg, problems with attention/concentration, memory), and behavioral/emotional disturbances (eg, depression, anxiety, irritability). A practical component of the CPG is the Clinical Symptom Management section, offering pharmacologic and nonpharmacologic, consensus-based and common practice options for symptom management. The mild TBI CPG contains 2 algorithms that inform the critical decision points in the management of symptoms related to a history of mild TBI depending on whether the patient presents for an initial visit, or if the visit is related to management of persisting or new onset symptoms.

In addition to supporting the mild TBI CPG development, the DVBIC also produced clinical recommendations as clinical practice tools that expand the recommendations outlined in the VA/DoD CPG for mild TBI. Clinical recommendations are developed by DVBIC in collaboration with subject matter experts from the DoD, VA, and academia to provide consensus-based guidance where evidence is lacking. Based on the commonly occurring symptoms experienced by service members and veterans with a history of TBI, the DVBIC has clinical recommendations and a host of related training products targeting assessment and treatment indicators for headache, sleep, visual disturbances, dizziness, neuroendocrine dysfunction, and cognitive rehabilitation.[19]

## RESEARCHING THE LONG-TERM EFFECTS OF TRAUMATIC BRAIN INJURY

In 2013, in the annals of the federal government addressed the issues of mild TBI for 2 reasons: funding of the Chronic Effects of Neurotrauma Consortium (CENC) and the establishment of the National Research Action Plan. The National Research Action Plan was launched in response to President Obama's Executive Order, "Improving Access to Mental Health Services for Veterans, Service Members, and Military Families," dated August 31, 2012. The DoD, VA, Department of Health and Human Services, and Department of Education were directed to formulate the strategic roadmap to address the research issues surrounding TBI and behavioral health. The focus was advancing the knowledge of the missing components of these military and national health problems. The recommendation from the National Research

Action Plan experts included developing new technologies to assess these conditions, creating repositories for biosamples and tissue, creating a more useful classification of TBI (to better test diagnostics and therapeutics), and creating a means to share research data.[20]

Started at the same time as the National Research Action Plan, the CENC is a coordinated, multicenter, research collaboration between the VA and DoD, jointly funded in 2013 to effectively address the diagnostic and therapeutic ramifications of TBI and its long-term effects.[21] The CENC brings together a nationwide group of researchers from VA, DoD, academia, and the private sector to address gaps in basic science, brain health, and neurodegeneration with the goal of contributing to the development of guidelines for the prevention, protection, and diagnostic and therapeutic interventions for identified service members and veterans at all levels of risk and susceptibility (**Fig. 2**).

CENC efforts are centered in Richmond, Virginia, and are anchored between the VA Polytrauma Rehabilitation Center and Virginia Commonwealth University. This nucleus provides the leadership and guidance to the member institutions. The CENC has 5 cores that direct and provide standardization and analyses to investigators executing CENC research efforts: Data and Study Management Core, Biorepository, Biostatistics, Neuroimaging, and Neuropathology. The cores provide data quality control as a dynamic process that identifies data collection errors early to avoid repetitive, large, and costly problems that would adversely affect study results and power.

The main research study, the Observational Study on Late Neurologic Effects of Operation Enduring Freedom/Operation Iraqi Freedom/Operation New Dawn Combat (referred to as Study 1) obtains a detailed history of the top 10 brain injuries a participant has sustained, followed by objective testing to include neuropsychological batteries, physical examinations, neuroimaging, and biomarker testing. To date, more than 1200 participants have been enrolled in this study.[22] In addition to the primary study, the CENC was directed to incorporate other research efforts into the consortium. These include neurootolith, retinal thickness, blast-related cohort follow-up, balance assessments, diffuse tensor imaging analyses and diffuse tensor imaging diffuse tensor imaging phantom creation. Several of these studies contribute patients

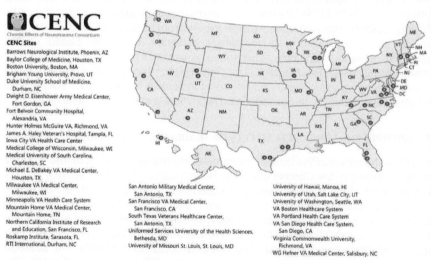

# CENC
Chronic Effects of Neurotrauma Consortium

**CENC Sites**

Barrows Neurological Institute, Phoenix, AZ
Baylor College of Medicine, Houston, TX
Boston University, Boston, MA
Brigham Young University, Provo, UT
Duke University School of Medicine, Durham, NC
Dwight D. Eisenhower Army Medical Center, Fort Gordon, GA
Fort Belvoir Community Hospital, Alexandria, VA
Hunter Holmes McGuire VA, Richmond, VA
James A. Haley Veteran's Hospital, Tampla, FL
Iowa City VA Health Care Center
Medical College of Wisconsin, Milwaukee, WI
Medical University of South Carolina, Charleston, SC
Michael E. DeBakey VA Medical Center, Houston, TX
Milwaukee VA Medical Center, Milwaukee, WI
Minneapolis VA Health Care System
Mountain Home VA Medical Center, Mountain Home, TN
Northern California Institute of Research and Education, San Francisco, FL
Roskamp Institute, Sarasota, FL
RTI International, Durham, NC

San Antonio Military Medical Center, San Antonio, TX
San Francisco VA Medical Center, San Francisco, CA
South Texas Veterans Healthcare Center, San Antonio, TX
Uniformed Services University of the Health Sciences, Bethesda, MD
University of Missouri St. Louis, St. Louis, MD

University of Hawaii, Manoa, HI
University of Utah, Salt Lake City, UT
University of Washington, Seattle, WA
VA Boston Healthcare System
VA Portland Health Care System
VA San Diego Health Care System, San Diego, CA
Virginia Commonwealth University, Richmond, VA
WG Hefner VA Medical Center, Salisbury, NC

**Fig. 2.** Chronic Effects of Neurotrauma Consortium sites. (*From* https://cenc.rti.org/Consortium-Members/Participating-Organizations. Accessed October 10, 2018; with permission.)

o Study 1. To date, the CENC has produced more than 32 peer-reviewed articles. Interim analyses of CENC results are featured in a special issue of *Brain Injury*, scheduled to be published in September 2018.

Although the CENC focuses on the long-term effects of mild TBI, another VA/DoD research collaboration covers all TBI severity levels. The prospective longitudinal study to "Improve Understanding of Medical and Psychological Needs (IMAP) in Veterans and Service members with Chronic Traumatic Brain Injury (TBI)," was initiated in May of 2015. This study complements the congressionally mandated 15-Year Longitudinal Study of the Effects of TBI (SEC 721. National Defense Authorization Act (NDAA) 2007), which was initiated in April of 2011 and currently is underway at Walter Reed National Military Medical Center.[23] The IMaP is based at the Tampa Polytrauma Rehabilitation Center with partnering sites at the Minneapolis, Richmond, and the San Antonio Polytrauma Centers and focuses on comorbid conditions associated with TBI, chronic effects, and long-term needs such as rehabilitation and activities of daily living services.

The clinical implication of this work is that knowledge translation of research findings from IMAP can help to improve the VA's ability to meet the long-term needs of veterans with TBI. Analysis and dissemination of findings help to educate the field on the types of enhancements needed in clinical care at PRCs to mitigate problems associated with chronic TBI, and the types of changes needed to provide the most appropriate TBI follow-up recommendations and services to veterans and service members with TBI.[24]

## SUMMARY

As with all diseases and disorders common to veterans, the VA is leading the world in identifying, developing, studying, and implementing real-world solutions that benefit veterans today and all Americans for the future. The VA's PSC represents a functional and effective partnership among the VA, DoD, other federal agencies and civilian institutions to provide state of the science care while pursuing research excellence to improve the care of service members, veterans, and the public at large. The PSC is particularly poised to lead veterans care in TBI with polytrauma now and in the future based on its logical, scientific, and dynamic processes, which seek to improve on the care as new evidence presents itself.

## REFERENCES

1. Jaffee M, Martin EM. Defense and Veterans Brain Injury Center: program overview and research initiatives. Mil Med 2010;175(7 Suppl):37–41.
2. Defense and Veterans Brain Injury Center. DoD worldwide TBI numbers. Available at: http://dvbic.dcoe.mil/files/tbi-numbers/worldwide-totals-2000-2017_feb-14-2018_v1.0_2018-03-08.pdf. Accessed February 14, 2018.
3. Pasquina PF, Cooper RA, editors. Care of the combat amputee. Washington, DC: Office of the Surgeon General, United States Army, US Government Printing Office, Borden Institute; 2009.
4. Salazar AM, Zitnay GA, Warden DL, et al. Defense and veterans head injury program: background and overview. J Head Trauma Rehabil 2000;15(5):1081–91.
5. Title 38 U.S.Code 7327. "Centers for research, education, and clinical activities on complex multi-trauma." Available at: https://www.law.cornell.edu/uscode/text/38/7327. Accessed April 9, 2018.
6. Cifu DX, Cohen SI, Lew HL, et al. The history and evolution of traumatic brain injury rehabilitation in military service members and veterans. J Phys Med Rehabil 2010;89:688–94.

7. Sweeney JK, Smutok MA. Vietnam head injury study: preliminary analysis of the functional and anatomical sequelae of penetrating head trauma. Phys Ther 1983; 63:2018–25.
8. Department of Veterans Affairs (VA). VA history in brief. Available at: https://www.va.gov/opa/publications/archives/docs/history_in_brief.pdf. Accessed April 3, 2018.
9. Cooper DB, Bowles AO, Kennedy JE, et al. Cognitive rehabilitation for military service members with mild traumatic brain injury: a randomized clinical trial. J Head Trauma Rehabil 2016;32(3):E1–15.
10. VA Polytrauma System of Care. Available at: https://www.polytrauma.va.gov/. Accessed April 3, 2018.
11. Schwab KA, Ivins B, Cramer G, et al. Screening for traumatic brain injury in troops returning from deployment in Afghanistan and Iraq: initial investigation of the usefulness of a short screening tool for traumatic brain injury. J Head Trauma Rehabil 2007;22:377–89.
12. Belanger HG, Vanderploeg RD, Sayer N. Screening for remote history of mild traumatic brain injury in VHA: a critical literature review. J Head Trauma Rehabil 2015;19:1–11.
13. Cicerone KD, Kalmar K. Persistent concussion syndrome: the structure of subjective complaints after mild traumatic brain injury. J Head Trauma Rehabil 2010;25:447–60.
14. Scholten J, Danford E, Leland A, et al. Templated interdisciplinary rehabilitation care plan documentation for veterans with traumatic brain injury. Prof Case Manag 2016;21(6):266–76.
15. Masel BE, DeWitt DS. Traumatic brain injury: a disease process, not an event. J Neurotrauma 2008;27(8):1529–40.
16. Malec JF, Hammond FM, Flanagan S, et al. Recommendations from the 2013 Galveston Brain Injury Conference for implementation of a chronic care model in brain injury. J Head Trauma Rehabil 2013;28(6):476–83.
17. Gause LR, Finn JA, Lamberty GJ, et al. Predictors of satisfaction with life in veterans after traumatic brain injury: a VA TBI Model Systems Study. J Head Trauma Rehabil 2017;32(4):255–63.
18. VA/DoD clinical practice guideline for management of concussion/mTBI, 2016. Available at: https://www.healthquality.va.gov/guidelines/Rehab/mtbi/mTBICPGFullCPG50821816.pdf. Accessed April 3, 2018.
19. Defense and Veterans Brain Injury Center: clinical tools for providers on mild TBI. Available at: http://dvbic.dcoe.mil/clinical-tools-providers-mild-tbi. Accessed April 3, 2018.
20. National Research Action Plan. Available at: https://obamawhitehouse.archives.gov/sites/default/files/uploads/nrap_for_eo_on_mental_health_august_2013.pdf. Accessed April 9, 2018.
21. The Chronic Effects of Neurotrauma Consortium (CENC). Available at: https://cenc.rti.org/. Accessed April 9, 2018.
22. Walker WC, Carne W, Franke LM, et al. The Chronic Effects of Neurotrauma Consortium (CENC) multi-centre observational study: description of study and characteristics of early participants. Brain Inj 2016;30(12):1469–80.
23. Report to Congress. Section 721 of the National Defense Authorization Act for Fiscal Year 2007 (public law 109–364), 7-year update. Available at: https://health.mil/Reference-Center/Reports/2017/07/19/Longitudinal-Study-on-Traumatic-Brain-Injury-Incurred-by-Members-of-the-Armed-Forces. Accessed April 9, 2018.
24. VA TBI model systems/IMAP newsletter. Caregiver needs. Issue 6, Summer 2017. Available at: https://www.polytrauma.va.gov/PolytraumaCenterDatabase/publications/NewsletterIssue06.pdf. Accessed April 9, 2018.

# Department of Veterans Affairs Polytrauma Rehabilitation Centers
## Inpatient Rehabilitation Management of Combat-Related Polytrauma

Michael Armstrong, MD[a],*, Julie Champagne, MD[b],
Diane Schretzman Mortimer, MD, MSN[c]

### KEYWORDS

• Polytrauma • Acute rehabilitation • Polytrauma rehabilitation center

### KEY POINTS

• Acute polytrauma rehabilitation at Department of Veterans Affairs (VA) Polytrauma Rehabilitation Centers (PSCs) provides veterans and active duty servicemembers with traumatic brain injury and other polytraumatic injuries comprehensive rehabilitation care using an interdisciplinary model.
• From admission to discharge, the interdisciplinary team strives to meet the medical, functional, and quality of life needs of the person served in preparation for discharge at maximal level of independence.
• Regardless of the final discharge destination, the PSC provides lifelong care management through the utilization of polytrauma case management and treatment team, the network of care established within the PSC, and the vast array of resources available through the broader VA health care system.

## INTRODUCTION

Traumatic brain injury (TBI) is often referred to as one of the signature injuries of Operation Iraqi Freedom and Operation Enduring Freedom (OIF/OEF).[1] Between 2000 and 2017, Department of Defense surveillance data identified more than 379,000 TBIs in

Disclosure Statement: The authors have nothing to disclose.
[a] Department of Physical Medicine and Rehabilitation, Minneapolis VA Health Care System, University of Minnesota, 1 Veterans Drive (117), Minneapolis, MN 55417, USA; [b] Polytrauma Transitional Rehabilitation, Minneapolis VA Health Care System, 1 Veterans Drive (117), Minneapolis, MN 55417, USA; [c] Department of Physical Medicine and Rehabilitation, Polytrauma Network Site, Minneapolis VA Health Care System, 1 Veterans Drive (117), Minneapolis, MN 55417, USA
* Corresponding author.
E-mail address: Michael.armstrong@va.gov

servicemembers across all branches of the United States military. Although a vast majority of the TBIs identified were mild in severity, more than 45,000 servicemembers suffered moderate to severe and penetrating TBIs worldwide.[2]

Blast exposure resulting from improvised explosive devices as well as other blast mechanisms have been the predominant cause of combat-related TBIs in OIF/OEF. Although advances in training, body armor, and military medicine have improved combat survival rates overall, significant blast exposure often results in concurrent trauma to other body systems in addition to TBI.[1,3] These traumas may include, but are not limited to, fractures and soft tissue injuries, amputations, vision and hearing loss, spinal cord injury, and posttraumatic stress disorder (PTSD). The combination of moderate to severe TBI with these additional combat-related injuries is the underlying definition of the term, *polytrauma*. To meet the rehabilitation needs of servicemembers and veterans suffering from the diverse conditions associated with polytrauma, the Department of Veterans Affairs (VA) required a new paradigm of care.

In response to the need for a new care paradigm, Congress passed Public Law 108-422, Section 302, and Public law 108-447 in 2004 paving the way for the development of the VA Polytrauma System of Care (PSC). By September 2005, the VA established 4 Polytrauma Rehabilitation Centers (PRCs) as the initial step in the implementation of the PSC.[4] These tertiary centers (located at the Hunter Holmes McGuire VA in Richmond, Virginia; the James A. Haley VA in Tampa, Florida; the Minneapolis VA Health Care System in Minneapolis, Minnesota; and the VA Palo Alto Health Care System in Palo Alto, California) had previously served as TBI lead centers under the Defense and Veterans Head Injury Program (later renamed the Defense and Veterans Brain Injury Center [DVBIC]).[5] In addition to their previous service as DVBIC TBI lead centers, each of the 4 VA facilities maintained Commission on Accreditation of Rehabilitation Facilities (CARF) accredited inpatient rehabilitation services, education, and research capabilities related to TBI and the specialty surgical, medicine, and mental health services strongly positioning them to meet the additional needs of polytrauma survivors. To further expand the reach of tertiary rehabilitation centers in the PSC, the VA opened a fifth PRC at the South Texas Veterans Health Care System in San Antonio, Texas, in 2011.[6]

Although their primary function is to serve as the regional referral centers for acute inpatient rehabilitation for TBI and polytraumatic injuries in the VA, PRCs also serve additional roles across the broader PSC. PRCs provide coordination, leadership, and training and education to their Polytrauma Network Sites (PNS) and Polytrauma Support Clinic Teams. In addition, PRCs serve as research centers for TBI and polytrauma, both locally and through their affiliations with other PSC sites and National Institute on Disability, Living, and Rehabilitation Research (NIDILRR) Traumatic Brain Injury Model Systems (TBIMS) sites, and as VA representatives within the 22-site DVBIC network.

## ACUTE REHABILITATION AT POLYTRAUMA REHABILITATION CENTERS

In general, acute inpatient rehabilitation is the provision of coordinated, patient-centered, interdisciplinary care by an array of rehabilitation professionals to meet the medical, functional, and quality-of-life needs of the person served. Acute rehabilitation has been shown to improve functional outcomes and reduce the financial burden of disabling neurologic conditions, such as TBI.[7–9] Individuals admitted to inpatient acute rehabilitation units require 24/7 medical and nursing care, receive at least 3 hours of therapy per day to address condition-specific disability, and cannot have their needs adequately met at a lower level of care.[10] This interdisciplinary acute inpatient rehabilitation model is the mainstay of care for moderate to severe TBI survivors with large functional deficit burdens and ongoing postacute medical needs as they transition from acute care medical systems.

Acute polytrauma rehabilitation at VA PRCs generally follows this description of acute inpatient rehabilitation, including the need for constant, daily medical and nursing care as well as a treatment plans consisting of at least 3 hours of therapy per day to address the disabilities related to the underlying condition.[11] In addition, PRCs also provide specialized rehabilitation programming, such as the Emerging Consciousness Program[12] for disorders of consciousness, where lengths of stay may extend far beyond community standards to allow for emergence and maximize an individual's opportunity for rehabilitation and further recovery. PRCs may also incorporate specialized military and Veteran-specific services within the rehabilitation continuum to meet the unique needs of a servicemember or veteran. Examples of these specialized services include assistive technology, mental health and PTSD care, military liaisons, transition case management, and caregiver support.

## POLYTRAUMA REHABILITATION CENTER PREADMISSION PROCESS

Referrals for admission to VA PRCs originate from a variety of sources and care settings. Veterans and servicemembers may be referred from the acute care hospital where the PRC is located, any other VA medical centers within the PRC's catchment area, or civilian hospitals in the community. ADSMs injured in combat are typically referred from Department of Defense Military Health System after returning to the continental United States for war-related injuires.[6]

Veterans and ADSMs are considered appropriate candidates for admission to acute inpatient rehabilitation at PRCs if they have TBI or polytrauma-related needs requiring inpatient rehabilitation and meeting the aforementioned requirements for care or require other specialized programming available at PRCs (eg, emerging consciousness program for disorders of consciousness, dynamic assessment program, and respite care program).[6]

Although the PRC medical director is ultimately responsible for making the initial determination regarding the type and level of rehabilitation services that are likely necessary for a referral to the PRC, PRC case management resources play a critical role in the coordination of the entire preadmission process. The PRC case manager typically serves as the point of contact for admission referrals, collects relevant clinical and administrative data regarding the referral, coordinates admission decisions and timelines with the medical director, maintains constant communication with PRC and referral site team members throughout the preadmission process, and assists with coordinating transportation for accepted referrals. In addition, PRC case managers perform patient and family outreach and education during the preadmission process. For referrals within the VA or military health systems, this outreach and communication often occur through the use of clinical video-telehealth to allow for face-to-face communication between the team, patient, and family.[13] During this process, case managers ensure that patients and families are given information regarding the expected type, length, and intensity of services to be provided. This process also ensures that patients and families can participate in developing appropriate goals and planning for eventual postdischarge needs. It is vital to start this process as early as possible, given the complexity of these patients.[6]

## THE POLYTRAUMA REHABILITATION CENTER ADMISSION

Multiple team members play a role in the admission process at the PRC. These professionals and their roles and responsibilities are summarized in **Table 1**.

**Table 1**
**Professionals involved in the Polytrauma Rehabilitation Center admission process**

| Professional | Responsibilities |
|---|---|
| PRC medical director | • Ensures that the medical admission is completed, including the history and physical, admission orders, and interim rehabilitation treatment plan |
| VA liaison for health care | • Facilitates the referral and admissions process for ADSMs<br>• Facilitates bidirectional communication with the patient and family, PRC team, and military treatment facility<br>• Helps address any transition issues that arise |
| VA polytrauma nurse liaison | • Facilitates the referral and admission process for ADSMs<br>• Provides education to the patient and family prior to transfer<br>• Collaborates with military treatment facility, PRC team and VA liaison for health care |
| PRC admissions coordinator | • Reviews clinical data with the PRC medical director<br>• Monitors the patient's medical and rehabilitation status until transfer occurs<br>• Informs the IDT of planned admission<br>• Documents preadmission screening information in the electronic medical record<br>• Confirms with referring facility that authorization for care has been provided by TRICARE or other payor as indicated<br>• Helps locate appropriate setting for referred patients who are not appropriate for PRC |
| PRC case manager | • Coordinates transfers in collaboration with the admissions coordinator<br>• Contacts family prior to admission to establish communication, begin orientation, and facilitate transition to PRC<br>• Coordinates travel to the PRC<br>• Coordinate preadmission communication with Department of Defense and VA liaison to ensure smooth transition of care<br>• Notifies local OEF/OIF/Operation New Dawn program manager of the admission |

*Data from* Veterans Health Administration. VHA handbook 1172.01: polytrauma system of care. Washington, DC: Department of Veterans Affairs; 2013.

Initial assessment of the acute polytrauma rehabilitation admission is a dynamic process performed by an interdisciplinary team (IDT), including the medical director, therapy disciplines, psychology, social work, registered dietician, pharmacist, and nursing. The admission history and physical performed by the medical director include review of acute care and past medical histories, including laboratory and imaging data; interview with the patient regarding current subjective symptoms; interview with the family regarding remote and recent health-related events; observation of current behaviors and functional status; and physical examination. Potential restrictions or activity limitation are considered and appropriately communicated to the team to maximize safety on the rehabilitation unit. Individual therapy disciplines review past therapy interventions and progress and assess current functional status, establish interim therapy goals, and evaluate the need for initial durable medical equipment.

Rehabilitation nursing plays a critical role in the admission assessment including assessment of common challenges in rehabilitation populations, such as pain, bowel and bladder changes, and sleep-wake cycle disturbances. Skin integrity is also an area of particular rehabilitation nursing expertise and is critical in the assessment of trauma and bedridden patients. Rehabilitation nurses perform comprehensive skin assessments and assess risk factors for skin breakdown, such as decreased sensation, altered mobility, agitation, nutritional deficiencies, and incontinence. Using these assessments, nursing staff implement interventions aimed at preventing skin breakdown on admission to acute rehabilitation.[14]

Due to the typically prolonged and often complicated acute care course for polytrauma patients prior to admission, a complete medication reconciliation is critical on arrival to the PRC to ensure continuity and safety. This tedious but indispensable process includes evaluation of medications the patient was taking on transfer to the PRC. The patient's preinjury medications also considered. Allergies are reviewed, confirmed, and documented. The PRC pharmacist plays an instrumental role in this process to ensure accurate medication reconciliation.

Although patient, family, and caregiver education begin prior to arriving at the PRC, the individual's learning style, educational, and psychosocial needs and readiness to learn are thoroughly assessed and documented during the admission process. Over the course of the inpatient stay, the patient, family, and caregivers receive individualized education as well as ongoing updates about the patient's medical condition, impairments, and treatment needs. To ensure families and caregivers are engaged in treatment planning and that information and education are delivered at the most appropriate times, the clinical team uses a process of readiness-based education outlined in the VA PRC Family Care Map.[15,16] Methods of education may include didactic presentations, informal and formal training during therapy sessions, patient and family meetings, and written information. PRCs may also provide family and counseling psychology services to assist families and caregivers to further support their needs and cope with the stressors associated with the loved one's injuries.

## POLYTRAUMA REHABILITATION CENTER INTERDISCIPLINARY REHABILITATION

The hallmark of acute polytrauma rehabilitation at PRCs is interdisciplinary care. The interdisciplinary model of care developed shortly after World War II as health care professionals attempted to address the severe and complex needs of returning injured soldiers. The challenge of caring for the complexity of trauma and medical conditions in these patients required a comprehensive and collaborative treatment approach involving multiple disciplines to achieve successful outcomes. This collaborative model would eventually grow to be a preferred treatment approach throughout all specialties of medicine, but ultimately became the central tenet of care for the field of physical medicine and rehabilitation.[17] Within the field of rehabilitation, the IDT includes the patient and family on the team to ensure the goals and treatment plans are patient-centric to maximize participation and engagement.

Effective IDTs require clear leadership, strong communication and respect between members, an appropriate mix of skills with diversified strengths, a patient-centered focus, and a clear and unified vision and are able to assist the patient in accomplishing their own goals of care. When effective teams are in place, IDT collaboration has been shown to improve patient compliance and satisfaction, lower cost, reduce mortality, decrease length of stay, and increase team member job satisfaction.[18,19]

Through a combination of PSC-directed education and training in the care of polytrauma injuries along with years of clinical experience in rehabilitation of TBI, the rehabilitation professionals at PRCs have the specialized expertise to address the complex needs of veterans and ADSMs admitted for acute polytrauma rehabilitation. The application of this specialized expertise within the collaborative interdisciplinary treatment model at the PRC allows the IDT to maximize rehabilitation outcomes. The individual IDT members, their primary roles, and their contributions to the collaborative are further described in **Table 2**.

The primary mechanism of coordination and communication between PRC IDT members occurs through formal IDT meetings or rounds. These weekly IDT meetings ensure the entire team is working toward common goals, predicting monitoring and communicating outcome measure progress, identifying and communicating barriers to care while planning actionable steps to overcome them, establishing discharge expectations, and facilitating discharge disposition planning.

In addition to weekly IDT meetings, the IDT holds frequent meetings with the patient and family and/or caregivers. These family conferences allow for formal communication between the team and the person served and are critical in the identification of patient center goals for rehabilitation. They also serve as a forum for sharing medical progress, prognosis, and outcome and discharge expectations. In addition, these formal meetings allow for an opportunity to engage the patient and family in education about the patient's condition and resultant disabilities.

In addition to family conferences, significant communication occurs between IDT members and the patient and family during individual treatment sessions. A significant goal in these sessions is the training of family and caregiver for the patient's eventual discharge and community reintegration needs. By discharge, the family and caregiver need to know how to safely and effectively use medications, prosthetic and orthotic devices, and durable medical equipment. Information regarding restrictions and precautions regarding issues, such as driving, swallowing, or general activity level, is provided. The team also helps the family or caregiver identify and access available resources in the home community.[6]

## POLYTRAUMA REHABILITATION CENTER REHABILITATION OUTCOME MEASUREMENT

The use of standardized outcome measures for rehabilitation in PRC programs assists in prognostication of outcomes, the measurement of success or failure of interventions, the monitoring progress toward IDT goals, and predicting discharge needs and timeframes.

During the initial IDT meeting shortly after admission, the IDT formulates a prediction regarding the progress that the patient is likely to make in rehabilitation. This prediction is an estimate based on the patient's injuries and current functional status. The prediction includes several formalized outcome measures, length of stay, and expected discharge location. On discharge from the program, the predicted outcomes are compared with actual. This process allows the team to continually engage in process and performance improvement activities.

Outcome measures also inform the treatment plan throughout the rehabilitation stay. Patients are considered to be making progress as standardized outcome measures demonstrate improvement. As progress continues, initial predictions may be modified and length of stay may be extended to allow for additional progress, more functional independence, and decreased burden of care on discharge. Conversely, if scores plateau or stagnate (absent of other explanations or issues) the IDT needs to consider discharging the patient whether or not the patient met all rehabilitation goals or completed the expected length of stay. Decisions regarding these multifaceted issues are made after thoughtful discussions with the IDT, patient, and family and in collaboration with other stakeholders.

**Table 2**
**Role of interdisciplinary team members**

| Discipline | Primary Role(s) | Team Collaboration |
|---|---|---|
| Patient and family | Integral members of the rehabilitation team; participate in all aspects of the rehabilitation process | Participate in developing patient-centered goals and the plan of care; provide feedback regarding the services received at the PRC |
| Physiatrist | Provides, coordinates, and leads the medical and rehabilitation care for polytrauma patients | Provides team leadership while closely interacting and collaborating with the IDT; provides medical updates and education on medical comorbidities and how they impact the patient's abilities to participate in the treatment plan |
| Nursing | Provides rehabilitation nursing cares; works directly with patient in managing bowel and bladder function; medication management, monitoring skin integrity; and provides ongoing education to the patient and family[14] | Reports patient behaviors, sleep, function and compliance with care for patient care hours outside of individual treatment sessions; assists with identifying appropriate cues for completing activities of daily living, homework, and exercises; relays family concerns to team |
| Occupational therapy | Evaluates and treats cognitive, motor, and visual impairments to maximize the patient's level of independence in activities of daily living and instrumental activities of daily living; treats impairments in upper extremities (gross and fine motor control, spasticity); evaluates wheel chair seating, power mobility, and assistive technology needs; performs home assessments | Contributes to developing strategies for patient motivation and sense of purpose; cotreats with other disciplines to address functional goals; assists team with establishing behavior plans; provides critical information regarding the patient's home environment |
| Physical therapy | Evaluates and treats functional limitations and participation deficits related to balance and mobility, coordination, vestibular disorders, pain and musculoskeletal impairments; evaluates for wheelchair and seating, power mobility, and assistive technology needs of the patient | Contributes to developing strategies for patient mobility and transfers; relays mobility and balance impairments, pain and musculoskeletal concerns to the team; develops walking programs, home exercise programs, and transfer strategies for the IDT |
| Speech and language pathology | Evaluates and treats dysphagia, speech and communication disorders, and cognitive impairments; trials appropriate assistive technology for memory and speech compensation | Collaborates with the patient and team to identify effective communication and cognitive compensatory strategies; provides feeding and dietary recommendations |

*(continued on next page)*

**Table 2**
*(continued)*

| Discipline | Primary Role(s) | Team Collaboration |
|---|---|---|
| Recreational therapy | Evaluates leisure interests (including adaptive sport) and promotes community integration in ways that enhance health, socialization, functional abilities, independence, and quality of life; focuses on safe mobility in the community, including awareness of environmental barriers, and use of public transportation | Provides critical information to the IDT regarding patient's behaviors and functional performance in the community; identifies patient's preferred healthy leisure activities during "off times" on the inpatient service |
| Rehabilitation psychology | Evaluates and treats mental or emotional issues related to adjustment to disability as well as primary mood disorders including PTSD; evaluates need for behavior plans for patients with organic brain disorders; provides family and couples counseling services at PRCs | Educates IDT on the patient's psychosocial issues and their impact on function and participation in therapies as well as effective strategies for interacting with the patient; implements behavior management plans |
| Psychiatry | Evaluates and treats mood and behavioral disorders | Collaborates with team to address problematic behaviors and other mood-related barriers to treatment; educates team how mental health issues effect function and participation as well as rationale for psychiatric medications |
| Pharmacy | Oversees the pharmacologic needs of the patient, including safety, cost, medication reconciliation, monitoring drug levels and side effects, and optimizes drug therapy for medical conditions | Collaborates with physicians, nurses, and other health care providers to prescribe, monitor, and optimize patients' drug therapy while reducing medication risks |
| Social work | Responsible for ensuring continuity of care through the admission, evaluation, treatment, and follow-up processes; serves as the point of contact for referral sources, patients, and families; facilitates and coordinates disposition planning and postdischarge resources | Alerts team to family questions and concerns and provides insight into stressors and dysfunctions in the family; serves as the IDT's central coordinator from admission through discharge |
| Neuropsychology | Completes neuropsychological assessment of brain function, behavior, mood and personality; provides cognitive rehabilitation, education, and therapy | Correlates test findings with the anatomic location of the brain injury and resultant functional impact; educates team on how these results impact strategies for cognitive remediation |

*(continued on next page)*

| Discipline | Primary Role(s) | Team Collaboration |
|---|---|---|
| **Table 2** *(continued)* | | |
| Vocational rehabilitation | Performs comprehensive assessments of vocational history, previous skill sets, interests, and barriers; services include interest testing, career exploration, return to school, veteran benefits, assessment and placement for inpatient compensated work therapy, resume writing, mock interviewing and job coaching; acts as a liaison between the patient and employer to discuss job duties, responsibilities, and recommendations for gradual return to work | Provides feedback to team on the patient's abilities, interest, and motivation for return to work or school |
| Driver rehabilitation | Performs comprehensive cognitive, physical and visual assessments as well as behind the wheel assessments to determine driving capabilities, safety, and need for adaptive equipment | Provides input on patient's performance behind the wheel, specific problem areas, and restrictions and recommendations for return to driving |
| Blind rehabilitation specialist | Evaluates vision needs and provides vision rehabilitation, living skills, orientation and mobility training, oculomotor and binocular vision training, and visual perceptual training | Provides feedback to team on visual impairments as well as the impact on function and level of independence |
| Assistive technology engineer or specialist | Evaluates, designs, customizes and manages assistive technology plans and related devices to maximize function; AT devices may include sensory aids, home and worksite modifications, environmental control systems, communication and cognitive aids, and computer access | Collaborates with IDT to recommend appropriate assistive devices, environmental augmentations to maximize independence |

*Data from* Refs.[20–23]

The Functional Status and Outcomes Database (FSOD) is the Department of Veterans Affairs standard outcomes management tool for rehabilitation. All veterans and Servicemembers with TBI and/or polytrauma receiving care at a PRC are entered into the FSOD. This database uses the Functional Independence Measure (FIM) as its central assessment tool. Patient-specific functional data are documented and tracked. The FSOD, which is stored at the Austin Information Technology Center, provides valuable information about service utilization and performance improvement efforts throughout the system of care.[6]

The FIM tool, which is widely used in rehabilitation settings, helps clinicians quantify goals, abilities, and outcomes relating to standardized measures of daily living and overall function. Scores range from dependent to fully independent. FIM's motor and cognitive components are further divided into subgroups that address self-care, sphincter control, transfers, locomotion, communication, and social cognition.[24]

In addition to the FIM, numerous other outcome measures and tools are used by the IDT during rehabilitation to measure progress and predict outcomes.

The Rancho Los Amigos Levels of Cognitive Functioning Scale is used to help describe cognitive and functional recovery after TBI. It provides numeric depictions of current cognitive status and approximations of how much assistance is required with activities of daily living in the setting of cognitive impairment. Using standardized language for these intricate issues allows for effective care planning.[25]

The Agitated Behavior Scale is a studied tool with proved validity and reliability for the objective assessment of agitation in patients with TBI. The Agitated Behavior Scale, which divides behaviors into categories of aggression, disinhibition, and lability, helps clinicians measure and track agitation extent and duration throughout the rehabilitation treatment course. This information can play a crucial role because agitation after TBI has been associated with decreased therapy participation, physical and emotional harm, difficulty achieving functional goals, and longer rehabilitation stays.[26,27]

The Glasgow Outcome Scale (GOS) and Glasgow Outcome Scale-Extended (GOS-E) are used to help quantify functional outcomes after TBI. The GOS is a functional assessment inventory that describes recovery on a 5-point scale ranging from death to good recovery. The GOS-E is divided into 8 outcome categories in an effort to provide additional information. Both scales are extensively used in TBI research studies.[28]

The Disability Rating Scale provides a quantitative index of disability. This 30-point scale, which was developed specifically for brain injury, evaluates functional dimensions from eye opening and verbalization to overall functioning and employability. Many clinicians find it to be more relevant than the GOS or GOS-E.[29]

The JFK Coma Recovery Scale-Revised is used to assess patients with disorders of consciousness. It involves observing for the presence or absence of responses to standardized auditory, visual, and tactile stimuli. Clinicians using this scale can differentiate between vegetative, minimally conscious, and emerged state of consciousness.[30]

The Disorder of Consciousness Scale also scores responses to standard stimuli like spoons, pictures, and juice. In contrast to the JFK Coma Recovery Scale-Revised, Disorder of Consciousness Scale can score responses as present or absent, localized, or generalized. Both scales are performed by clinicians at the bedside and can track progress over time through serial assessments.[31]

In addition to these outcome measures, the VA entered a partnership with NIDILRR TBIMS in 2008 to establish VA TBIMS sites at each of the 5 PRCs to collect longitudinal data on participating veterans and ADSMs with TBI. The VA data set for TBIMS not only includes the demographic, socioeconomic, preinjury health, injury characteristics, and function and disability measures in the NIDILRR TBIMS database but also additional measures specific to veterans and servicemembers, including more detailed military history and broader mental health and PTSD measures to capture the unique nature of this population. This longitudinal data, collected at admission and at 1-year, 2-year, 5-year, 10-year, and 20-year postinjury intervals, is used to enhance the understanding of TBI sequelae and outcomes both within the VA and in collaboration with NIDILRR TBMIS.[32]

Beyond these measures to evaluate individual TBI outcomes, PRCs assess the overall quality of the programming provided through CARF accreditation of their acute rehabilitation and TBI continuum of care programs. This accreditation, and its associated external survey processes, ensures PRCs provide high-quality rehabilitation care through regular evaluation of program content and delivery, outcomes and durability, employee education and competency, organizational resources and safety, leadership and communication, and patient and family satisfaction.[33]

## POLYTRAUMA REHABILITATION CENTER DISCHARGE

Discharge planning begins on admission to the PRC. Throughout the course of care, the IDT works closely with the patient and family to plan for anticipated postdischarge disposition location and their associated ongoing needs, including the need for post-acute rehabilitation services within the PSC continuum of care.

The decision to discharge is made in collaboration with the patient, family, referral source, and other stakeholders, as appropriate. Although planning is patient-centered and individualized, there are some criteria that typically provide rationale for discharge from acute rehabilitation. First, discharge is appropriate when patients have met rehabilitation goals. Second, patients have achieved maximum benefit from the specific level of care, as evidenced by lack of improvement on subjective and objective measures. Discharge is also fitting when the patient is no longer able or willing to participate in the rehabilitation program.

Discharge planning includes ensuring that there are sufficient resources to maximize the potential for safety. A home evaluation may be conducted so the team can make recommendations for home modifications and required equipment. Resources for follow-up medical and rehabilitation care are also identified.

Throughout the PRC admission, the family is provided ongoing educational support with structured opportunities during daily care and therapy sessions. This education allows them to become comfortable and skilled in managing a patient's ongoing care needs. By discharge, the caregiver should be able to demonstrate competence in managing these issues. The caregiver's physical, emotional, and financial limitations are also addressed and supported by the IDT. Information about local and national resources for education, advocacy, and support is reviewed.

Intensive case management is a hallmark of the discharge process from the PRC. When transitioning to another level of care after discharge, extensive communication and handoffs occur between the PRC team and the receiving facility or team. This process, which is coordinated by the polytrauma case manager and can involve many of the same individuals who facilitated the admission (see **Table 1**), ensures that the patient experiences the smoothest and safest possible transition.

Polytrauma case managers are also central to the transition that occurs when ADSMs discharge from the PRC. The discharge location can range from an additional treatment facility, a military unit, or another location to continue convalescence. The PRC IDT provides the receiving facility or team with instructions about the medical plan, adaptive devices, and equipment. Recommendations regarding activity level, including potential return to active duty, are also provided. Legal documents, such as guardianship and power of attorney forms, are forwarded to the appropriate point of contact.[6]

An integrated discharge summary is completed for each individual served in the PRC. The summary includes medical, functional, and psychosocial status of the patient at the time of discharge; progress and treatment; goals achieved; activity restrictions; current medications; adaptive and prosthetic equipment; discharge setting; family and support system needs; education provided; continued care needs; and the follow-up services arranged. The Individualized Rehabilitation and Community Reintegration Care Plan is a document that facilitates, records, and tracks interdisciplinary communication and care planning for the treatment team, patient, and family.

The Individualized Rehabilitation and Community Reintegration Care Plan is completed by the assigned case manager for every patient receiving polytrauma rehabilitation and, in addition to the integrated discharge summary, is used at the time of discharge to facilitate communication of the ongoing treatment plan to the patient, family, and receiving team if additional care is required.[34]

## POLYTRAUMA REHABILITATION CENTER POSTDISCHARGE

Post-PRC discharge destinations for veterans and ADSMs vary based on medical need, postacute rehabilitation goals, functional level, family and/or caregiver support, active duty service obligations, and the location and accessibility of the patient's home. Depending on these factors, the discharge plan for veterans may include transition to other postacute rehabilitation programs within the PSC, including the Polytrauma Transitional Rehabilitation Program (PTRP) for residential rehabilitation, subacute inpatient or outpatient rehabilitation programs at a PNS, or at a community facility or home with outpatient services and case management. For ADSMs, the discharge plan may also include transition back to a military treatment facility or a return to service with the military unit.

PTRPs are CARF-accredited residential inpatient rehabilitation programs located at each of the 5 PRC sites. Each PTRP program has a minimum of 10 beds and provides 24/7 nursing supervision. Rehabilitation services are provided both in group milieu and 1-to-1 treatment formats. The overarching goal of PTRP is to help participants return to the most appropriate, least restrictive community setting, by targeting skills necessary for return to home, school, work, or military service. PTRPs challenge participants through a wide range of individual and group therapeutic activities and living skills practices both in house and in the community. They offer interactive therapy programs designed to address the individual needs and goals of each participant and to improve physical, cognitive, communicative, behavioral, psychological, and social functioning after injury.

When the intensity of services provided by PTRP or other subacute inpatient rehabilitation units at a PNS or in the community is not required at discharge, the PSC provides specialized outpatient rehabilitation programs and clinics to provide ongoing care. These programs and services are available PNSs and Polytrauma Support Clinic Teams at more than 100 facilities over regions spanning the entirety of VA health system. At each of these sites, a team of rehabilitation specialists with expertise in TBI and polytrauma are available to provide post-PRC discharge care plans, complete comprehensive assessments and develop further plans of care based on progress.

For veterans or ADSMs with severe injuries or for those who develop needs beyond the scope of the local treatment team, a return to the PRC for admission and reassessment may be necessary. Otherwise known as the PRC dynamic assessment, these admissions provide an opportunity to address new emerging complications, manage social or caregiver issues or barriers, and support and expand education for family and caregivers. They also provide an opportunity to assess the durability of PRC rehabilitation outcomes and update the ongoing treatment and provide new treatments or technology as they emerge. Dynamic assessment admissions are offered annually or more frequently as condition warrants.

In addition to the ongoing support of the family and caregiver available through the VA and PSC, eligible veterans may also receive up to 30 days of respite care per year to provide their family a reprieve from those with heavy caregiver burdens. Although this care is typically provided in the home, at a community nursing home, or within a VA Medical Center Community Living Center, respite care may also be provided within PRC units when a veteran requires greater medical oversight or when TBI management expertise is required for patient safety. These respite stays also serve as an opportunity to reassess the veteran's medical and functional status as well as update treatment plans.[35]

Regardless of the final discharge destination from the PRC or their level of function and degree of reintegration in the community, veterans receive life-long TBI and polytrauma services from PSC case managers and their associated treatment team.

## SUMMARY

Acute polytrauma rehabilitation at VA PRCs provides veterans and ADSMs with TBI and other polytraumatic injuries comprehensive rehabilitation care using an interdisciplinary model. From admission to discharge, the IDT strives to meet the medical, functional, and quality-of-life needs of the person served in preparation for discharge at maximal level of independence. Regardless of the final discharge destination, the PSC provides lifelong care management through the utilization of polytrauma case management and treatment team, the network of care established within the PSC, and the vast array of resources available through the broader VA health care system.

## REFERENCES

1. Swanson TM, Isaacson BM, Cyborski CM, et al. Traumatic brain injury incidence, clinical overview, and policies in the US military health system since 2000. Public Health Rep 2017;132(2):251–9.
2. Defense and Veterans Brain Injury Center. DoD Worldwide Numbers Numbers for TBI. Available at: http://dvbic.dcoe.mil/dod-worldwide-numbers-tbi. Accessed March 17, 2018.
3. Greer N, Sayer N, Kramer M, et al. Prevalence and epidemiology of combat blast injuries from military cohort 2001-2014. VA evidence-based synthesis program reports. Department of Veterans Affairs; 2016.
4. Veterans Health Administration. VHA handbook 1172.1: polytrauma rehabilitation procedures. Washington, DC: Department of Veterans Affairs; 2005.
5. Defense and Veterans Brain Injury Center. History. Available at: http://dvbic.dcoe. mil/hiostory. Accessed March 17, 2018.
6. Veterans Health Administration. VHA handbook 1172.01: polytrauma system of care. Washington, DC: Department of Veterans Affairs; 2013.
7. Eapen BC, Allred DB, O'Rourke J, et al. Rehabilitation of moderate-to-severe traumatic brain injury. Semin Neurol 2015;35(01):e1–13.
8. Zhu XL, Poon WS, Chan CC, et al. Does intensive rehabilitation improve the functional outcome of patients with traumatic brain injury? A randomized control trial. Brain Inj 2007;21(7):681–90.
9. Cowen TD, Meythaler JM, DeVivo MJ, et al. Influence of early variables in traumatic brain injury on functional independence measure scores and rehabilitation length of stay and charges. Arch Phys Med Rehabil 1995;76(9):797–803.
10. Kahn F, Amatya B, Galea MP, et al. Neurorehabilitation: applied neuroplasticiy. J Neurol 2017;264:603–15.
11. Mas MF, Mathews A, Gilbert-Baffoe E. Rehabilitation needs of the elder with traumatic brain injury. Phys Med Rehabil Clin N Am 2017;28(4):829–42.
12. Veterans Health Administration. Polytrauma system of care. Available at: https://www.polytrauma.va.gov/about/Ermerging_Consciousness.asp. Accessed March 17, 2018.

13. Darkins A, Cruise C, Armstrong M, et al. Enhancing access of combat-wounded Veterans to specialist rehabilitation services: the VA Polytrauma Telehealth Network. Arch Phys Med Rehabil 2008;89:182–7.
14. Bines AS. Rehabilitation nursing. In: Zollman FS, editor. Manual of traumatic brain injury: assessment and management. 2nd edition. New York: Demos; 2016. p. 234–41.
15. Veterans Health Administration. PRC Family Care Map. Available at: https://www.polytrauma.va.gov/fcm. Accessed March 17, 2018.
16. Ford J, Wise M, Krahn D, et al. Family care map: sustaining family-centered care in polytrauma rehabilitation centers. J Rehabil Res Dev 2014;51(8):1311–24.
17. Strasser D, Uomoto J. The interdisciplinary team and polytrauma rehabilitation. Arch Phys Med Rehabil 2008;89:179.
18. Scheffer BK, Rubenfeld MG. Critical thinking: a tool in search of a job. J Nurs Educ 2006;45(6):195–6.
19. Nancarrow S, Booth A, Ariss S, et al. Ten principles of good interdisciplinary team work. Hum Resour Health 2013;11:19.
20. The American Occupational Therapy Association, Inc. About occupational therapy. Available at: https://www.aota.org/About-Occupational-Therapy. Accessed March 17, 2018.
21. American Physical Therapy Association. About physical therapists. Available at: https://www.movefowardpt.com/AboutPTsPTAs/defalut.aspx. Accessed March 17, 2018.
22. American Psychological Association. Clinical neuropsychology. Available at: www.apa.org/ed/graduate/specialize/neuro.aspx. Accessed March 17, 2018.
23. Veterans Health Administration. Rehabilitation and prosthetics services. Available at: https://www.prosthetics.va.gov/blindrehab/BRS_Coordinated_Care.asp. Accessed March 17, 2018.
24. Uniform Data System for Medical Rehabilitation. Guide for the uniform data set for medical rehabilitation. Buffalo (NY): State University of New York; 1996.
25. Hagen C, Malkmus D, Durham P. Levels of cognitive functioning. In: Rancho Los Amigos Hospital, editor. Rehabilitation of the head-injured adult: comprehensive management. Downey (CA): Rancho Los Amigos Hospital; 1979.
26. Bogner J, Barrett RS, Hammond FM, et al. Predictors of agitated behavior during inpatient rehabilitation for traumatic brain injury. Arch Phys Med Rehabil 2015;96:S274–81.
27. Corrigan JD. Development of a scale for assessment of agitation following traumatic brain injury. J Clin Exp Neuropsychol 1989;11:261–77.
28. Wilson JT, Pettigrew LE, Teasdale GM. Structured interviews for the glasgow outcome scale and the extended glasgow outcome scale: guidelines for their use. J Neurotrauma 1998;15:573–85.
29. Rappaport M, Hall KM, Hopkins K, et al. Disability rating scale for severe head trauma: coma to community. Arch Phys Med Rehabil 1982;63:118–23.
30. Giacino JT, Kalmar K, Whyte J. The JFK coma recovery scale-revised: measurement characteristics and diagnostic utility. Arch Phys Med Rehabil 2004;85:2020–9.
31. Pape TL, Heinemann AW, Kelly JP, et al. A measure of neurobehavioral functioning after coma. Part 1: theory, reliability, and validity of disorders of consciousness scale. J Rehabil Res Dev 2005;42:1–17.
32. Nakase-Richardson R, Stevens LF, Tang X, et al. Comparison of the VA and NIDILRR TBI model systems cohorts. J Head Trauma Rehabil 2017;32(4):221–33.
33. CARF International. Available at: www.carf.org/home/. Accessed March 17, 2018.

34. Scholten J, Danford E, Leland A, et al. Templated interdisciplinary rehabilitation care plan documentation for Veterans with traumatic brain injury. Prof Case Manag 2016;21:266–76.
35. Veterans Health Administration. Geriatrics and extended care – Respite care. Available at: https://va.gov/GERIATRICS/Guide/LongTermCare/REspite_Care. asp. Accessed March 17, 2018.

# Evolution of Care for the Veterans and Active Duty Service Members with Disorders of Consciousness

Michelle Peterson, DPT[a],*, Blessen C. Eapen, MD[b],
Mary Himmler, MD[a], Pawan Galhotra, PT[c], David Glazer, MD[d]

## KEYWORDS

• Traumatic brain injury • Disorders of consciousness • Rehabilitation • Polytrauma

## KEY POINTS

• A formalized emerging consciousness program that collects and reviews data, educates interdisciplinary team members including family members, and coordinates clinical care and other support services can improve long-term function and outcomes.

• Serial assessments are important to establish an accurate diagnosis, monitor change, and provide prognostic information in order to give patients' families reliable information to help them in making decisions about the selection of care, treatment provided, and end-of-life decisions.

• Program review that includes reviewing data for trends that may affect programming, monitoring latest publications to incorporate applicable research findings, and sharing processes with similar programs is an essential element to maximizing outcomes.

## INTRODUCTION

The Polytrauma Rehabilitation Centers (PRCs) of the Veterans Health Administration (VHA) are located at the Department of Veterans Affairs (VA) Palo Health Care System in Palo Alto, California; the James A. Haley VA Medical Center in Tampa, Florida; the Minneapolis VA Health Care System in Minneapolis, Minnesota; the McGuire VA

Disclosure Statement: The authors have nothing to disclose.
[a] Physical Medicine and Rehabilitation Service, Polytrauma Rehabilitation Center (4K), Minneapolis VA Health Care System, One Veterans Drive, Minneapolis, MN 55417, USA; [b] Department of Physical Medicine and Rehabilitation, VA Greater Los Angeles Health Care System, 11301 Wilshire Boulevard, Los Angeles, CA 90073, USA; [c] Physical Medicine and Rehabilitation Service, Polytrauma Rehabilitation Center, Palo Alto Health Care System, 3801 Miranda Avenue (PSC 117), Palo Alto, CA 94304, USA; [d] Physical Medicine and Rehabilitation Service, Polytrauma Rehabilitation Center, Hunter Holmes McGuire VA Medical Center, 1201 Broad Rock Boulevard, Richmond, VA 23249, USA
* Corresponding author.
E-mail address: Michelle.Peterson@va.gov

Phys Med Rehabil Clin N Am 30 (2019) 29–41
https://doi.org/10.1016/j.pmr.2018.08.006
1047-9651/19/© 2018 Elsevier Inc. All rights reserved.

Medical Center in Richmond, Virginia; and the South Texas Veterans Health Care System in San Antonio, Texas. The Emerging Consciousness Program (ECP) within the PRCs was developed in response to the increasing numbers of service members returning from recent US military conflicts with severe neurologic injury resulting in disorders of consciousness (DOC).[1] Veterans and service members with severe and complex injuries, including DOC, require a very high level of integrated and coordinated clinical care and significant support services. The mainstay of treatment in the PRC's ECP is the holistic interdisciplinary team (IDT) approach with patients and families at the center of the treatment program.[2] The ECP PRC National Work Group was developed to address ongoing continuing improvement as issues arise and evidence changes to assure optimal care is provided to our service members and veterans. The work group consists of both clinician and leadership personnel involved in the ECP at each PRC. This article addresses programmatic changes that have occurred in the ECP since its inception in 2006.

## EMERGING CONSCIOUSNESS PROGRAM DESCRIPTION AND EXPANSION

The PRC ECP is a 90-day program dedicated to supporting the recovery of patients with DOC. The original 4 PRCs were located at the VA Palo Alto Health Care System in Palo Alto, California; James A. Haley VA Medical Center in Tampa, Florida; the Minneapolis VA Health Care System in Minneapolis, Minnesota; and the Hunter Holmes McGuire VA Medical Center in Richmond, Virginia. In 2011, the addition of the South Texas Veterans Health Care System in San Antonio, Texas helped balance out the geographic regions and improved access and increased the number of patients who could be admitted to the ECPs.

Gray and Burnham[3] found the subgroup of patients with DOC who have a slower rate of recovery significantly benefitted from longer periods of rehabilitation programming. When the ECP was initially developed, a 60-day time frame was proposed. Prior admissions data were reviewed and demonstrated several individuals had emerged in the third month of programming, so the program length was set at 90 days. In 2013, Nakase-Richardson and colleagues[4] reported 122 persons were admitted to the VHA ECPs from January 2004 to October 2009. Since October 2009 through September 2017, an additional 165 veterans and service members have been provided ECP treatment resulting in a total of 287 persons served. The emergence rate has remained fairly consistent, 64% and 66%, respectively, for the first- and second-decade groups.

The ECP admission criteria is listed in **Table 1**. The authors have refined their inclusion criteria to include the subset of Rancho Los Amigos (RLA) IV who have not met their emergence criteria. In the past, the programs used the RLA score of less than IV. The VHA ECP work group had noted that some patients who would be described

| Table 1 | |
|---|---|
| Emerging consciousness program admission criteria | |
| **Inclusion** | **Exclusion** |
| • Veteran or service member | • Diminished responsiveness due to acute reversible |
| • Acquired brain injury | processes, such as central nervous system infection |
| • Timeline within 2 y of injury | • Progressive neurologic conditions, such as |
| • Ongoing impairment in | terminal brain tumors |
| consciousness | • Need for mechanical ventilation |
| | • Medical instability affecting ability to safely |
| | transfer to the program |

as RLA IV were in a minimally conscious state (MCS) as well. The continuum to emerging awareness could at times include RLA IV, and the group made the decision to include RLA IV patients who have not yet met the criteria for emergence from MCS. Table 2 provides descriptions of the RLA scale of cognitive function levels I to IV.[5] The rationale for this decision stems from the following discussion from several other work groups who have provided guidance for patients in DOC over the years, including the Multi-Task Force of the American Academy of Neurology and the Aspen Neurobehavioral Conference Workgroup. DOC can be categorized by 2 dimensions, arousal (level of consciousness) and awareness (content of consciousness).[6] Arousal is determined by the presence of eye opening and brainstem responses, whereas awareness refers to the ability to form an integrated response based on internal and external stimuli. Table 3 provides clarification among the subgroups in DOC. A person in a coma or RLA I has neither arousal nor awareness. A person in a vegetative state (VS) has emerging arousal but no awareness. Behaviors of eye opening or reflexive posturing are consistent with RLA II. A person in an MCS has arousal and emerging awareness, which can include both RLA III as well as some RLA IV behaviors. These patients may orient toward sound, smile, inconsistently follow commands, or have random verbalizations. When the arousal and awareness level of an individual meets the threshold set by the program, then the individual is deemed emerged from consciousness. The emergence criteria used by the ECP is based on consensus recommendations by Giacino and colleagues,[7] functional communication or functional object use. The definitions of these two criteria are described in Table 4.

All the ECPs have experienced admission of a patient presumed to be in a DOC based on referral site documentation who has then been determined to be emerged based on team evaluations using the PRCs' ECP outcome measures and emergence criteria. The PRC ECP National Work Group recognizes the importance of accurate diagnosis as well as some of the difficulties in obtaining an accurate diagnosis. Accuracy for simple yes/no situational orientation questions can be challenging for patients in early recovery from brain injury with posttraumatic confusion/amnesia. Individuals in DOC may have confounding motor impairments, cognitive impairments (such as apraxia, impaired attention, and decreased initiation), or language processing deficits (such as aphasia) that may limit their ability to respond correctly. Nakase-Richardson and colleagues[8] found in their study that confused patients answered simple orientation and situational orientation questions inaccurately 22% to 31% of the time. It is important to include observations and response interpretations from all IDT members, as different specialties may have different viewpoints about the response. It is

| Table 2 | | |
|---------|---|---|
| **Rancho Los Amigos scale of cognitive levels (I–IV)** | | |
| Level I | No response | There is no response to external stimuli, and patients appear asleep. |
| Level II | Generalized response | Responses to external stimuli are nonspecific and nonpurposeful. |
| Level III | Localized response | Responses present to stimuli are specific but inconsistent and may follow simple commands for motor action. |
| Level IV | Confused-agitated response | Responses are bizarre, nonpurposeful, incoherent, or inappropriate. |

*Data from* Bushnik T. The level of cognitive functioning scale. The Center for Outcome Measurement in Brain Injury; 2000. Available at: http://www.tbims.org/combi/lcfs. Accessed January 17, 2018.

**Table 3**
**Disorder of consciousness diagnostic subgroups**

| Coma | No arousal or awareness | Absent sleep/wake cycle, motor function may include reflex and postural responses, no response to auditory or visual stimulation, no verbalizations |
|---|---|---|
| Vegetative state | Some level of arousal but no awareness | Sleep/wake cycle present, may posture or withdraw to noxious stimuli or occasional nonpurposeful movement, responses to auditory or visual stimuli are reflexive or brief in duration, no verbalizations |
| MCS | Arousal with some level of awareness to oneself or environment | Sleep/wake cycle present, movement localizes to noxious stimuli, automatic movements or purposeful movements may be present, localization to sound or inconsistent command following are noted, sustained fixation and pursuit may be present, verbalizations may occur |

*Data from* Giacino JT, Ashwal S, Childs N, et al. The minimally conscious state: definition and diagnostic criteria. Neurology 2002;58:349–53; and Multi-Society Task Force on PVS. Medical aspects of the persistent vegetative state (1). N Engl J Med 1994;330:1499–508.

important for the accuracy of the DOC diagnosis and determining emergence from DOC. IDT members often discuss the emergence criteria and actively debate the presence of confounding variables that may interfere with an accurate diagnosis. The ECP National Work Group realizes that this may be an area for future refinement.

## EMERGING CONSCIOUSNESS PROGRAM OUTCOME MEASURES

In 2009, the VHA PRCs held an ECP planning meeting at the James A. Haley VA Medical Center in Tampa. The conference included members from the PRCs ECP and several distinguished experts in DOC. Aims accomplished at this meeting were the evaluation of the ECP outcome measurement process, therapeutic approach and care continuum, and the establishment of future research priorities.

Guidance provided at this meeting led to the sites systematically collecting and using data to help with diagnosis, intervention, and prognosis. The ECP continues to collect the following measures: Coma Recovery Scale-revised (CRS-R); Functional Independence Measure (FIM); and Disability Rating Scale (DRS). **Table 5** briefly describes the constructs of these measures. Although the list has not changed since the planning meeting, the frequency of administration of one of the measures has changed.

The ECP uses the CRS-R to determine DOC diagnosis and to monitor the change in state (coma, VS, MCS, emergence.) Before the 2009 planning meeting, the scale was

**Table 4**
**Emergence criteria**

| Functional Communication | Accurate yes/no response to 6 of 6 basic situational orientation questions on 2 consecutive evaluations |
|---|---|
| Functional Object Use | Generally appropriate use of 2 objects on 2 consecutive evaluations |

*Data from* Giacino JT, Ashwal S, Childs N, et al. The minimally conscious state: definition and diagnostic criteria. Neurology 2002;58:349–53.

| Table 5 | |
|---------|---|
| **Emerging consciousness program outcome measures** | |
| CRS-R | 6 subscales (auditory, visual, motor, oromotor, communication, and arousal functions) arranged in a hierarchal manner for a total of 23 items |
| FIM | 18 items in the motor and cognitive/social domains |
| DRS | 8 items in the 3 domains of impairment level (eye opening, communication ability, motor response), disability level (feeding, toileting, grooming), and handicap level (level of functioning, employability) capturing level of disability |

*Data from* Refs.[22–24]

administered on a weekly basis throughout the length of the program or until the individual emerges. After the summit, the frequency of administration changed to 2 to 3 per week. Benefits of increased frequency of administration are improved accuracy of diagnosis and increased data for determining consistency and rate of change. Fluctuations of behaviors based on a variety of factors in the individual with DOC may lead to an early misdiagnosis. Serial administration of the CRS-R (6 assessments within the first 10 days of admission) showed improved diagnostic accuracy.[9] In monitoring responsiveness, more data points are beneficial to study variability and consistency. When scores are graphed, the slope of the line can be used to demonstrate rate of change. No change would be represented by a horizontal line, and this visual aid could be helpful in discussions with families about long-term needs and expected level of change. Variation in scoring can assist with identifying optimal testing schedules and intervention times. The CRS-R is the only scale recommended, with minor reservations, by the American Congress of Rehabilitation Medicine to assess individuals with DOC.[10] Several sites do administer other DOC scales, but those measures are not consistent across the PRCs.

The FIM allows for assessment of progress from the PRCs' ECP throughout the duration of inpatient rehabilitation for those who have emerged. FIM data are collected at the time of admission and discharge for all individuals enrolled in the ECP. If an individual emerges, the FIM frequency changes to weekly administration until hospital discharge.

The DRS can measure general functional change over the course of recovery, from the PRC ECP and acute rehabilitation programs through the polytrauma system of care continuum and is administered at admission and discharge. This measure offers the ECP the ability to monitor changes of individuals with DOC after discharge from the authors' facility and is one of the measures collected in the Veteran Affairs Brain Injury Model System (VA TBIMS) collaborative, which is described later in this article.

## EMERGING CONSCIOUSNESS PROGRAM TEAM MEMBERS

Services are provided by an IDT of professionals who have experience in brain injury rehabilitation. New team members are mentored by existing staff. Since the authors' last publication, the PRCs have expanded services in the areas of assistive technology (AT), education, and integrative medicine. **Box 1** provides the current list of ECP team members.

One cannot minimize the importance of family member or care giver collaboration with the ECP team. Family members or care givers are considered additional team members. Those close to the veteran or service member are often the first to report

Box 1
Emerging consciousness program professions

Physiatrist

Psychologist

Social worker

Rehabilitation nurse

Rehabilitation engineer

Pharmacist

Nurse educator

Chaplain

Physical therapist

Occupational therapist

Speech language pathologist

Recreational therapist

Blind rehabilitation therapist

Dietician

Nurse case manager

signs of responsiveness. Individuals often respond to a familiar voice or may visually fixate on familiar faces.[11,12] The IDT recognizes the importance of these observations and tailors activities to include those observed by the family. The IDT includes family members in treatment sessions to allow for observations of response, which provides opportunities to improve communication and education for both staff and family members.

The AT laboratories were developed to effectively support veterans and service members with cognitive, sensory, and physical disabilities and to enhance their independence, comfort, and overall quality of life through the use of AT. The addition of this service has provided improved customization of specialty wheelchairs for this population and has improved the options available to engage and monitor patients. The use of simple switches may assist patients with a particular task. Initially patients demonstrate inconsistent use of such devices, but continued practice may provide a route to determine ultimate emergence via functional object use. Use of technology to monitor change in different ways is being attempted. One such device that has been trialed is an eye-gaze system. Commercially, these glasses are donned by a consumer as they walk through a retail outlet. The glasses track observations by the consumer and relay the environment and focus on a video monitor. Retailers can view what the consumer observes. This information allows the retailer to present products in a systematic manner to visually appeal to the consumer. These glasses have been trialed on several patients with DOC to observe eye movements, which allows the clinician to determine where the individual is focusing and how much time is spent on a specific target. Clinicians can determine if motion in the environment, object in the environment, or neither result in eye movements. Response time from command to obtaining visual target can also be captured. Although one can argue that clinicians are able to determine the response without the glasses, they do allow for some quantification that is not yet clinically available. Several issues do limit the use of the glasses in this opulation: initial calibration, expense, risk of breaking the glasses. This device is one xample of how AT has added to clinical and possible research ideas for monitoring nd treating DOC.

Although all disciplines prioritize education of family members, the addition of a pol-trauma nurse educator has allowed for expansion of these services. Most sites have developed a family burden of care checklist as well as brain injury educational mate-ial. **Table 6** lists the components of the burden of care checklist that are tailored to amily member/caregiver needs. During IDT rounds, the team determines which disci-pline is best suited to provide specific education. Although most educational materials are currently site specific, there has been a discussion on further collaboration to stan-dardize and broaden the education available for families and caregivers. The sites have started to discuss the development of an EC toolkit that can facilitate training of residents and new staff in the VHA.

The VHA has been incorporating integrative health into the national system of care. More research is needed to determine the effects of use of integrative health for the DOC population. The ECP is able to include integrative health interventions to patient's with DOC. Family members can direct the team in deciding what options they would like to see trialed. A few of the integrative services currently offered are healing touch, aromatherapy, and acupuncture. Treatment depends on the resources available at each site. If a family member chooses one of these services, the team will monitor changes as with any other intervention; families will then have information to determine if they wish to continue with the treatment.

## EMERGING CONSCIOUSNESS PROGRAM PATHWAY

The primary goal for the program is to promote increased arousal and awareness while managing medical stability and preventing secondary complications. The program

| Table 6 Burden of care checklist | |
|---|---|
| Mobility | Durable medical equipment, including any type of lift or wheelchair along with sitting schedules, optimal positioning, and pressure relief Home exercise programs, including splint management, range of motion, and structured environmental interventions |
| Nutrition | PEG tube management, including care, schedule, rate, and checking residuals Hydration |
| Medical Management | Respiratory care, including tracheostomy management or any respiratory treatment Wound care, including dressing changes; a large focus on prevention Disease management, which educates about what would be a neurologic decline as well as how to manage storming if present |
| Medication | Types, including the side effects and signs of inappropriate dosing Schedule Delivery |
| Hygiene/ADLs | Dressing Bathing Grooming, such as, but not limited to, oral care and shaving Eating and aspiration precautions Sleep Continence programs and incontinence cares |

*Abbreviations:* ADLs, activities of daily living; PEG, percutaneous endoscopic gastrostomy.

has evaluation/admission, intervention, and discharge assessments to help establish a baseline, assess health stability, monitor changes based on interventions, evaluate equipment needs, and reinforce educational components for family members, all to help with the transition to the next phase of recovery.

The evaluation period following admission is important in establishing the initial DOC diagnosis and baseline behaviors, which help to identify future change in responsiveness. Evaluation includes a review of history, recent structural imaging, and serial testing. Variables, such as the length of time after the injury, age, level of consciousness, rate of change of responsiveness, and imaging findings, can contribute to prognostic information. Information is collected throughout the patients' stay to help provide a more complete picture. As an integral part of the ECP team, family members/caregivers are included in ongoing assessments and conversations to help with prognosis discussions and transitions.

The evaluation period typically lasts from 1 to 3 weeks and is a time to optimize medical stability to facilitate neural recovery. Medications that interfere with responsiveness are eliminated if possible. Health stability is a major focus of treatment, and monitoring for medical complications and neurologic sequelae (**Box 2**) continues throughout the length of the program. Establishing an accurate baseline is also an important variable to consider when determining the need for further diagnostic imaging. For a review of different types of diagnostic imaging, the reader is referred to Dr Eapen and colleagues'[13] article "Disorders of Consciousness."

Following the evaluation period, the team determines which pharmacologic and nonpharmacologic interventions may prevent comorbidities and promote recovery of consciousness. The ECP recognizes the severity of injury sustained by patients with DOC as well as the emotional and psychological toll on the patients' family unit. A discussion of the role of the family psychologist is reiterated.

One medication that all sites often trial is amantadine, which is one of the most commonly prescribed medications for patients with prolonged DOC. A randomized control study from Giacino and colleagues[14] found that amantadine accelerated the pace of functional recovery during active treatment in patients with posttraumatic disorders of consciousness. Other medications may be trialed at individual sites, but current evidence is not as supportive as for amantadine. The reader is referred to the article "Disorders of Consciousness" by Eapen and colleagues[13] for review of the

---

**Box 2**
**Medical complications and neurologic sequelae**

Spasticity

Paroxysmal sympathetic hyperactivity

Seizure

Endocrine abnormalities

Abnormal intracranial pressures

Intracranial infections

Nonintracranial infections

Pressure ulcers

Venous thromboembolism/pulmonary embolus

Heterotopic ossification

pharmacologic effects of amantadine and discussion of other pharmaceuticals used in the DOC population.

Neurostimulation as a restorative treatment of DOC is an emerging field. Limited studies using both invasive (deep brain stimulation) and noninvasive (transcranial magnetic stimulation and transcranial direct current stimulation) techniques are now being published.[13,15] At this time, the ECP does not include these treatments in the formal program. More research is needed to delineate the safest and best modality, preconditions, timing, and optimal dosage. The PRC ECP work group will continue to monitor the field in this area and incorporate as the research and evidence warrants.

Nonpharmacologic interventions include preventing the comorbidities associated with bedrest, regulating the environment, and establishing structure and tailored sensory stimulation programs. As with many of the therapeutic options available in neurologic rehabilitation in general, studies proving efficacy are limited. However, most programs provide this typical standard of care. Evidence suggests that individuals admitted early to formalized programs have better outcomes.[16] The primary focus of these interventions in the ECP has changed little during the past 10 years. The one change that did occur was the result of another discussion sparked at the EC summit. The discussion centered around how to measure tailored sensory stimulation.

Immobility and bed rest result in negative changes to multiple organ systems[17,18] (**Table 7**). Development of a range-of-motion program including splint use and contracture prevention is important. A sitting and standing program is crucial to normalizing the gravitational pressures that can improve cardiovascular, pulmonary, and bowel/bladder function. The reticular activating system (RAS) modulates certain postural reflexes and muscle tone, helps control breathing and heartbeat, and regulates brain arousal and consciousness. Upright positioning increases demand on the RAS, which may improve the level of arousal and improve responsiveness.

Regulating the environment is an important factor to consider; too much environmental stimulation can overstimulate and/or fatigue the individual leading to decreased responsiveness.[19] Monitoring and metering the extraneous noise in all sensory domains (touch, auditory, vision) are important and can be difficult to control in a hospital environment with all of the noise of overhead paging, monitoring devices, bantering of visitors, and so forth. Opportune times for family and caregiver education includes nursing care sessions and therapy treatment sessions; patients who may be starting to process information can also benefit from this type of education. Schedules help normalize routine and establish sleep/wake cycles; patients will benefit from getting up in the morning, enjoying some outdoor time, and reestablishing roles and rituals while balancing fatigue and stimulation levels.

Behavioral observation is a large component in structuring therapy sessions. Outcome measures and multiple sensory domains are used to assess patients during

| Table 7 Potential complications associated with immobilization | | |
|---|---|---|
| **Musculoskeletal** | **Cardiovascular** | **Respiratory** |
| Decreased muscle strength and atrophy | Increased heart rate | Decreased overall ventilation |
| Decreased endurance | Decreased cardiac reserve | Regional changes in ventilation and perfusion |
| Contracture | Orthostatic hypotension | Atelectasis |
| Osteoporosis | Deep vein thrombosis | — |

a treatment session; if a clear and purposeful response is observed, the team can begin to structure tailored stimulation protocol for those patients. The protocol captures the sensory modality identified as a strength of the individual, and then principles of neuroplasticity (**Table 8**) are applied. The team starts to monitor the consistency of responses to command (able to lick upper lip several times in a row), improvement in the response (tongue protrusion greater with lip licking), and transfer capacity of the response (individual can lick both upper and lower lips to command.)

In order to capture change in these individualized protocols, the EC summit was helpful in identifying the technique of individualized quantitative behavioral assessment.[20] This process applies the principles of single-subject experimental design to capture the individual's unique injury presentation. Therapists create a series of command following items thought to be within the individual's repertoire of movement based on previous performance and systematically record positive/negative responses to random presentation of these items. This information allows direct comparison of performance from session to session and day to day. Variability in performance is common in this population. This type of session-session, day-day monitoring is helpful and an adjunct to information from the CRS-R.

The ECP psychologists play a vital role in assisting families with the ambiguous loss that occurs with the trauma or event leading to DOC. Dr Pauline Boss[21] has developed the theory of ambiguous loss, which has been very useful for the ECP. Ambiguous loss is defined as a situation in which a loved one is perceived as physically present while psychologically absent or physically absent but kept psychologically present because their status is unclear. With DOC, a person is physically present but psychologically absent to their family. Because the authors' society promotes quick solutions, families

| Table 8 Principles of experience-dependent neuroplasticity | |
|---|---|
| **Principle** | **Example in DOC** |
| Use it or lose it | Promoting purposeful responses in patients in an impaired state of consciousness will prevent degradation of neural circuitry for that response. |
| Use it and improve it | Promoting a purposeful response in patients in an impaired state of consciousness can strengthen the response. |
| Specificity | Incorporating purposeful responses into a functional task may lead to the production of new neural connections. |
| Repetition matters | Repetition of purposeful responses requires sufficient dosing to promote plasticity. |
| Intensity matters | Continued challenge to the demands of the purposeful response is required to promote plasticity. |
| Time matters | There may be an optimal time window in which therapy can have improved effectiveness in inducing neuroplasticity, and the processes driving the neuroplasticity may occur at different time periods. |
| Salience matters | Training experience needs to be meaningful to patients to optimize plasticity; family members can have a pivotal role with this principle. |
| Age matters | Training-induced plasticity is reduced with aging. |
| Transference | Effective environmental management may lead to improvement in other purposeful responses in addition to the criterion response. |
| Interference | Ineffective environmental management may lead to interference with acquisition of the response itself and/or other similar responses. |

*Data from* Kleim JA, Jones TA. Principles of experience-dependent neural plasticity: implications for rehabilitation after brain damage. J Speech Lang Hear Res 2008;51:S225–39.

are often hopeful the patients' situation will be remediated, fixed, or cured. After emergence, family members often express that their loved one is not the person they married or knew. At the same time, comments about who the person was in the past come through as well. Family members attempt to interpret behaviors in relation to the person they knew such as providing rationale for smiles or frowns. Psychologists work with the families to find ways to understand the loss and realize most of their feelings are normal in situations that deny resolution. The psychologists work hard on trying to help family members develop a new identity of their loved one, which is a combination of the past and present self, then try to help restore roles, rules, and rituals of that individual, including a role of being a parent or spouse.

When a family chooses to avoid working with psychology, the team can be negatively affected. The family members often attempt to control what they can, such as who can visit their loved one, what type of therapy the patients can receive, which medications the patients can take, who will or will not be the guardian if anyone is selected at all, and so forth. The authors' ECP teams are taught to recognize maladaptive behaviors of family members/caregivers and avoid power struggles. When formal psychology is not accepted by the family, the team members try to educate caregivers by using recommendations provided by the psychologist.

## EMERGING CONSCIOUSNESS PROGRAM OUTCOME MANAGEMENT AND FOLLOW-UP

In 2008, National Institute of Disability, Independent Living, and Rehabilitation Research and the VA began a collaborative relationship between the VA TBIMS and the VA PRCs to allow the PRCs to longitudinally assess the rehabilitation and functional outcomes of individuals with traumatic brain injury (TBI). A mirrored database for the PRCs was created to collect the same data as the TBIMS national database with additional data items chosen by the PRCs. Tracking the outcomes of the EC population was added to this database. Data are collected on discharge, 1 year, 2 years, 5 years, and 10 years. Study elements (**Box 3**) address the long-term physical and mental effects on the individual with a DOC, the health care needs after the completion

---

**Box 3**
**Veterans Affairs Traumatic Brain Injury Model System national database inclusions**

Demographic information

Preinjury history

Long-term medical outcomes

Long-term social outcomes

Community integration outcomes

Daily living outcomes

Employment outcomes

Information related to the degree of disability associated with traumatic brain injury

Information related to the resources required

ECP enrollment

*Data from* Nakase-Richardson R, Stevens LF, Tang X, et al. Comparison of the VA and NIDILRR TBI model system cohorts. J Head Trauma Rehabil 2017;32(4):221–33.

of inpatient rehabilitation, current long-term care rehabilitation programs and services options, and the effects on family members of the individual with a DOC. This partnership allows for veteran and service member studies to guide VA policy and programming, promotes collaboration with other agencies, and allows for comparisons with other TBI rehabilitation systems of care. Since October 2009, the VA TBIMS has published several articles using these data. Specific articles looking at long-term outcomes, life span system management, and comparisons between VA TBIMS and TBIMS EC populations will be, it is hoped, explored in the future.

The VHA is also starting to incorporate innovative ways to use telehealth. At inception, the PRCs have been able to virtually communicate to assist with management of patients within the system of care. The focus now includes the use of telehealth for communication from site to individual, which will provide opportunities for the ECP to develop new life span system management models.

## SUMMARY

VHA PRC ECP programming modifications and additions during the past decade have enhanced patient care and improved family/caregiver training and education. The system of care continues to explore interventions that may further improve patient care and outcomes. The ECP continues to adapt based on the most updated information. The DOC population continues to provide unique challenges to rehabilitation systems by requiring specialized testing procedures, structured environments, prevention of comorbidities, and long-term follow-up needs. Further research is needed in many areas. Over the next 10 years, the EC programs will continue to make strides in assistive technology, education, telehealth, and research to improve programming.

## REFERENCES

1. McNamee S, Howe L, Nakase-Richardson R, et al. Treatment of disorders of consciousness in the veterans health administration polytrauma centers. J Head Trauma Rehabil 2012;27(4):244–52.
2. Eapen BC, Jaramillo CA, Tapia RN, et al. Rehabilitation care of combat related TBI: veterans health administration polytrauma system of care. Curr Phys Med Rehabil Rep 2013;1(3):151–8.
3. Gray DS, Burnham RS. Preliminary outcome analysis of a long-term rehabilitation program for severe acquired brain injury. Arch Phys Med Rehabil 2000;81(11):1447–56.
4. Nakase-Richardson R, McNamee S, Howe L, et al. Descriptive characteristics and rehabilitation outcomes in active duty military personnel and veterans with disorders of consciousness with combat- and noncombat-related brain injury. Arch Phys Med Rehabil 2013;94:1861–9.
5. Bushnik T. The level of cognitive functioning scale. The Center for Outcome Measurement in Brain Injury; 2000. Available at: http://www.tbims.org/combi/lcfs. Accessed January 17, 2018.
6. Laureys S, Boly M, Moonen G, et al. Coma. Encyclopedia of Neuroscience 2009; 2:1133–42.
7. Giacino JT, Ashwal S, Childs N, et al. The minimally conscious state: definition and diagnostic criteria. Neurology 2002;58:349–53.
8. Nakase-Richardson R, Yablon SA, Sherer M, et al. Emergence from minimally conscious state: insights from evaluation of posttraumatic confusion. Neurology 2009;73:1120–6.

9. Wannez S, Heine L, Thonnard M, et al. The repetition of behavioral assessments in diagnosis of disorders of consciousness. Ann Neurol 2017;81:883–9.

10. Seel RT, Sherer M, Whyte J, et al. Assessment scales for disorders of consciousness: evidenced-based recommendations for clinical practice and research. Arch Phys Med Rehabil 2010;91:1795–813.

11. del Guidice R, Blume C, Wislowska M, et al. Can self-relevant stimuli help assessing patients with disorders of consciousness? Conscious Cogn 2016;44:51–60.

12. Tacikowski P, Ehrsson HH. Preferred processing of self-relevant stimuli occurs mainly at the perceptual and conscious stages of information processing. Conscious Cogn 2016;41:139–49.

13. Eapen BC, Georgekutty J, Subbarao B, et al. Disorders of consciousness. Phys Med Rehabil Clin N Am 2017;28:245–58.

14. Giacino JT, Whyte J, Bagiella E, et al. Placebo-controlled trial of amantadine for severe traumatic brain injury. N Engl J Med 2012;366:819–26.

15. Schnakers C, Monti MM. Disorders of consciousness after severe brain injury: therapeutic options. Curr Opin Neurol 2017;30:573–9.

16. Timmons M, Gasquoine L, Sciback JW. Functional changes with rehabilitation of very severe traumatic brain injury survivors. J Head Trauma Rehabil 1987;2:64–73.

17. Dittmer DK, Teasell R. Complications of immobilization and part 1: musculoskeletal and cardiovascular complications. Can Fam Physician 1993;39:1428–37.

18. Teasell R, Dittmer DK. Complications of immobilization and bed rest. Part 2: other complications. Can Fam Physician 1993;39:1440–2, 1445–6.

19. Wood RL. Critical analysis of the concept of sensory stimulation for patients in vegetative states. Brain Inj 1991;4:401–10.

20. Day KV, DiNapoli MV, Whyte J. Detecting early recovery of consciousness: a comparison of methods. Neuropsychol Rehabil 2017;1–9. https://doi.org/10.1080/09602011.2017.1309322. Online.

21. Boss P. Introduction: loss and ambiguity. In: Loss, trauma, and resilience: therapeutic work with ambiguous loss. 1st edition. New York: Norton, W. W. & Company, Inc; 2006. p. 2–20.

22. Giacino JT, Kalmar K, Whyte J. The JFK coma recovery scale-revised: measurement characteristics and diagnostic utility. Arch Phys Med Rehabil 2004;85(12):2020–9.

23. Wright J. The FIM(TM). The Center for Outcome Measurement in Brain Injury; 2000. Available at: http://www.tbims.org/combi/FIM. Accessed January 17, 2018.

24. Rappaport M. The disability rating and coma/near-coma scales in evaluating severe head injury. Neuropsychol Rehabil 2005;15(3–4):442–53.

# A Model of Care for Community Reintegration
## The Polytrauma Transitional Rehabilitation Program

Edan Critchfield, PsyD, ABPP-CN[a],*, Kathleen M. Bain, PhD[b],
Crystal Goudeau, PT, DPT[b], Christopher J. Gillis, OTR[b],
Maria Teresa Gomez-Lansidel, QTR, ABLS[b], Blessen C. Eapen, MD[c,1]

KEYWORDS

- Community reintegration • Polytrauma • Transitional rehabilitation • Brain injury
- Veterans

KEY POINTS

- Polytrauma injuries affect numerous body systems, resulting in physical, cognitive, and psychosocial limitations with possible lifelong rehabilitation needs.
- An interdisciplinary approach to rehabilitation is essential to effectively meet the complex and often overlapping needs of patients with polytrauma injuries.
- The Department of Veterans Affairs Polytrauma Transitional Rehabilitation Program (PTRP) provides interdisciplinary residential care to maximize functional independence and quality of life on community reintegration.
- Challenges when providing community reintegration rehabilitation include patient lack of accurate awareness for limitations, premorbid substance abuse, and family adjustment to injury.

## INTRODUCTION

As the result of recent conflicts, the military has seen a significant rise in the number of severe polytrauma injuries. The Veterans Health Administration defines polytrauma as "two or more injuries, one of which may be life threatening, sustained in the same

Disclosure Statement: The authors have nothing to disclose.
[a] Polytrauma Transitional Rehabilitation Program (PTRP), South Texas Veterans Healthcare System (STVHCS), 4949 Gus Eckert Road, San Antonio, TX 78240, USA; [b] Polytrauma Transitional Rehabilitation Program (PTRP), South Texas Veterans Healthcare System (STVHCS), 4949 Gus Eckert Road, San Antonio, TX 78240, USA; [c] Department of Physical Medicine and Rehabilitation, VA Greater Los Angeles Health Care System, 11301 Wilshire Boulevard, Los Angeles, CA 90073, USA
[1] Present address: 8939 Rocky Ridge, San Antonio, TX 78255.
* Corresponding author. 4949 Gys Eckert Road, San Antonio, TX 78240.
E-mail address: Edan.critchfield@va.gov

incident that affect multiple body parts or organ systems and result in physical, cognitive, psychological, or psychosocial impairments and functional disabilities."[1] In 2005, the Veterans Health Administration created the Polytrauma System of Care to meet the rising need for interdisciplinary care of veterans and active duty service members with polytrauma injuries.[2] The Polytrauma System of Care is a tiered continuum of rehabilitation care for service members and veterans that includes the Polytrauma Rehabilitation Center, the Polytrauma Network Site, and the Polytrauma Transitional Rehabilitation Program (PTRP).[1] The PTRP is a unique residential rehabilitation program embedded at each of 5 polytrauma centers (Minneapolis, Minnesota; Palo Alto, California; Richmond, Virginia; San Antonio, Texas; and Tampa, Florida) that is designed to foster effective community reintegration with a focus on return-to-duty, return-to-work, return-to-school, and/or management of complex life skills and psychological adjustment in an ecologically valid setting.[3]

During the height of the Operation Iraqi Freedom/Operation Enduring Freedom military conflict, the PTRP focused rehabilitation care primarily on those with polytraumatic injuries associated with moderate to severe traumatic brain injury (TBI). As combat referrals have declined, however, the PTRPs have extended services to those with other causes, such as stroke, anoxic brain injury, amputation, or mild TBI/postconcussive syndrome.[3]

PTRP admission decisions are made by a committee of team members tasked with interviewing potential applicants, reviewing their medical records, and determining appropriateness for the PTRP milieu. In specific, the admissions committee looks to identify whether an applicant has specific treatment needs/goals, has motivation to engage in rehabilitation, and has a clear disposition toward which to gear community reintegration. Specific admission criteria vary to some degree between PTRPs, given that each location has evolved to meet the needs of its community. See **Box 1** for review of admission criteria for the San Antonio PTRP.[4] Aggregate PTRP demographic data reported in Duchnick and colleagues[3] indicated 60% of patients were on active duty; the average age was 30, with an average length of rehabilitation that ranged from 60.3 days to 168.8 days.

The management of this complex patient population requires a holistic treatment approach provided by an interdisciplinary team of providers who are in frequent

---

**Box 1**
**San Antonio Polytrauma Transitional Rehabilitation Program admission criteria**

Residents admitted to PTRP must meet the following criteria:
1. At least 18 years of age
2. Medically stable
3. Have impairments that restrict community reintegration (impaired in areas, such as employment, school, independent living, cognition, and/or psychological adjustment secondary to TBI)
4. Have discernible goals that would benefit from a 24 hours per day, 7 days per week, structured, and supportive living setting
5. Do not exhibit behaviors posing risk/safety threat to self or others or exhibit behaviors that require alternate mental health services
6. Have the potential to successfully participate in groups and to benefit from therapy sessions
7. Need no more than supervision for basic activities of daily living
8. Can actively participate in medication self-administration program
9. Willing to participate in the program and to adhere to facility rules
10. No current substance abuse or dependence

communication to ensure consistent coordination of interventions across all disciplines (**Box 2**). Delivery of rehabilitation services includes evaluation and individual or group treatment within a clinic or residential setting as well as treatments extended into the community to ensure generalizability of skills obtained. For each patient, 1 team member is designated as a "lead therapist." The role of the lead therapist is to act as a clinical liaison between the patient and the treatment team. The lead therapist meets at least weekly with the patient to discuss progress toward treatment goals, plan therapeutic weekend passes, and facilitate any communication with the interdisciplinary treatment team. Although each patient presents personal characteristics that have an impact on recovery, treatment needs generally include some combination of physical, cognitive, psychological, and physical rehabilitation.

## COGNITIVE NEEDS

Polytrauma injuries can lead to a host of cognitive impairments that radically disrupt a person's ability to function independently, perform familiar roles, and complete daily routines. Cognitive dysfunction is of particular concern in patients who have experienced moderate TBI or severe TBI. The high rates of unemployment, substance abuse, social isolation, and incarceration among people with moderate to severe TBI are a testament to the potential negative effect of the injury on a patient's ability to be successful in the community.[5–8] Given their location in the cranium, the frontal and temporal lobes of the cerebral cortex are especially susceptible to damage in moderate to severe TBI. Damage to these cortical regions may result in persistent global cognitive impairments, namely with dysfunction in attention, memory, and executive functioning skills.[9,10]

| Box 2 |
| --- |
| **Polytrauma transitional rehabilitation program interdisciplinary team** |
| Physiatrist |
| Occupational therapist |
| Speech and language therapist |
| Physical therapist |
| Kinesiotherapist |
| Clinical pharmacist |
| Recreational therapist |
| Vision therapist |
| Neuropsychologist |
| Clinical psychologist |
| Family psychologist |
| Psychiatrist |
| Chaplain |
| Dietician |
| Case manager/social worker |
| Rehabilitation nursing |

According to the enablement/disablement model of rehabilitation, functional cognitive limitations result in decreased quality of life and decreased community participation.[11] A patient's successful reintegration into the community can hinge on cognitive proficiency. For example, to maintain employment, most people must have a working memory robust enough to encode instructions made by their employer, and they must have the executive function skills to successfully sequence these instructions. Similarly, to be independent in self-care tasks, one must have the visual perceptual skills to successfully put on clothing at the start of the working day. Preinjury roles and routines can become arduous to individuals with persistent cognitive impairments.

Therapeutic intervention for cognitive deficits often is initiated in the PTRP residential setting and then transitioned into the community. Generally, the treatment team addresses cognitive rehabilitation from 2 angles: restorative treatment and compensatory treatment. Restorative techniques are designed to restore premorbid cognitive strengths through exposure to material in the area of the deficit. Compensatory techniques, on the other hand, are designed to circumvent deficits by using new patterns of cognitive activity or compensatory mechanisms for impaired neurologic systems.[12]

Cognitive rehabilitation goals are usually hierarchical in nature, in that basic cognitive skills (eg, attention and orientation) are addressed before more complex skills (eg, planning and organization). Similarly, procedural, familiar tasks (eg, dressing) are addressed before more unstructured, novel tasks (eg, demonstrating appropriate social skills in a hospital common room). Rehabilitation staff, notably occupational therapists and speech language pathologists, provide training for basic self-care tasks, often with the use of memory compensation techniques, such as checklists or cuing systems. These therapists also provide retraining exercises to address specific cognitive skills and assist patients in relearning social skills through techniques such as rehearsal.

As a patient transitions from the PTRP to outpatient community care, the clinical staff, including occupational therapists, speech therapists, recreational therapists, and physical therapists, typically provide training and assist in the development of compensatory techniques for engagement in home management tasks, financial management tasks, care of others, health management, community mobility, and shopping. Staff also recommend environmental adaptations to assist with cognitive functioning (such as labeling drawers, placing calendars in plain view, and using alarms on a phone). Additionally, outpatient clinicians can assist patients in developing effective schedules and routines for employment pursuits and leisure exploration. Some therapists consult with employers and/or educational systems to adapt the work and school environment to facilitate a patient's functions in these settings. In the outpatient setting, care generally is conducted from a compensatory perspective. Success in the community is driven by the patient (and patient caregiver's) ability to use new strategies/mechanisms to successfully create purposeful everyday routines and maintain meaningful social roles.

## PSYCHOLOGICAL NEEDS

Changes in neurologic and physical functioning after TBI are often apparent to both patients and providers, and they typically follow an upward trajectory of incremental improvement over time. In contrast, emotional changes after TBI may be more difficult to identify and may not follow a linear course of recovery. Despite being the least visible, psychiatric sequelae of head injury can include persistent and disabling symptoms with significant implications for the success of community reintegration efforts.[13]

Broadly, 3 phases must be considered when addressing emotional functioning in individuals who have experienced a TBI: premorbid, acute/postacute, and long-term/adjustment-related. Many survivors of TBI have premorbid psychiatric disorders and there is some evidence that the presence of a disorder prior to injury increases the risk of experiencing a disorder after injury.[14,15] It is important for rehabilitation providers to obtain a thorough history of patients' past mental health diagnoses, treatments received, and efficacy of those treatments. This information can help providers monitor for resurgence or exacerbation of premorbid emotional symptoms as well as provide useful indicators for treatments that are more likely to be helpful.

In the acute and postacute phases of brain injury recovery, complex neurochemical cascades related to the injury itself can produce short-term emotional symptoms. This cascade of neurometabolic changes involves alterations in both the structure and function of neurons, leading to impaired neurotransmission and vulnerability to delayed cell death and dysfunction.[16] Neuroanatomic and neurometabolic changes often occur in frontal and anterior temporal regions, contributing to affective instability, whereas alterations in dopaminergic pathways can produce symptoms of apathy.[17] These symptoms may represent obstacles to patients' full engagement in rehabilitation services and, therefore, should be identified and addressed swiftly. In addition to acute neurometabolic changes, physical damage to discrete brain regions in moderate to severe TBI is associated with emotional and personality changes after injury. Specifically, lesions to brain regions involved in emotion processing (eg, anterior temporal poles, amygdala, and orbitofrontal cortex) can produce chronic symptoms of emotional dysregulation, social disinhibition, and altered mood state.[18]

Finally, exposure to new psychosocial stressors or exacerbation of preexisting stressors may contribute to emotional distress and psychiatric disorders in survivors of TBI. For some patients, resuming independent management of complex activities of daily living after an extended period of recovery in inpatient settings can be a difficult adjustment, and the demand to complete these activities in the face of newly acquired physical and/or cognitive limitations may increase adjustment-related distress.[19] Alterations in family dynamics and dysfunctional family relationships can contribute to depression.[20] Reductions in social problem-solving skills and opportunities for socializing are common and can limit community participation, resulting in social isolation.[21] Unemployment or underemployment after injury is also common and may introduce significant financial stressors. Furthermore, some patients may struggle with spiritual concerns related to their injuries (eg, survivor guilt).[5]

Although all team members play a role in monitoring patient mood states and behaviors, the rehabilitation psychologist takes the lead in obtaining a mental health history, identifying symptoms as they emerge, and developing an appropriate treatment plan. The psychologist's expertise in assessment is crucial for appropriate diagnosis, because it can be difficult to distinguish among symptoms of grief/bereavement, depression, and adjustment disorder. Similarly, somatic symptoms of depression (eg, sleep disturbance, fatigue, changes in appetite, or impaired concentration) may overlap with symptoms attributable to head injury itself, complicating diagnosis. In addition to providing evidence-based treatments for mood, anxiety, and trauma-related disorders, psychologists also may treat sleep disorders and chronic pain. Furthermore, they may take the lead in designing behavioral modification plans for problematic behaviors (eg, inappropriate behaviors toward others), disseminating plans to the rehabilitation treatment team, and monitoring their effectiveness. When concerns related to family dynamics are present, the family psychologist may be called on for additional assessment and intervention. The team chaplain also plays an important role in helping patients cope with spiritual concerns related to injury and postinjury adjustment.

## PHYSICAL NEEDS

The physical injuries commonly associated with polytrauma injuries are a combination of sensory, motor, neurologic, and orthopedic injuries that collectively affect independent functional movement. These injuries are often a result of a TBI and include the possible sequelae of dizziness, headaches, vision deficits, limb weakness, hemiplegia, spasticity, ataxia, and/or other motor coordination deficits.[5,6] TBI can be unique from other neurologic incidents, such as stroke, in that there are often other comorbidities, such as traumatic orthopedic fractures to the face, pelvis, and/or limbs, spinal cord injuries, and traumatic amputations. In the transitional rehabilitation setting, therapists often find themselves treating both acute injuries from the current trauma and chronic injuries that predated the traumatic event. If patients have had a long acute care stay, their acute injuries may have already transitioned into chronic injuries. Headaches are a common chronic pain complaint post-TBI.[22] In a systematic review of chronic pain after a TBI, 57.8% of 1670 patients complained of chronic headache. The review also noted links between TBI and complex regional pain syndrome, painful heterotopic ossification, and peripheral neuropathies.[23] When pain has transitioned into the chronic stage, its treatment necessitates an interdisciplinary approach in which the psychosocial aspects of treatment are as important as the physical and medical approaches to treatment. These physical deficits can cause a barrier to community reintegration through difficulty with safe and independent gait and mobility, decreased activity tolerance, difficulty with chronic pain, and reduced capacity to manage the increased sensorimotor demands that accompany multisensory/multitasking environments, such as crowded malls, grocery stores, parks, and businesses.

In acute care, the focus of rehabilitation of these physical deficits is primarily on independence with basic mobility and self-care through individualized rehabilitation sessions. If a patient were to return home after acute rehabilitation and not continue with transitional rehabilitation, the patient may be physically independent at a wheelchair or walker level within the home for mobility but may not have the stamina, balance, or mobility to integrate successfully back into the community where there are increased physical and sensorimotor demands.[24,25] Outpatient therapy is limited with addressing a patient's needs in the clinic setting. Transitional rehabilitation bridges this gap by providing rehabilitation not only in the austere environment of the clinic setting but also out in the multitasking, multisensory environment of the community.

The primary focus of physical rehabilitation in a transitional rehabilitation setting is achieving the highest level of functional independence possible. This includes helping patients return to their previous level of physical conditioning or helping them to discover and pursue goals at whatever new physical level they currently possess. The extent or length of physical rehabilitation in the transitional setting is individualized and based on a patient's goals. A patient's goals may include the physical ability to return to a certain type of work (a soldier returning to active duty or an electrician being able to climb up a ladder or crawl under a house), a return to or new development of an interest or hobby (having the balance to return to fly fishing, endurance to return to running, or coordination to be able to bowl), or the ability to multitask (holding a conversation while ambulating down a grocery aisle and remembering what one is shopping for or being able look at one's phone screen and walk at the same time safely). Other patients may simply have the goal of being independent with ambulation and daily tasks at home for a defined period of time to allow a caregiver or spouse to work or leave the house for errands. At PTRP, the individual and the interdisciplinary team can work to decrease and overcome barriers to community reintegration. This may include developing compensatory strategies, maximizing use of spared modalities, and practicing effective use of durable medical equipment and orthoses. Examples may include using a functional electrical stimulation device for ambulation to allow an individual to walk for longer distances or with a cane instead of a walker or acquiring motor-assisted wheels for a wheelchair to increase an individual's endurance for managing hills and ramps while attending school. Another example may be teaching scanning strategies on a timed schedule to find items in the grocery store. The length of treatment and prognosis of transitional physical rehabilitation is determined by a patient's goals, and the solutions can be as individualized and unique as the patients.

## CLINICAL CHALLENGES

Whether due to a neurologic process (ie, anosognosia) or a psychological defense mechanism (ie, denial), inaccurate understanding or lack of appreciation for cognitive and physical limitations after polytrauma injuries can present a challenge for community reintegration.[26] From a rehabilitation perspective, patients who lack insight and awareness of their deficits are less likely to participate in rehabilitation or to use compensatory strategies in the community, which can limit their community reintegration potential.[27] It is important to recognize that an overestimate of ability can also present a safety risk and potentially result in reinjury. Contrary to individuals with moderate to severe brain injuries who may lack an appreciation for their deficits, individuals with mild TBIs may have an exaggerated sense of their deficits and lack an accurate appreciation of their abilities.[28]

One of the goals for community reintegration rehabilitation is to help patients to build an accurate assessment of their abilities and limitations. This can be done through various interventions, which often include comparing patients' predicted performance to their actual performance on tasks or setting up controlled failure interventions to highlight functional deficits.[29] Conversely, in working with patients with mild TBI who overestimate their disabilities, providing observation of their ability level in the community can help provide them with evidence of adequate cognitive or psychological ability.

A relationship exists between alcohol and substance misuse and polytrauma injuries. In part, individuals who misuse alcohol and substances are at a greater risk of acquiring injuries but also individuals who have sustained polytrauma injuries are at a greater risk of developing alcohol and substance use disorders.[30,31] Also, of increased concern within this population is the increased risk for seizures post–severe TBI, a risk that is heightened when combined with alcohol use.[32] Despite the recognized need to address drug and alcohol use within community reintegration programs, however, treatment remains challenging due to many of these patients' poor insight/awareness and increased impulsivity. Additionally, risk for alcohol/substance use remains elevated due to factors, such as ongoing pain, psychological comorbidities, limited access to follow-up care, and often a wealth of unproductive free time postinjury.[33]

Helping a patient's family adjust to changes that are inherent after polytrauma injuries poses another significant challenge within community reintegration rehabilitation. Family members play a critical role throughout the rehabilitation process. Acutely, this might mean providing significant assistance with basic activities of daily living or wound care. It is not uncommon during this period for parents to revert back to an earlier developmental stage of parenting or for a spouse to take on a role as a caregiver rather than a companion.[34] Although the extra support might be necessary during the acute phase of rehabilitation, within the context of community reintegration too much family support can restrict growth. Often this is due to family members not allowing the patient to struggle with functional challenges and thus inadvertently hindering recovery. To address this, it is recommended that family members observe rehabilitation sessions in the community to get a better idea of a patient's functional ability. Family therapy is also vital to provide education about rehabilitation and to aid in the family unit's adjustment to injury.

## POLYTRAUMA TRANSITIONAL REHABILITATION PROGRAM COMMUNITY REINTEGRATON OUTCOMES

Successful community reintegration and individual patient progress are assessed using the clinical staff rating of the Mayo-Portland Adaptability Inventory, 4th revision (MPAI-4) at both admission and discharge.[35] The MPAI-4 is a standardized measure of 34 domains of functioning that examines physical and cognitive ability, psychosocial adjustment, and participation. Aggregate outcome data across PTRP sites have demonstrated statistically and clinically meaningful change across all MPAI-4 domains.[3]

Functional outcomes are also collected at 6 months postdischarge to assess patient involvement in productive activities. Based on 2016 6-month follow-up data presented by the San Antonio PTRP, 30% of patients were employed, 30% regularly engaged in volunteer activities, 20% were enrolled in college, and 50% of patients were independently driving[36] (**Box 3**). These functional outcomes are consistent with similar rehabilitation programs that have found at follow-up 62% of patients were engaged in general productive activity,[37] 35.4% had returned to work,[38] and 40% were able to drive.[39]

### Clinical Case Presentation

This clinical case is presented to demonstrate the complexity of rehabilitation for polytrauma injuries, the interplay of PTRP disciplines and an example of successful community reintegration.

Sergeant (SGT) BE is a 26-year-old, right-handed, white man on active duty within an Army Special Forces unit who was injured when an improvised explosive device exploded beneath his vehicle in Afghanistan. Injuries included depressed left temporoparietal fracture and subarachnoid hemorrhage, requiring left hemicraniectomy and ventriculoperitoneal shunt. He sustained a severe TBI characterized by a loss of consciousness of 7 days and posttraumatic amnesia of approximately 3 weeks. From the site of the blast, he was evacuated to Landstuhl, Germany, where he remained for 2 months for medical stabilization. Given his family was from New Mexico, Sgt BE was transferred to the San Antonio PTRP for community reintegration.

---

**Box 3**
**San Antonio Polytrauma Transitional Rehabilitation Program functional outcomes (2016)**

Productivity at 6 months postdischarge
- 30% Employed
- 30% Volunteering
- 20% Enrolled in college
- 50% Driving (legally)

---

On admission 87 days postinjury, Sgt BE presented to the PTRP with a primary goal of remaining on active duty and returning to driving. Initial neuropsychological evaluation of the patient revealed global impairment with a prominent expressive aphasia, which limited communication to physical gestures and simple yes/no responses. He presented with a significant lack of awareness for his functional deficits (managing finances, driving, and so forth) which was exacerbated by his slowed processing speed, impulsivity, and impaired memory. As a result of his right-sided hemiparesis, he arrived at PTRP at a wheelchair level for independent community mobility and a platform walker for independent household ambulation. He also had limited functional use of his Right Upper Extremity due to increased tone. Psychologically, he denied any problems with anxiety, depression, or adjustment to injury. Despite his communication deficits, he was quite vocal of his desire to have no contact with the PTRP psychologist given his concerns that talking to a psychologist would jeopardize his ability to remain on active duty.

The interdisciplinary treatment team worked to address his deficits, with the primary focus across all disciplines on the patient's lack of awareness. Developing an accurate awareness of limitations was addressed through repeated education on the sequelae of his injury, controlled failure exercises, and interventions where he compared his predicted performance on tasks to his actual performance. Speech therapy addressed expressive language deficits and use of assistive technology (ie, iPad) to communicate his needs. As is frequently the case with the active duty military population, rehabilitation of physical deficits came easier for Sgt BE given his premorbid fitness routine and motivation to return to the military's fitness standards. Although he was resistant to meet with psychology, his religious upbringing helped him develop a relationship with the PTRP chaplin, who was able to help him process his life changes and introduce the idea of developing options should he not be retained by the military. Cotreatments with occupational, physical, and recreation therapy focused on regaining the mobility and fine motor control necessary to resume leisure activities, such as fishing, shooting, and playing soccer. The PTRP family psychologist worked closely with the patient's mother and his fiancée to define their respective roles as care providers and to resist the urge to speak for the patient in conversation both privately and in the community. Family therapy was critical in helping his mother and fiancée develop an accurate understanding of Sgt BE's limitations and how this might have an impact on his long-term care needs.

At discharge after 97 days of rehabilitation, Sgt BE's treatment had transitioned almost entirely from the clinic setting into the community. Mobility improved to independent ambulation with a knee and ankle brace, with use of single-point cane only for uneven ground. Right upper extremity tone had improved to allow for use of right upper extremity to complete functional tasks with cleaning, opening doors, and preparing food in the kitchen. Expressive language and cognitive deficits had improved to a level where Sgt BE was able to make his own medical decisions, and with oversight he could manage his finances. Goals for returning to driving had not been met but were planned on being addressed further on an outpatient basis. After intervention from the family psychologist, the patient's mother decided to return home to New Mexico and his fiancée stepped in to provide assistance/support, as needed. Finally, the patient's military command had not initiated a medical evaluation board but encouraged the patient to develop a back-up plan should he be medically retired.

At his 6-month follow-up, Sgt BE had married his fiancée and the couple were living together in an apartment. Given limited dexterity with his upper extremity, the patient reported that a medical evaluation board had been initiated and he had accepted that he would likely be medically retired from the Army. With continued cognitive recovery, he was cleared to drive and discussed plans to take a college class the following semester. Given his dedication to the Special Forces community, he volunteered weekly with their medical liaison to provide support for other injured service members. Overall, although it is difficult to communicate the numerous complexities of this case, transitional rehabilitation was able to help Sgt BE increase his awareness of deficits, improve his communication, and achieve more independence with mobility, allowing him to be more successful with reintegration back into his community.

## SUMMARY

With the escalation of military conflicts in recent years, there has been a corresponding increase in the number of severe polytrauma injuries. The Department of Veterans Affairs PTRP was established as an integral part of the Polytrauma System of Care to extend the rehabilitation of veterans and active duty service members past the acute phase and into the community setting. Community reintegration is a return to productivity through functional independence and resumption of social roles at premorbid or new levels postinjury. Effective community reintegration is best achieved with a diverse interdisciplinary team that can use a collaborative approach to treat patients' physical, cognitive, and psychological deficits. Barriers, such as lack of awareness of deficits or exaggeration of deficits, can present a significant challenge for community reintegration. Substance abuse can also present as a premorbid and continuing challenge with rehabilitation. Strong family support is vital to helping patients reach their maximal recovery potential and helps combat these challenges. Recovery with polytrauma injuries, especially with moderate to severe brain injuries, is often lifelong, with the transition from inpatient to outpatient treatment continuing for ongoing maintenance of needs.

## REFERENCES

1. VHA Handbook 1172.01, Polytrauma System of Care - ViewPublication.asp. Available at: http://www.va.gov/vhapublications/ViewPublication.asp?pub_ID=2875. Accessed April 2, 2013.
2. Eapen BC, Jaramillo CA, Tapia RN, et al. Rehabilitation care of combat related TBI: veterans health administration polytrauma system of care. Curr Phys Med Rehabil Rep 2013. https://doi.org/10.1007/s40141-013-0023-0.
3. Duchnick JJ, Ropacki S, Yutsis M, et al. Polytrauma transitional rehabilitation programs: Comprehensive rehabilitation for community integration after brain injury. Psychol Serv 2015;12(3):313–21.
4. Department of Veterans Affairs, South Texas Veteran's Healthcare System, PTRP11P-14-TO11, Polytrauma Transitional Rehabilitation Program Admission Policy and Procedure.
5. Cuthbert JP, Harrison-Felix CH, Corrigan JD, et al. Unemployment in the United States after traumatic brain injury for working-age individuals: Prevalence and associated factors 2 years postinjury. J Head Trauma Rehabil 2015;30(3):160–74.
6. Hoofien D, Gilboa A, Vakil E, et al. Traumtic brain injury (TBI) 10-20 years later: a comprehensive outcome study of psychiatric symptomatology, cognitive abilities and psychosocial functioning. Brain Inj 2001;15(3):189–209.
7. Corrigan JD. Substance abuse as a mediating factor in outcome from traumatic brain injury. Arch Phys Med Rehabil 1995;76:302–9.
8. Farrer TJ, Hedges DW. Prevalence of traumatic brain injury in incarcerated groups compared to the general population: a meta-analysis. Prog Neuro-Psychopharmacology Biol Psychiatry 2011;35:390–4.

9. Mahar C, Fraser K. Barriers to successful community reintegration following acquired brain injury (ABI). Int J Disabil Management 2012;6:49–67.
10. Stuss DT. Traumatic brain injury: relation to executive dysfunction and frontal lobes. Curr Opin Neurol 2011;24(6):584–9.
11. Brandt EN, Pope AM. Enabling America: assessing the role of rehabilitation science and engineering. Washington, DC: National Academy Press; 1997.
12. Harley JP, Allen C, Braciszewski TL, et al. Guidelines for cognitive rehabilitation. NeuroRehabilitation 1992;2:62–75.
13. Jorge RE, Arciniegas DB. Mood disorders after TBI. Psychiatr Clin North America 2014;37(1):13–29.
14. Whelan-Goodinson R, Ponsford J, Johnston L, et al. Psychiatric disorders following traumatic brain injury: their nature and frequency. J Head Trauma Rehabil 2009;24(5):324–32.
15. Whelan-Goodinson R, Ponsford JL, Schönberger M, et al. Predictors of psychiatric disorders following traumatic brain injury. J Head Trauma Rehabil 2010;25(5):320–9.
16. Giza CC, Hovda DA. The new neurometabolic cascade of concussion. Neurosurgery 2014;75(4):S24–33.
17. McAllister TW. Neurobiological consequences of traumatic brain injury. Dialogues Clin Neurosci 2011;13(3):287–300.
18. Beer JS, Lombardi MV. Insights into emotion regulation from neuropsychology. In: Gross JJ, editor. Handbook of emotion regulation. New York: Guilford Press; 2007. p. 69–86.
19. Groom KN, Shaw TG, O'Connor ME, et al. Neurobehavioral symptoms and family functioning in traumatically brain-injured adults. Arch Clin Neuropsychol 1988;13(8):695–711.
20. Gould KR, Ponsford JL, Johnston L, et al. The nature, frequency, and course of psychiatric disorders in the first year after traumatic brain injury: a prospective study. Psychol Med 2011;41:2099–109.
21. Sander AM, Struchen MA. Interpersonal relationships and traumatic brain injury. J Head Trauma Rehabil 2011;26(1):1–3.
22. Linder SL. Post-traumatic headache. Curr Pain Headache Rep 2007;5(11):396–400.
23. Nampiaparampil D. Prevalence of chronic pain after traumatic brain injury: a systematic review. J Am Med Assoc 2008;300(6):711–9.
24. Walker WC, Pickett TC. Motor impairments after severe traumatic brain injury: a longitudinal multicenter study. J Rehabil Res Development 2007;44(7):975–82.
25. O'Dell D, Nolde-Lopez G. Physical complications. In: Reyst H, editor. The essential brain injury guide. Heidi Reyst, Brain Injury Association of America; 2016. p. 160–84.
26. Vanderploeg RD, Belanger HG, Duchnick JD, et al. Awareness problems following moderate to severe traumatic brain injury: prevalence, assessment methods, and injury correlates. J Rehabil Res Development 2006;44:937–50.
27. Ownsworth T, Clare L. The association between awareness deficits and rehabilitation outcome following acquired brain injury. Clin Psychol Rev 2006;26:783–95.
28. Lange RT, Iverson GL, Rose A. Post-concussion symptom reporting and the "Good-Old-Days" bias following mild traumatic brain injury. Arch Clin Neuropsychol 2010;25:442–50.
29. Flemming JM, Ownsworth T. A review of awareness intervention in brain injury rehabilitation. Neuropsychological Rehabil 2006;16(4):474–500.

30. Corrigan JD, Bogner J, Holloman C. Lifetime history of traumatic brain injury among persons with substance use disorders. Brain Inj 2012;(2):139–50.
31. Grossbard J, Malte CA, Lapham G, et al. Prevalence of alcohol misuse and follow-up care in a national sample of OEF/OIF VA patients with and without TBI. Psychiatr Serv 2017;68:1.
32. Vaaramo K, Puljula J, Tetri S, et al. Predictors of new-onset seizures: a 10-year follow-up of head trauma subjects with and without traumatic brain injury. J Neurol Neurosurg Psychiatry 2014;85:598–602.
33. Graham DP, Cardon AL. An update on substance use and treatment following traumatic brain injury. Ann New York Acad Sci 2008;1141:148–62.
34. Godwin EE, Schaaf KW, Kreutzer JS. Practical approaches to family assessment and intervention. In: Zasler ND, Katz DI, Zafonte RD, editors. Brain injury medicine. New York: Demos Medical Publishing, LLC; 2013. p. 1329–48.
35. Malec J. The Mayo-Portland adaptability inventory. 2005. Available at: http://www.tbims.org/combi/mpai. Accessed March 13, 2018.
36. Critchfield E, Lemmer J, Caya L, et al. Polytrauma Transitional Rehabilitation Program (PTRP): 2016 Year In Review. Poster presented at: Texas Brain Injury Alliance Conference, 2016; Austin, TX, December 11, 2015.
37. Harrick L, Krefting L, Johnston J, et al. Stability of functional outcomes following transitional living programme participation: 3-year follow-up. Brain Inj 1994;8:439–47.
38. Lippert-Gruner M, Wedekind C, Klug N. Functional and psychosocial outcome one year after severe traumatic brain injury and early-onset rehabilitation therapy. J Rehabil Med 2002;34:211–4.
39. Olver JH, Ponsford JL, Curran CA. Outcome following traumatic brain injury: a comparison between 2 and 5 years after injury. Brain Inj 1994;10(11):841–8.

# Comprehensive Care for Persons with Spinal Cord Injury

Timothy Lavis, MD[a,b,]*, Lance L. Goetz, MD[a,b]

## KEYWORDS

- Spinal cord injury • Primary care • Preventive care • Surveillance

## KEY POINTS

- Spinal cord injury results in multiple secondary comorbidities, which vary based on injury severity and other characteristics.
- Persons with spinal cord injury are at lifelong risk for many complications, most of which are at least partially preventable with proper medical care.
- The Veterans Health Administration Spinal Cord Injury and Disorders System of Care offers evaluations to all persons in their registries.
- Persons with spinal cord injury are often by necessity heavy users of the health care system.

## OVERVIEW

The care of veterans and active duty service members with spinal cord injury (SCI) in the Veterans Health Administration (VHA) takes place in a unique system, which encompasses not only acute rehabilitation but also lifelong primary and acute care focused on the complications associated with SCI. The system is set up to allow veterans with SCI to receive care from a specialized an interdisciplinary team of medical professionals, which includes medical providers, therapists from multiple disciplines, social workers, psychologists, dieticians, rehabilitation engineers, prosthetists, and nurses who work primarily with individuals who have spinal cord injuries. Even when acute rehabilitation is completed outside the Veterans Administration (VA) system, veterans often will enter the VA system shortly after to take advantage of this specialized treatment team and the level of care they earned through their service.

The authors have nothing to disclose.
a Spinal Cord Injury and Disorders Service, Hunter Holmes McGuire VA Medical Center, 1201 Broad Rock, Boulevard, Richmond, VA 23249, USA; b Department of Physical Medicine and Rehabilitation, Virginia Commonwealth University, 4th Floor, 1223 E Marshall Street, Richmond, VA 23298, USA
* Corresponding author. Spinal Cord Injury and Disorders Service, Hunter Holmes McGuire VA Medical Center, 128, 1201 Broad Rock, Boulevard, Richmond, VA 23249.
E-mail address: timothy.lavis@va.gov

Phys Med Rehabil Clin N Am 30 (2019) 55–72
https://doi.org/10.1016/j.pmr.2018.08.010
1047-9651/19/Published by Elsevier Inc.

pmr.theclinics.com

The VA Spinal Cord Injury and Disorders (SCI&D) System of Care is set up in a hub and spoke structure, with currently 24 spinal cord "hub" centers across the United States.[1] These centers work with smaller "spoke" centers, where a more limited level of specialized care is obtained. Because of the complexities of care for individuals and complications associated with SCI, it is recommended within the VA system that prolonged hospitalizations and specialized medical procedures take place at one of the SCI centers, to allow for optimal care on medical units staffed and set up specifically to take care of persons with SCI.

The SCI&D System of Care, which is detailed in VHA Handbook 1176.01, has been mentioned as deserving of recognition.[2] The VHA regulations direct the structure of the SCI&D system, population served, services provided, and staffing within the SCI&D system.[3] Once veterans are enrolled, they are eligible for lifelong care through this VA System, including admission to an SCI center for rehabilitation, primary care services, elective and nonelective surgical procedures, as well as respite care and hospice services.

One of the cornerstones of the care provided to veterans with spinal cord injuries is the annual evaluation. All veterans with SCI are eligible for, offered, and encouraged to receive, a comprehensive annual evaluation at an SCI center, usually the center associated with the local VA "spoke" clinic. VA SCI&D centers provide what has been described as a "one-stop-shopping" approach during a single outpatient day or brief inpatient stay if needed, during which veterans with SCI have encounters with nursing, SCI medicine clinicians, psychologists, physical, occupational, recreation, and kinesiotherapists, social workers, and other specialized allied health providers, such as dietitians. Referrals to any other needed providers can be made after these assessments.

Outlined in later discussion are relevant areas of assessment and related complications that are evaluated as part of the SCI annual evaluation process.

## CHANGING DEMOGRAPHICS OF SPINAL CORD INJURY

Persons with SCI remain largely (around 80%) men and 90% adult at time of onset. The last 30 years have seen a relative decrease in percentage of injuries from vehicular causes and an increase in persons with spinal stenosis cause, including progressive myelopathy and ground level falls.[4,5] This aging population brings with it additional medical concerns.

## GENERAL

Providers annually elicit any medication changes, major illnesses, hospitalizations, emergency room visits, and operative procedures since the last annual examination. A general "internal medicine" review of systems is performed to screen for excess fatigue, rash, itching, nasal congestion, bleeding, changes in hearing, tinnitus, vertigo, headaches, autonomic symptoms such as dizziness, changes in sweating, diplopia, or blurred vision, shortness of breath, cough, wheezing or chest pain, palpitations, and others. The SCI medicine specialist recognizes that, because of the unique pathophysiology of SCI, symptoms can mean different things than they would in persons without SCI. For example, a stuffy nose, although perhaps benign in the general population, could represent a symptom of autonomic dysreflexia (AD) in a person with SCI.

## NEUROMUSCULOSKELETAL

The provider should query regarding details of insult or injury, including date, cause, spine or other fractures, surgeries, and coinjuries. In addition, any changes in neurologic (sensory, motor, or autonomic) function as well as any decline in mobility since the prior annual evaluation should be noted. The general neurologic examination documents muscle stretch reflexes, the presence or absence of pathologic reflexes, bulk, atrophy, tone, clonus, gross and fine motor coordination, gait, and overall function, so that changes can be identified, if present, on future evaluations. The neurologic portion of the rectal examination is of both prognostic and functional importance and includes objective evaluation of voluntary anal contraction, light touch, pinprick, deep anal pressure, tone, anal wink, and bulbocavernosus reflex (BCR).

SCI centers within the VA SCI&D System of Care perform the International Standards for Neurological Classification After Spinal Cord Injury (ISNCSCI)[6] examination at each annual evaluation. Posttraumatic syringomyelia (PTS) is a feared complication of SCI that can result in neurologic deterioration with functional decline, progressive respiratory compromise, and death. Clinically significant PTS occurs in at least 3% to 4% of persons with SCI and can manifest as early as 1 month or as late as many years after SCI.[7] Changes can occur slowly and be very subtle, especially slight dermatomal sensory changes. Other potential issues can include recurrent spinal stenosis, radiculopathies, or compression neuropathies.

## SPASTICITY

Spasticity, part of the upper motor neuron syndrome, manifests as increased tone or tightness in muscles, clonus, muscle jerks, and hyperreflexia. Incidence estimates vary, but roughly half of persons with SCI report it.[8] It is more likely to occur in persons with higher injuries. The SCI provider should assess its timing, severity, effect on which functional activities, sleep, or whether it causes discomfort, in which case treatment may be indicated. Treatments include stretching, modalities, medications, nerve or muscle blockade, or intrathecal medication delivery. The annual evaluation offers the opportunity to assess whether spasticity is adequately controlled, or conversely, overtreated and in need of adjustment.

## FUNCTIONAL EVALUATION

The functional assessment is at the core of the physiatric examination. History and musculoskeletal examination, sources of pain, past and current functional status, level of independence with mobility (eg, gait, wheelchair propulsion, transfers), activity of daily (or nightly) living (ADLs), and equipment needs are assessed. Proper prescription, use, and maintenance of devices for mobility, ADLs, and skin protection are critical for optimal function and prevention of injuries or other complications. For example, in a manual wheelchair user with paraplegia, proper transfer technique is critical to prevention of shoulder injuries.[9]

## PAIN

Pain can be classified as acute, subacute, chronic, neuropathic, musculoskeletal, visceral, and above, at, or below the level of injury. Pain is an important problem for many persons with SCI, as 50% or more of persons with SCI live with chronic pain of one, or often more than one, type.[10,11] A critical determination for the clinician is, does the person's current pain medication regimen enhance (or impair) the person's ability to function, including performance of ADLs and participating in work or recreation. Choice of medical or nonmedical management options depends on a multitude of factors beyond the scope of this discussion.

Current recommendations recommend limiting opiate use to brief periods as needed following acute trauma and some surgical procedures. Debate continues regarding the efficacy of opioids for chronic non–cancer pain, with evidence to support or refute their use.[12] Recently published guidelines[13] for long-term opioid use involve completion of patient provider agreements, or "contracts," queries of state prescription monitoring programs, periodic screening for use of illicit and prescription agents, and other interventions to mitigate risks of adverse outcomes such as overdose or medication diversion.

## RESPIRATORY FUNCTION

Respiratory complications are a leading cause of mortality in SCI. Respiratory causes are the leading cause of mortality during the first year after injury and remain a leading cause in the subsequent years following injury.[14] Individuals with SCI are particularly vulnerable to complications from respiratory infections, and the rate of fatal pneumonia is significantly higher in persons with SCI compared with those without SCI.[15] Pneumonia accounts for 70.1% of the deaths secondary to respiratory disease in those with SCI.[4] In persons with complete tetraplegia, respiratory complications following SCI are associated with 3 main components of respiratory function: hypoventilation, secretion management, and atelectasis.[4] The 3 muscle groups that are involved in respiratory function are the diaphragm, the intercostals, and the abdominal muscles. The diaphragm receives innervation from cervical levels C3, C4, and C5. Therefore, individuals with neurologic level of injury above C3 can experience complete diaphragm paralysis. Persons with SCI within C3–C5 levels can experience varying degrees of diaphragm impairment, which often leads to decreased inspiratory weakness and a decrease in vital capacity. The diaphragm typically contributes approximately 65% of the vital capacity in non–spinal cord injured subjects.[16] Veterans with neurologic impairment of the diaphragm may require ventilator assistance for breathing, particularly when the level of injury is above C3. Patients with upper cervical injuries will often require ventilator management, particularly in the acute phase. An important aspect of rehabilitation care in the SCI&D System of Care is ventilator management and weaning when appropriate. The VA SCI&D centers are able provide care to veterans requiring ventilatory support, with programs to maximize efforts to wean veterans from ventilators. For veterans who are unable to wean from the requirement of ventilator support, the SCI&D system works with veterans to obtain the appropriate medical equipment, including portable ventilators to maximize their independence in the community. The thoracic spinal cord, levels T1–T11, provides neurologic input to the intercostal muscles of the rib cage. The external intercostal muscles can also assist with forced inhalation.[4] In addition to inspiration, expiration is also an important aspect of the pulmonary process that can be affected following SCI. Exhalation is primarily a passive process; however, forceful expiration and cough are important processes whereby impairment can lead to clinical difficulties. The intercostal muscles and abdominal muscles play important roles in exhalation. The abdominal muscles also play a key role in cough and secretion management. The abdominal muscles receive innervation from the lower half of the thoracic spinal cord (T7–T12); therefore, individuals with a level of injury within this region also can experience varying levels of difficulty in clearing respiratory secretions, which lead to mucous plugging. An injury above T7 will lead to severe impairment in this process.

Atelectasis and mucous plugging are common complications associated with respiratory impairment following SCI, particularly paraplegia above the T7 level and tetraplegia in the acute setting. Atelectasis can make patients with SCI susceptible to pneumonia, which can then lead to an increase in pulmonary secretions that can result in further mucous plugging leading to pneumonia. Overburdened residual respiratory muscles can fatigue acutely, resulting in respiratory failure. Aggressive secretion management is very important in this population due to impairment in the ability to produce effective cough. There are many techniques and devices that can be used to assist with pulmonary toilet in the hospital or home setting, such as assisted cough, mechanical insufflation-exsufflation, incentive spirometry, chest vibration or percussion, and postural maneuvers. Nebulized bronchodilators and mucolytic medications can also be helpful in secretion management.

Secondary to the high morbidity and mortality of lower respiratory infections for individuals with SCI, the VA System of Care has developed health care reminders in the electronic medical record to notify providers if veterans have received their yearly influenza vaccines as well as a pneumococcal vaccine regardless of age. These vaccines are recommended for these veterans who receive care in the VA system.

## SLEEP APNEA

The prevalence of sleep-disordered breathing has been shown to range from 27% to 62% following SCI.[17–20] The most common type has been associated with obstructive sleep apnea; however, central sleep apnea patterns have also been seen, particularly in high tetraplegia. Very often patients with SCI will not complain of daytime issues with their sleep, so it is important to have a high clinical suspicion in this patient population, and focused questions related to sleep disturbances should be part of their annual medical examination. In tetraplegia, there has been an association with neck circumference, age, and body mass index and time after injury.[18,19] There is also a high utilization of potentially sedating medications used for spasticity, such as baclofen and diazepam, as well as for pain, and these should be monitored closely and reviewed with patients to be minimized as clinically appropriate.

## CARDIOVASCULAR AND METABOLIC DYSFUNCTION

Cardiovascular disease remains a leading cause of death in the general population and of those with SCI. Coronary heart disease is the leading cause of deaths attributable to cardiovascular disease in the United States.[21] Although some studies have shown the prevalence of myocardial infarction in men injured at least 20 years is similar to the general population, it remains a major source of mortality in the SCI population.[22] Patients with SCI should be monitored at least annually for obesity, cholesterol levels, blood pressure, glucose intolerance/diabetes, and tobacco use by their primary providers. The VA annual evaluation includes an electrocardiogram for individuals over 40 years of age, due to the risk of abnormal or even asymptomatic presentation of coronary artery disease in individuals with SCI.[23] With regard to lipid metabolism, although levels of low-density lipoprotein have been shown to be similar in the SCI population and the non-SCI population, levels of high-density lipoprotein (HDL) are shown to be lower in the SCI population than the general population.[24] Higher levels of HDL have been shown to be protective to the risk of coronary heart disease.[25]

Obesity has also been shown to be a risk factor for ischemic heart disease, and patients with SCI, secondary to decreased energy expenditure from decreased muscle mass and sedentary lifestyles, are at particular risk, especially in higher injuries. Physical activity has been shown to account for nearly 30% of total daily energy expenditure.[26] Individuals with SCI, particularly tetraplegia, have lower levels of physical activity than non-SCI individuals. Those with tetraplegia have lower levels of daily energy expenditure and aerobic activity than those with paraplegia.[27,28] It is also important to note that due to body composition changes following SCI, resulting in decreased proportion of lean body mass, obesity may be underestimated in the spinal cord population.

Hypertension has been strongly associated with cardiovascular disease and should be monitored in veterans with SCI. Although hypotension is typically seen following SCI, particularly in higher-level injuries, hypertension is often seen in subsets of individuals, particularly those with incomplete SCI, those with premorbid and associated vascular comorbidities. The presence of hypertension is also common in individuals with SCI associated with aortic disease or aortic repair.[29]

Relative hypotension is often seen following SCI, with an inverse relationship between blood pressure and level of injury.[30] This hypotension does not result in tachycardia response; however, persons with thoracic injuries below T5 typically have higher resting heart rates than those with tetraplegia or without SCI.

Veterans with SCI are also monitored closely for glucose intolerance and diabetes. It is recommended in the VA system that hemoglobin A1c be monitored at least on a yearly basis. The prevalence of diabetes in veterans with SCI is similar to that of other veterans, but may occur at a younger age in the SCI population.[31] Studies have also shown that individuals with tetraplegia have an increased risk of carbohydrate metabolism disorders than those with paraplegia.[32] Veterans with diabetes reported increased comorbidities and slower healing foot sores than those without diabetes.[31]

## AUTONOMIC DYSFUNCTION

Autonomic dysreflexia, or "AD," formerly termed autonomic hyperreflexia, can perhaps be thought of as "spasticity of the autonomic nervous system." AD results in sudden hypertension that may often increase to crisis levels. It occurs due to an exaggerated autonomic response to a noxious stimulus that is generally not perceived by the person with SCI due to their sensory impairment. AD is a syndrome that is unique to persons with SCI, except for unusual cases reported in persons with multiple sclerosis. It usually occurs in persons at or above T6 level of injury and is rarely reported with lower injuries.[33,34] Symptoms classically include a pounding headache, sweating, and vasodilation with flushing above the injury, vasoconstriction and clamminess below the injury, blurry vision, and anxiety or a sense of impending difficulties.[33] Elevated blood pressure, with or without reflex bradycardia, but without any symptoms can occur, which is known as "silent AD." Increased time after injury decreases AD symptoms, increasing the likelihood of silent AD, thought to be due to decreased baroreceptor sensitivity.[35]

The most common causes of AD are bladder-related issues, such as overdistension, irritation or infection, and instrumentation from procedures. Lower urinary tract (LUT) causes, such as bladder irritation, infection, overdistension, and instrumentation, are the most common. Other causes include rectal impaction, hemorrhoids, genital stimulation, fractures, acute abdomen, and a variety of less common causes. Any person at risk, indeed any person with SCI and elevated blood pressure, should have a careful history taken to elicit potential symptoms and sources of AD.

Orthostatic hypotension is a common problem, especially in persons with higher cervical SCI. Many individuals experience this in the acute phase with resolution after a few weeks. Others may have chronic or intermittent difficulties with symptomatic low blood pressure. Inciting causes, such as urinary tract infections (UTIs), hyponatremia, or other conditions, should be explored. Treatments include compression stockings, abdominal binders, liberalizing sodium intake, midodrine, or fludrocortisone.

## GENITOURINARY/NEUROGENIC BLADDER

Many investigators have noted that, before World War II, urinary tract complications were the leading cause of death in persons with SCI. Due to improved tools available for urinary tract management and surveillance, urinary tract complications are no longer a leading cause of death following SCI.

The goals of genitourinary tract management after SCI include prevention of infection, injuries or trauma, optimizing social continence and function, and preventing upper tract deterioration.

The provider should elicit the person's type of urinary management, which may include spontaneous voiding, use of indwelling urethral or suprapubic catheter, intermittent catheterization, external (also referred to as "condom," "Texas," or "Posey") catheter, and combinations of the above. For persons using intermittent catheterization, frequency and timing of intermittent catheterization, fluid intake and volumes obtained should be noted. Voiding complaints including urgency with or without incontinence, dysuria, frequency, hesitancy, and changes in bladder function from prior examination and amount of assistance needed (Functional Independence Measure score) should be queried.

UTI is the most frequent infection after SCI, with an average of 2.5 episodes per year.[36] The number and severity of UTIs experienced by the person should be assessed. The diagnosis of UTI depends primarily on the presence of new or worsened symptoms.[37,38] Many persons with SCI who use urinary catheters for management have bacterial colonization of their bladder. The standard of care is to avoid treating asymptomatic bacteriuria with antimicrobial agents.[39] Symptoms of UTI include cloudy or malodorous urine, fevers, chills, nausea, vomiting, new onset or changes in spasticity from baseline, leaking around indwelling catheter or between intermittent catheterizations.[40] Persons with SCI vary widely in their ability to predict UTI by symptoms, and symptoms vary widely in their value in predicting significant UTI.[40,41]

A history of recurrent infections, urinary tract stone disease, or vesicoureteral reflux with hydronephrosis suggests suboptimal management due to elevated bladder storage pressures, inadequate emptying, or both. Prostatitis, epididymitis, or orchitis may all occur, may suggest the need to search for similar issues, and may also prompt need for cystoscopy, urodynamic studies, or functional renal studies. Biochemical tests of urinary tract status performed at annual evaluations at VA SCI&D centers include serum creatinine or cystatin C, urinalysis (UA) with microscopy, and a properly collected urine culture. UA and culture are commonly performed as part of annual evaluations; however, routine collection of urine may lead to unnecessary treatment of asymptomatic bacteriuria.[39]

UA may reveal bacteriuria, quantitative pyuria, and red blood cells. The standard of care for persons with SCI does not recommend antimicrobial treatment of asymptomatic bacteriuria. Many persons are asymptomatic despite significant pyuria as well.

Persons with extensive muscle atrophy may have a low serum creatinine even in the presence of renal dysfunction, so the trend over time may be more revealing. Results of 24-hour urine collection for creatinine clearance estimation can also be affected. Cystatin C has several advantages over serum creatinine. It is made by all nucleated cells and is not affected by muscle mass.[42] Normative ranges have been established.[43] Its value can be affected by inflammatory processes, however. Yearly renal and bladder ultrasound is the initial imaging test of choice and can reveal hydronephrosis, renal or bladder calculi, complex renal cysts or masses, and bladder trabeculation or distension. Cystatin C has several advantages over serum creatinine. It is made by all nucleated cells and is not affected by muscle mass.[42] Normative ranges have been established.[43] Its value can be affected by inflammatory processes, however. Yearly renal and bladder ultrasound is the initial imaging test of choice and can reveal hydronephrosis, renal or bladder calculi, complex renal cysts or masses, and bladder trabeculation or distension.

Evidence to guide the frequency of diagnostic testing, especially cystoscopy, is limited. The risk of bladder cancer in persons with SCI has been estimated to be 16 times higher than the general population,[44] which emphasizes its critical importance. Available practice guidelines for management of neurogenic LUT dysfunction do not specify recommended intervals for cystoscopy. At the authors' center, they recommend at least every 5 to 10 years in persons with indwelling catheters and when clinically indicated (for example, for workup of hematuria). One large center[45] performs cystoscopy annually in all persons with SCI after 10 years after injury and more frequently if the person is having problems such as recurrent UTIs.

Urodynamic testing is often indicated as a baseline assessment for persons with SCI, especially those with suprasacral lesions. Follow-up urodynamic testing has been recommended as often as every 1 to 2 years,[44] but resource capacity issues generally limit the practicality of this approach. Urodynamics should be considered when a change in management is contemplated.

Vince and Klausner[44] reviewed available guidelines for recommendations regarding upper urinary tract surveillance. Renal ultrasound was the most common recommended imaging, at intervals varying from 6 to 24 months. The authors perform yearly renal and bladder ultrasound to screen for hydroureteronephrosis, upper urinary tract or LUT stone disease, masses, which can guide need for computed tomography or cystoscopy. The bladder on ultrasound may be dilated, trabeculated/thickened, or collapsed around an indwelling catheter. If stone disease is known or suspected, computed tomography using a renal protocol is indicated.

In addition, the authors perform genital and testicular examination and prostate examination (if prostate specific antigen [PSA] is needed, it is done with other laboratory tests before digital rectal exam) to evaluate for epididymitis, orchitis, torsion, or indwelling catheter traction injury or hypospadias. In women, long-term Foley catheters are not recommended, because dilation of the relatively short bladder neck and urethra can occur with intractable leakage.

Recommendations for PSA testing after SCI are the same as for the general population. However, in persons with SCI and neurogenic bladder, elevated PSA levels may occur due to LUT infection or inflammation rather than malignancy. Lynne and colleagues[46] reported higher serum, but lower seminal PSA levels in men with SCI.

## NEUROGENIC BOWEL DYSFUNCTION

Neurogenic bowel dysfunction remains a major life-limiting problem and an area of least competence for persons with SCI.[47] Management goals include optimal social function, especially minimizing incontinence and interference with life activities, and prevention of complications, such as abdominal pain, impaction, bowel obstruction, and hemorrhoids. Important historical variables include premorbid bowel habits, current frequency of bowel movements, level of assistance needed (FIM score), frequency of characteristics of incontinent episodes, effects on social function such as leaving the house, stool consistency (eg, Bristol stool scale score), medications/supplements, diet, fluid intake, and changes in bowel function from prior visits. Sensation of need for a bowel movement, ability to prevent stool leakage (continence), and voluntary anal sphincter contraction are relevant measures of autonomic and motor function.[48]

Oral medications are prescribed to modulate stool consistency. Guideline recommendations help to determine goals. For persons with upper motor neuron, or "spastic" type function, a soft but formed stool is recommended. For persons with lower motor neuron or "flaccid" bowel dysfunction, a firm-formed (but not excessively scybalous) stool is the goal.[49] Guideline-recommended management includes a timed bowel emptying with suppositories and/or digital rectal stimulation for persons with reflex bowel function, and timed manual removal for persons with flaccid bowel function. Some persons may use enemas, but these are generally discouraged, because they do not lend themselves to establishment of a bowel "rhythm" and are thought to potentially cause a "lazy, enema-dependent" bowel.[50]

Persons with SCI require at least the same, if not a higher level of screening for colorectal cancer. However, some persons may not receive it, potentially because of physical access issues. False positive fecal occult blood tests occur frequently because of bowel care interventions, such as manual stool removal, digital rectal stimulation, as well as a high rate of hemorrhoids in this population. Other common gastrointestinal symptoms experienced by persons with SCI include oropharyngeal pain or swallowing difficulty (possibly due to cervical instrumentation or osteophytes), diarrhea, constipation, change in appetite, heartburn, weight gain, and unintentional weight loss.

## NEUROGENIC SKIN

Monitoring of the skin for pressure injury on a regular basis is a very important part of care following SCI. Pressure injury is a very serious complication of SCI, which can lead to significant, lifelong issues. Pressure injury of the skin can have significant impact on an individual's overall quality of life. It can have impacts physically, socially, and psychologically. The National Pressure Ulcer Advisory Panel defines a pressure injury as localized damage to the skin and underlying soft tissue usually over a bony prominence or related to a medical or other device. The injury can present with intact skin or an open ulcer and may be painful. The injury occurs as a result of intense and/or prolonged pressure or pressure in combination with shear.[51]

The primary factors leading to pressure injury are pressure and shear.[52] In addition, there are many other contributing factors to development of pressure injuries in persons with SCIs. These factors include friction, moisture, immobility, impaired sensation, medical comorbidities, nutrition, as well as economic, social, and psychological factors.[53] Of the numerous contributing risk factors in the literature, the direct contributive effects of each factor are not known and likely are variable in the contributive involvement with each individual who develops a pressure wound.

The incidence of pressure injury in SCI patients is high, even during their initial rehabilitation course. Pressure injury was seen in 23.7% of patients during acute rehabilitation.[54] As individuals age with SCI, the incidence and prevalence of pressure injury increase.[55,56] Pressure injury remains one of the most common reasons for rehospitalization in persons with SCI.[57] Data have shown an incidence of pressure injury at 15% at 1 year following injury, increasing to almost 30% at 20 years after injury.[58] The most common locations of pressure ulcers after 2 years of injury are the ischium, trochanter, and sacrum.[58]

Because of the elevated risk of pressure injuries in persons with SCI, it is important for individuals to be educated on appropriate pressure relief techniques when sitting in wheelchair and when in bed. Support surfaces are very important, and careful consideration should be used when selecting these for individuals to use. Part of the annual evaluation for veterans within the VA System of Care is evaluation of their seating systems and appropriateness of fit. Veterans should ideally be assessed in their wheelchairs during the face-to-face visit to ensure continued appropriate fit and alignment of the patient. Adjustments and new prescriptions should be obtained with changes significant in weight, which can affect weight distribution while sitting. These changes, in addition to other comorbidities, may affect a person's ability to perform appropriate weight shifts and transfers; chronic shoulder problems, which are common in the SCI population, must be taken into consideration as well. For individuals who have difficulty performing manual weight shifts, power mobility with reclining and tilting of the patient for weight relief should be considered. Pressure mapping using specialized equipment can be used during wheelchair assessment to help in identifying areas of high pressure, which may be at increased risk of breakdown, as well as to help to ensure areas of concern; previous wounds are maintained at appropriate pressures in the sitting position. Backup cushions are often indicated. A flat or ineffective cushion can result in a severe pressure ulcer and prolonged hospital stays.

Support surfaces for sleeping are also important in the prevention as well as treatment of pressure injury. There are many types of overlays and specialty mattresses that can be used to improve weight distribution while sleeping. The individual's ability to turn independently during the night and transfer in and out of bed should be considered as well as history of previous wounds when deciding the most appropriate support surface for the individual.

## AVOCATIONAL

Recreational activities and therapeutic exercise can confer numerous benefits for persons with SCI, including improvements in health, well-being, and socialization. As with employment, persons with SCI may face multiple barriers to exercise and recreation. Baseline fitness is generally lower than able-bodied counterparts. Persons with SCI may need specialized adaptations to allow maximal participation. Examples include ramps for bowling, hand cycles, upper extremity aids for shooting sports, and computer adaptations. Innervated muscle available for spontaneous exercise is variably reduced based on level and completeness of injury, and resulting degree of obligatory sarcopenia. Electrically stimulated exercise can increase caloric expenditure and cardiac output in persons who lack innervated muscle. Electronically stimulated exercise is generally not feasible as a method of weight loss, but can improve insulin and lipid profiles.[59,60]

At annual evaluation, SCI providers, working in partnership with physical, occupational, and recreation therapists, assess current avocational status, fitness, and risk factors, and make recommendations for exercise and recreation. Special attention should be given to autonomic issues, such as risk for exercise-induced hypotension and upper extremity overuse and misuse and thermoregulation.[61]

## EMPLOYMENT

Employment, which may be the most important marker of successful rehabilitation,[62] has been demonstrated to be associated with improvement in multiple domains of quality of life, satisfaction, and health.[63,64] Studies of persons with SCI followed at both private sector (NIDILRR Model Systems) centers and VA centers have been consistent in demonstrating very low rates of competitive employment, approximately 33% (ie, 67% unemployed) in postacute and chronic populations.[65] Persons with physical and cognitive disabilities face an array of potential barriers, including health ssues,[66,67] transportation, accessibility, employer attitudes, and need for job accommodations.[66,67] Recent research has demonstrated superiority of the individual placement and support (IPS) model, an evidence-based approach, to usual care, in obtaining competitive employment for veterans with SCI.[65] Many persons with SCI want to work, but historically have faced many barriers, including the perception by themselves and their health care providers that they are unable to work. The IPS model s a "zero-exclusion" approach that emphasizes integration of the vocational rehabilitation specialist with the interdisciplinary rehabilitation team, honoring veteran preferences regarding employment, ongoing benefits counseling, rapid job search in the person's local community, competitive employment in the community rather than sheltered work, and employer negotiation as needed to carve out the right job fit.[68,69] Many veterans with SCI have successfully returned to competitive employment, often part time, using this approach.[69] Armed with this knowledge, SCI clinicians should reassure their patients of the possibilities and benefits of employment and make referrals to vocational rehabilitation specialists. Several VA SCI centers have VR specialists embedded in their teams, greatly enhancing the ease of referrals.

## SEXUALITY

Persons with SCI rate sexual function as a high priority and desire information, but historically, many persons report that they did not receive any or adequate information during rehabilitation. Despite this, many persons report being sexually active following injury.

Sexuality assessment requires a team approach to evaluate interests and attitudes regarding sexual function, mobility and ADL status, and other issues. The American Occupational Therapy Association recognizes sexual activity as an ADL equal to other ADLs, such as dressing or bathing. The PLISSIT (Permission, Limited Information, Specific Suggestions, Intensive Treatment) model, developed in the 1950s,[70] is still widely used.[70] Some persons may benefit from referral to an American Association of Sexuality Educators, Counselors and Therapists–accredited provider for specialized issues. By providing information in a straightforward, nonjudgmental manner and maintaining confidentiality, providers normalize the discussion, giving the person "permission" to enter into an open and honest dialogue regarding their sexual function and concerns.[71]

The ISNCSCI examination and reflex function are critical to guide the practitioner in counseling regarding sexual function. Special attention should be directed to sensory level, T10–L2 and sacral dermatomes, anal sphincter tone, anal wink, BCR, and hip flexor reflex. The presence of the BCR and hip flexor reflexes, along with a sensory level above T10, predicts success with reflex ejaculation using optimized vibration.[72]

Men with SCI should be assessed for erectile function and ejaculatory function. Anejaculation with intercourse is present in roughly 95% of persons with motor complete SCI. However, biological parenthood for men is usually possible regardless of level or severity of injury. Penile vibratory stimulation (PVS) is successful in 86% of men with injuries at T10 or rostral, whereas electroejaculation approaches 100% regardless of injury level.[73] Insemination using PVS can frequently be done in the home setting[74] if AD is not too severe or mitigated with medications. For others, intrauterine insemination, in vitro fertilization, or intracytoplasmic sperm injection may be necessary, which is costlier. However, Brackett and colleagues[75] note that surgical sperm retrieval in SCI men is rarely indicated.

Many medications taken by persons with SCI can interfere with sexual function. Antispasticity medications, such as baclofen or benzodiazepines, can impair reflex erections. Antimuscarinic anticholinergic bladder medications, some blood pressure medications, and other classes of medications can cause dry mouth and impair vaginal lubrication. Selective serotonin reuptake inhibitors and opiate pain medications are well known to impair libido. In general, the lowest necessary dose and duration should be used. Treatments for erectile dysfunction include phosphodiesterase type 5 inhibitors, intracavernosal injections of alprostadil alone or in combination with other agents such as phentolamine and papaverine ("bi-, tri-, or quad mix"), intraurethral alprostadil suppositories, vacuum erection devices, or combinations of these approaches. Implantable penile prostheses, although a last resort, have a high satisfaction rate with a lower risk profile than older devices.[76]

In women with SCI, long-term fertility status is generally preserved. Women with SCI may lose menses temporarily but regain them and need the same level of counseling regarding birth control as noninjured women. There are special risks with use of birth control, including intrauterine devices and oral contraceptives. Women can become pregnant and raise children successfully regardless of injury level or severity. Women should be counseled regarding special medical and rehabilitation needs during pregnancy. Fertility history, gynecologic history, current functioning with regard to bladder management, genital lubrication, and neurologic function should be assessed.

## MENTAL HEALTH ISSUES

A spinal cord injury has a significant impact on the life of a person, from the aspect of physical and mental health. It is very important that those with SCI are regularly assessed and treated as needed by a mental health provider in the acute rehabilitation phase as well as part of their regular health care evaluations. The prevalence of depressive disorders after SCI is estimated at 22%.[77] Some studies have suggested a slightly higher level of 30% in the rehabilitation phase of treatment.[78] In comparison to depression in the general population, where women have shown higher incidence and prevalence than men, this gender difference was not noted in persons following SCI.[79] Depressive mood has also been associated with higher levels of pain following SCI, and with chronic pain following traumatic SCI prevalence, ranging from 26% to 96%; this association is very relevant in this population.[80,81] A higher prevalence of depressive mood disorders is also reported in nontraumatic SCI versus traumatic SCI.[82] Routine screening for depression should be done on the initial visit and annually thereafter for individuals with SCI.[83] In the VA system during the yearly annual evaluations, veterans are screened by psychologists in the SCI interdisciplinary team.

Suicide risk is a significant problem in the mental health of persons with SCI that also must be addressed on a consistent basis, both in the acute stages and in subsequent follow-up. Suicide risk may be specifically important in the VA population because suicide rates among veterans have been shown to be higher than the general population.[84] Suicide rates among the general population were 15.2/100,000, and 35.3/100,000 among veterans.[84] The suicide rate among persons with SCI has been reported at 46/100,000.[85] Although this rate has decreased since the 1970s, it continues to exceed both the general population and the population of veterans without SCI. The rate of suicide appears to be highest 1 to 5 years after injury.[86] The suicide rate remaining high for the first 5 years after injury shows the importance of maintaining engagement of the individual following completion of acute rehabilitation, and a reason annual follow-up examinations with an interdisciplinary team are strongly encouraged within the VA System of Care. Suicide risk assessments, including discussion regarding depression and suicide ideation, should be completed during annual assessments. Assessments early after injury should address prior mental health diagnosis and previous suicide attempts, because these individuals should be considered at high risk and receive continued close follow-up. It is equally important to provide easy access to mental health treatment for individuals at high risk for suicide and may also be an excellent area for utilization of telehealth, emergency hotlines, and peer support. Within the VA System of Care, expansion of and access to mental health care have been identified as priorities in the treatment of veterans.

## COMORBID TRAUMATIC BRAIN INJURY OR "DUAL DIAGNOSIS"

Estimates of the incidence of concurrent traumatic brain injury (TBI) in persons with SCI vary from 47% to 74% depending on factors such as cause and source.[87,88] In the largest study of veterans with SCI, Budd and colleagues[89] reported probable TBI exposure described by 77.6% of participants, with 38% reporting sustaining more than one injury. Self-reported TBIs classified as moderate/severe comprised 49.5% of injuries. Persons with self-reported TBI performed lower on FIM Cognitive and Chart Cognitive Independence subscales. The presence of comorbid TBI can impact SCI rehabilitation efforts and psychosocial function in important ways, including prolonging lengths of rehabilitation.[86] SCI psychology providers facilitate referrals to neuropsychology for testing and for colleagues in Polytrauma and/or Mental Health during annual evaluations.

## SUMMARY

Persons with SCI are often by necessity heavy users of the health care system. The intent of the annual evaluation is that use of this type of model can improve access to care, identify issues early, and help to prevent costly complications, such as pressure ulcers, UTIs, sepsis, and renal deterioration.

## REFERENCES

1. VA's Spinal Cord Injuries and Disorders System of Care. Available at: https://www.sci.va.gov/VAs_SCID_System_of_Care.asp. Accessed May 1, 2018.
2. Ho CH. Primary care for persons with spinal cord injury - not a novel idea but still under-developed. J Spinal Cord Med 2016;39(5):500–3.
3. VHA Handbook 1176.01. Washington, DC: Department of Veterans Affairs, Veterans Health Administration; 2011.
4. Devivo MJ, Chen Y. Epidemiology of traumatic spinal cord injury. In: Kirshblum S, Campagnolo D, editors. Spinal cord injury medicine. 2nd edition. Philadelphia: Lippincott Williams and Wilkins; 2011. p. 72–84.
5. De Vivo MJ, Go BK, Jackson AB. Model SCI system overview of the National Spinal Cord Injury Statistical Center database. J Spinal Cord Med 2002;25:335–8.
6. ASIA Neurological Standards Committee. International standards for neurological classification of spinal cord injury. Atlanta (GA): American Spinal Injury Association; 2011.
7. Schurch B, Wichmann W, Rossier AB. Post-traumatic syringomyelia (cystic myelopathy): a prospective study of 449 patients with spinal cord injury. J Neurol Neurosurg Psychiatry 1996;60(1):61–7.
8. Noreau L, Proulx P, Gagnon L, et al. Secondary impairments after spinal cord injury: a population-based study. Am J Phys Med Rehabil 2000;79(6):526–35.
9. Consortium for Spinal Cord Medicine. Preservation of upper limb function following spinal cord injury: a clinical practice guideline for health-care professionals. Washington, DC: Paralyzed Veterans of America; 2005.

10. Cardenas DD, Bryce TN, Shem K, et al. Gender and minority differences in the pain experience of people with spinal cord injury. Arch Phys Med Rehabil 2004;85(11):1774–81.
11. Störmer S, Gerner HJ, Grüninger W, et al. Chronic pain/dysaesthesiae in spinal cord injury patients: results of a multicentre study. Spinal Cord 1997;35(7): 446–55.
12. Meske DS, Lawal OD, Elder H, et al. Efficacy of opioids versus placebo in chronic pain: a systematic review and meta-analysis of enriched enrollment randomized withdrawal trials. J Pain Res 2018;11:923–34.
13. The Opioid Therapy for Chronic Pain, Work Group. VA/DoD clinical practice guideline for opioid therapy for chronic pain. 2017.
14. DeVivo MJ, Krause JS, Lammertse DP. Recent trends in mortality and causes of death among persons with spinal cord injury. Arch Phys Med Rehabil 1999; 80(11):1411–9.
15. Burns SP. Acute respiratory infections in persons with spinal cord injury. Phys Med Rehabil Clin N Am 2007;18(2):203–16, v-vi.
16. Lanig IS, Peterson WP. The respiratory system in spinal cord injury. Phys Med Rehabil Clin N Am 2000;11(1):29–43, vii.
17. Short DJ, Stradling JR, Williams SJ. Prevalence of sleep apnoea in patients over 40 years of age with spinal cord lesions. J Neurol Neurosurg Psychiatry 1992; 55(11):1032–6.
18. McEvoy RD, Mykytyn I, Sajkov D, et al. Sleep apnoea in patients with quadriplegia. Thorax 1995;50(6):613–9.
19. Stockhammer E, Tobon A, Michel F, et al. Characteristics of sleep apnea syndrome in tetraplegic patients. Spinal Cord 2002;40(6):286–94.
20. Berlowitz DJ, Brown DJ, Campbell DA, et al. A longitudinal evaluation of sleep and breathing in the first year after cervical spinal cord injury. Arch Phys Med Rehabil 2005;86(6):1193–9.
21. Benjamin E, Virani S, Callaway C. Heart disease and stroke statistics-2018 update. Available at: http://www.acc.org/latest-in-cardiology/ten-points-to-remember/2018/02/09/11/59/heart-disease-and-stroke-statistics-2018-update. Accessed May 1, 2018.
22. LaVela SL, Evans CT, Prohaska TR, et al. Males aging with a spinal cord injury: prevalence of cardiovascular and metabolic conditions. Arch Phys Med Rehabil 2012;93(1):90–5.
23. Bauman WA, Raza M, Spungen AM, et al. Cardiac stress testing with thallium-201 imaging reveals silent ischemia in individuals with paraplegia. Arch Phys Med Rehabil 1994;75(9):946–50.
24. Bauman WA, Spungen AM. Metabolic changes in persons after spinal cord injury. Phys Med Rehabil Clin N Am 2000;11(1):109–40.
25. National Cholesterol Education Program (NCEP) Expert Panel on Detection, Evaluation, and Treatment of High Blood Cholesterol in Adults (Adult Treatment Panel III). Third report of the national cholesterol education program (NCEP) expert panel on detection, evaluation, and treatment of high blood cholesterol in adults (adult treatment panel III) final report. Circulation 2002;106(25):3143–421.
26. Buchholz A, Pencharz P. Energy expenditure in chronic spinal cord injury [review]. Curr Opin Clin Nutr Metab Care 2004;7(6):635–9.
27. Figoni SF. Exercise responses and quadriplegia. Med Sci Sports Exerc 1993; 25(4):433–41.
28. Gass GC, Watson J, Camp EM, et al. The effects of physical training on high level spinal lesion patients. Scand J Rehabil Med 1980;12(2):61–5.

29. Sabharwal S. Essentials of spinal cord medicine. 1st edition. New York: Demos Medical Publishing; 2014.
30. Mathias CJ. Orthostatic hypotension: causes, mechanisms, and influencing factors. Neurology 1995;45(4 Suppl 5):S6–11.
31. Lavela SL, Weaver FM, Goldstein B, et al. Diabetes mellitus in individuals with spinal cord injury or disorder. J Spinal Cord Med 2006;29(4):387–95.
32. Bauman WA, Adkins RH, Spungen AM, et al. The effect of residual neurological deficit on oral glucose tolerance in persons with chronic spinal cord injury. Spinal Cord 1999;37(11):765–71.
33. Consortium for spinal cord medicine. Acute management of autonomic dysreflexia: individuals with spinal cord injury presenting to health-care facilities. Washington, DC: Paralyzed Veterans of America; 2001.
34. Sabharwal S. Cardiovascular dysfunction in spinal cord disorders. In: Lin V, editor. Spinal cord medicine: principles and practice. 2nd edition. New York: Demos Medical; 2010. p. 241–55.
35. Huang Y-H, Bih L-I, Liao J-M, et al. Blood pressure and age associated with silent autonomic dysreflexia during urodynamic examinations in patients with spinal cord injury. Spinal Cord 2013;51(5):401–5.
36. Darouiche RO. Infection and spinal cord injury. In: Lin V, editor. Spinal cord medicine: principles and practice. 2nd edition. New York: Demos; 2010. p. 263–9.
37. Goetz LL, Cardenas DD, Kennelly M, et al. International spinal cord injury urinary tract infection basic data set. Spinal Cord 2013;51(9):700–4.
38. Cardenas DD, Hooton TM. Urinary tract infection in persons with spinal cord injury. Arch Phys Med Rehabil 1995;76(3):272–80.
39. Skelton F, Grigoryan L, Holmes SA, et al. Routine urine testing at the spinal cord injury annual evaluation leads to unnecessary antibiotic use: a pilot study and future directions. Arch Phys Med Rehabil 2018;99(2):219–25.
40. Linsenmeyer TA, Oakley A. Accuracy of individuals with spinal cord injury at predicting urinary tract infections based on their symptoms. J Spinal Cord Med 2003;26(4):352–7.
41. Massa LM, Hoffman JM, Cardenas DD. Validity, accuracy, and predictive value of urinary tract infection signs and symptoms in individuals with spinal cord injury on intermittent catheterization. J Spinal Cord Med 2009;32(5):568–73.
42. Dharnidharka VR, Kwon C, Stevens G. Serum cystatin C is superior to serum creatinine as a marker of kidney function: a meta-analysis. Am J Kidney Dis 2002;40(2):221–6.
43. Levey AS, Fan L, Eckfeldt JH, et al. Cystatin C for glomerular filtration rate estimation: coming of age. Clin Chem 2014;60(7):916–9.
44. Vince RA, Klausner AP. Surveillance strategies for neurogenic lower urinary tract dysfunction. Urol Clin North Am 2017;44(3):367–75.
45. Linsenmeyer T. Neurogenic bladder following spinal cord injury. In: Kirshblum S, editor. Spinal cord medicine. 2nd edition. Philadelphia: Lippincott Williams and Wilkins; 2011. p. 234.
46. Lynne CM, Aballa TC, Wang TJ, et al. Serum and semen prostate specific antigen concentrations are different in young spinal cord injured men compared to normal controls. J Urol 1999;162(1):89–91.
47. Boss BJ, Pecanty L, McFarland SM, et al. Self-care competence among persons with spinal cord injury. SCI Nurs 1995;12(2):48–53.
48. Goetz LL, Emmanuel A, Krogh K. International standards to document remaining autonomic function in persons with SCI and neurogenic bowel dysfunction: illustrative cases. Spinal Cord Ser Cases 2018;4:1.

49. Consortium for Spinal Cord Medicine. Neurogenic bowel management in adults with spinal cord injury. Washington, DC: Paralyzed Veterans of America; 1998.

50. Stiens SA, Bergman SB, Goetz LL. Neurogenic bowel dysfunction after spinal cord injury: clinical evaluation and rehabilitative management. Arch Phys Med Rehabil 1997;78(3 Suppl):S86–102.

51. NPUAP Pressure Injury Stages. 2016. Available at: http://www.npuap. org/resources/educational-and-clinical-resources/npuap-pressure-injury-stages/. Accessed May 1, 2018.

52. Kirshblum SC, O'Connor K, Rader CQ. Pressure ulcers and spinal cord injury. In: Kirshblum S, Campagnolo D, editors. Spinal cord medicine. 2nd edition. Philadelphia: Lippincott Williams and Wilkins; 2011. p. 242–63.

53. Krouskop TA, Garber SL, Noble PC. The effectiveness of preventive management in reducing the occurrence of pressure sores. J Rehabil Res Dev 1983;20:74–83.

54. Chen D, Apple DF, Hudson LM, et al. Medical complications during acute rehabilitation following spinal cord injury–current experience of the Model Systems. Arch Phys Med Rehabil 1999;80(11):1397–401.

55. Charlifue S, Jha A, Lammertse D. Aging with spinal cord injury. Phys Med Rehabil Clin N Am 2010;21(2):383–402.

56. Chen Y, Devivo MJ, Jackson AB. Pressure ulcer prevalence in people with spinal cord injury: age-period-duration effects. Arch Phys Med Rehabil 2005;86(6): 1208–13.

57. Cardenas DD, Hoffman JM, Kirshblum S, et al. Etiology and incidence of rehospitalization after traumatic spinal cord injury: a multicenter analysis. Arch Phys Med Rehabil 2004;85(11):1757–63.

58. McKinley WO, Jackson AB, Cardenas DD, et al. Long-term medical complications after traumatic spinal cord injury: a regional model systems analysis. Arch Phys Med Rehabil 1999;80(11):1402–10.

59. Gorgey AS, Martin H, Metz A, et al. Longitudinal changes in body composition and metabolic profile between exercise clinical trials in men with chronic spinal cord injury. J Spinal Cord Med 2016;39(6):699–712.

60. Gorgey AS, Mather KJ, Cupp HR, et al. Effects of resistance training on adiposity and metabolism after spinal cord injury. Med Sci Sports Exerc 2012;44(1): 165–74.

61. Nash MS, Horton J, Cowan R, et al. Recreational and therapeutic exercise after spinal cord injury. In: Kirshblum S, Campagnolo D, editors. Spinal cord medicine. 2nd editon. Philadelphia: Lippincott Williams and Wilkins; 2011. p. 427–47.

62. Krause JS, Sternberg M, Maides J, et al. Employment after spinal cord injury: differences related to geographic region, gender, and race. Arch Phys Med Rehabil 1998;79(6):615–24.

63. Meade M, Reed K, Saunders L, et al. It's all of the above: benefits of working for individuals with spinal cord injury. Top Spinal Cord Inj Rehabil 2015;21(1):1–9.

64. Leduc BE, Lepage Y. Health-related quality of life after spinal cord injury. Disabil Rehabil 2002;24(4):196–202.

65. Ottomanelli L, Goetz LL, Suris A, et al. Effectiveness of supported employment for veterans with spinal cord injuries: results from a randomized multisite study. Arch Phys Med Rehabil 2012;93(5):740–7.

66. Goetz LL, Ottomanelli L, Barnett SD, et al. Relationship between comorbidities and employment among veterans with spinal cord injury. Top Spinal Cord Inj Rehabil 2018;24(1):44–53.

67. Meade MA, Forchheimer MB, Krause JS, et al. The influence of secondary conditions on job acquisition and retention in adults with spinal cord injury. Arch Phys Med Rehabil 2011;92(3):425–32.
68. Bond GR. Supported employment: evidence for an evidence-based practice. Psychiatr Rehabil J 2004;27(4):345–59.
69. Ottomanelli L, Goetz LL, Barnett SD, et al. Individual placement and support in spinal cord injury: a longitudinal observational study of employment outcomes. Arch Phys Med Rehabil 2017;98(8):1567–75.
70. Annon JS. The PLISSIT model: a proposed conceptual scheme for the behavioral treatment of sexual problems. J Sex Educ Ther 1976;2:1–15.
71. Consortium for Spinal Cord Medicine. Sexuality and reproductive health in adults with spinal cord injury: a clinical practice guideline for health-care professionals. Washington, DC: Paralyzed Veterans of America; 2010.
72. Bird VG, Brackett NL, Lynne CM, et al. Reflexes and somatic responses as predictors of ejaculation by penile vibratory stimulation in men with spinal cord injury. Spinal Cord 2001;39(10):514–9.
73. Brackett NL, Ibrahim E, Iremashvili V, et al. Treatment for ejaculatory dysfunction in men with spinal cord injury: an 18-year single center experience. J Urol 2010; 183(6):2304–8.
74. Biering-Sørensen F, Sønksen J. Sexual function in spinal cord lesioned men. Spinal Cord 2001;39(9):455–70.
75. Ibrahim E, Lynne CM, Brackett NL. Male fertility following spinal cord injury: an update. Andrology 2016;4(1):13–26.
76. Zermann D-H, Kutzenberger J, Sauerwein D, et al. Penile prosthetic surgery in neurologically impaired patients: long-term followup. J Urol 2006;175(3 Pt 1): 1041–4 [discussion: 1044].
77. Williams R, Murray A. Prevalence of depression after spinal cord injury: a meta-analysis. Arch Phys Med Rehabil 2015;96(1):133–40.
78. Craig A, Tran Y, Middleton J. Psychological morbidity and spinal cord injury: a systematic review. Spinal Cord 2009;47(2):108–14.
79. Kalpakjian CZ, Albright KJ. An examination of depression through the lens of spinal cord injury. Comparative prevalence rates and severity in women and men. Womens Health Issues 2006;16(6):380–8.
80. Craig A, Tran Y, Siddall P, et al. Developing a model of associations between chronic pain, depressive mood, chronic fatigue, and self-efficacy in people with spinal cord injury. J Pain 2013;14(9):911–20.
81. Dijkers M, Bryce T, Zanca J. Prevalence of chronic pain after traumatic spinal cord injury: a systematic review. J Rehabil Res Dev 2009;46(1):13–29.
82. Saurí J, Chamarro A, Gilabert A, et al. Depression in individuals with traumatic and nontraumatic spinal cord Injury living in the community. Arch Phys Med Rehabil 2017;98(6):1165–73.
83. Consortium for Spinal Cord Medicine. Depression following spinal cord injury: A clinical practice guideline for primary care physicians. Washington, DC: Paralyzed Veterans of America; 1998.
84. National Academies of Sciences, Engineering, and Medicine, Health and Medicine Division, Board on Health Care Services, Committee to Evaluate the Department of Veterans Affairs Mental Health Services. Evaluation of the department of veterans affairs mental health services. Washington, DC: National Academies Press (US); 2018. Available at: http://www.ncbi.nlm.nih.gov/books/NBK499503/. Accessed May 18, 2018.

85. Cao Y, Massaro JF, Krause JS, et al. Suicide mortality after spinal cord injury in the United States: injury cohorts analysis. Arch Phys Med Rehabil 2014;95(2): 230–5.
86. DeVivo MJ, Black KJ, Richards JS, et al. Suicide following spinal cord injury. Paraplegia 1991;29(9):620–7.
87. Macciocchi S, Seel RT, Thompson N, et al. Spinal cord injury and co-occurring traumatic brain injury: assessment and incidence. Arch Phys Med Rehabil 2008;89(7):1350–7.
88. Budisin B, Bradbury CCLB, Sharma B, et al. Traumatic brain injury in spinal cord injury: frequency and risk factors. J Head Trauma Rehabil 2016;31(4):E33–42.
89. Budd MA, Dixon TM, Barnett SD, et al. Examination of traumatic brain injury exposure among veterans with spinal cord injury. Rehabil Psychol 2017;62(3):345–52.

# Upper Extremity Amputation and Prosthetics Care Across the Active Duty Military and Veteran Populations

Jill M. Cancio, OTD, OTR/L, CHT[a,b], Andrea J. Ikeda, MS, CP[a,b],
Shannon L. Barnicott, MS, OTR[a], Walter Lee Childers, PhD, CP[a,b],
Joseph F. Alderete, MD[c], Brandon J. Goff, DO[a,*]

## KEYWORDS

- Upper extremity amputation • Upper extremity amputation rehabilitation
- Upper extremity prosthesis • Upper extremity osseointegration
- Upper extremity amputation surgical considerations

## KEY POINTS

- Given the invaluable functions of the upper extremity (UE) in daily life, replacement of a missing limb through prosthetic substitution is challenging.
- Goals of UE amputation surgery are to: preserve length and useful sensibility, prevention of symptomatic neuromas and adjacent joint contractures, facilitate early prosthetic fitting, and promote early return to functional activities.
- Design of UE prostheses is broadly categorized by the power source: body powered; externally powered; hybrid; or passive, in which the terminal device (TD) requires no power.
- The goal of preprosthetic training is to prepare the patient and his or her limb to receive a correct fitting and functional prosthesis.
- Fitting of a UE prosthesis should occur as early as possible so that the individual can begin training and performing bimanual tasks.

---

Disclosure Statement: The views expressed herein are those of the authors and do not reflect the official policy or position of the Brooke Army Medical Center, the US Army Medical Department, the US Army Office of the Surgeon General, the Department of the Army, the Department of the Air Force, and Department of Defense, or the US Government.
[a] Center for the Intrepid, Department of Rehabilitation Medicine, Brooke Army Medical Center, 3551 Roger Brooke Drive, JBSA Fort Sam Houston, San Antonioa, TX 78234, USA; [b] Extremity Trauma and Amputation Center of Excellence, 2748 Worth Road, Suite 29, JBSA Fort Sam Houston, San Antonioa, TX 78234, USA; [c] Center for the Intrepid, Department of Orthopaedic Surgery, Brooke Army Medical Center, 3551 Roger Brooke Drive, JBSA Fort Sam Houston, San Antonioa, TX 78234, USA
* Corresponding author. Center for the Intrepid, Brooke Army Medical Center, 3551 Roger Brooke Drive, JBSA Fort Sam Houston, San Antonio, TX 78234.
E-mail address: brandon.j.goff.mil@mail.mil

## INTRODUCTION

The hand has been described as the most individual and personal part of the human being.[1] The hand and arm are exceptionally dexterous, exquisitely sensitive, and proficient in performing tasks and functions. Given the countless functions of the upper extremity (UE), replacement of a missing limb through prosthetic substitution is challenging. Prosthetic and rehabilitation needs of injured Service members from recent military conflicts have brought UE amputation to the forefront, which has led to an increase in attention and resource allocation. During the height of conflict, the advanced rehabilitation centers in the Department of Defense (Center for the Intrepid at Brooke Army Medical Center, Military Amputee Treatment Center at Walter Reed National Military Medical Center, and Comprehensive Combat and Complex Casualty Care at Naval Medical Center San Diego) were ideal settings for UE amputee care because the entire rehabilitation team was on site working jointly in the care and management of UE amputees without limitation from insurance payers. This article provides an overview of the care of the UE amputee including surgical considerations, prosthetic design and fitting, and preprosthetic and post-prosthetic rehabilitation considerations.

## SURGICAL CONSIDERATIONS

Goals of UE amputation surgery are to:

- Preserve functional length
- Preserve useful sensibility
- Prevent symptomatic neuromas
- Prevent adjacent joint contractures
- Minimize and shorten sequelae of injury
- Facilitate early prosthetic fitting
- Promote early return of the patient's activities of daily living (ADLs)

From a surgical perspective, the rehabilitation professional must understand typical and atypical flap coverage; conventional levels and modern adaptations; preparation for advanced prosthetics, such as myoelectric devices and the necessary targeted muscle reinnervation (TMR); and advanced alternatives for limb optimization, such as UE replantation, transplantation, and osseointegration. Unlike in the lower limb, where myoplasty versus myodesis is important in optimal osseous coverage, these techniques are largely equivalent in the UE.[2]

### Proximal Upper Extremity and Shoulder Level

Typical reasons for limb ablation at the shoulder include tumor, trauma, and infection. This focuses on performing either a glenohumeral disarticulation or a forequarter amputation. Most of the time, a shoulder disarticulation (proper) is avoided with an ultra-high transhumeral amputation, keeping a small part of the humeral head and neck preserving cosmesis. When tumor, trauma, or infection proves amenable, this is preferred.[3] The forequarter amputation is extremely morbid in terms of body dysmorphism and function. It is reserved for tumor or life-threatening infections where the axillary artery and brachial plexus have been contaminated or when it is not prudent to leave these structures behind because of the risk of local recurrence. The entire forelimb is removed, in some cases with chest wall, and scapula, humerus, and a portion of the clavicle (**Fig. 1**).

The procedure is tailored to the patient and pathophysiology often requiring modifications of the classic approaches. In the case of high-energy trauma, the amputation

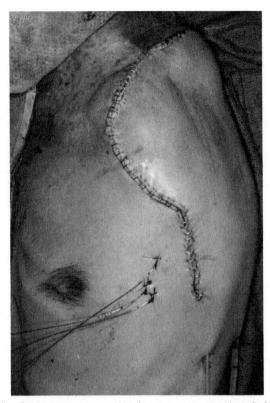

**Fig. 1.** Posterior flap forequarter amputation for sarcoma tumor–invaded humerus, scapula, and brachial plexus. Also visible are regional catheters for postoperative analgesia at plexus level.

about the shoulder can either be performed early or late secondary to patient wishes in the face of a flail limb. Early post-traumatic amputations, both shoulder disarticulation and forequarter, are predicated on the amount of tissue that is viable and free of contamination. There are several flaps that must be maintained and dictate the operative technique. The ultrashort transhumeral amputation is based on an intact "chevron" region (skin and muscle of the deltoid region). The ability to bias a chevron-shaped flap of skin, subcutaneous tissue, and deltoid muscle full thickness to bone makes the ultrashort transhumeral amputation an attractive option. The true shoulder disarticulation is performed using a lateral chevron region flap, a posterior flap, or an axillary-based flap of durable undersurface tissue. When possible, the axillary flap is advantageous because there is no muscle to atrophy over the osseous structures and durable padding is available for an articulating or cosmetic prosthesis. The forequarter amputation is based on a posterior periscapular flap or anterior pectoralis flap. Often in the face of neoplasm as an indication for amputation, the absolute necessity to achieve wide margin means that these classic flaps may not be available and regional rotation or free flaps a must. The latissimus dorsi rotational flap, either ipsilateral or contralateral, is a workhorse for rotation into the defect for coverage. Finally, free tissue from the amputated limb is sometimes necessary for coverage in the irradiated tumor patient.[4,5]

### Humeral Level and Elbow Disarticulation

Humeral amputations are defined by a level distal to the deltoid insertion. Typically, this is 7 cm below the shoulder joint. Most amputations from midhumeral distal should focus on the balance between placing the limb in space with an appropriate length fulcrum and enough soft tissue coverage to allow comfortable fitting in a prosthesis. There is no classic flap for a transhumeral amputation and soft tissue coverage is predicated on available tissue. Incisions directly over the bony residual should be avoided and a posterior-to-anterior flap is created because of the length and bulk of the distal triceps. Debate remains between long transhumeral amputation versus elbow disarticulation. A disarticulation maintains the rotational control of the humeral condyles and native soft tissue attachments but its bulk may inhibit a prosthetic elbow in shorter individuals. When a long humeral osteotomy is elected an angulation osteotomy of Marquardt and Neff or proximal shortening osteotomy is used to preserve length and rotational control.[6,7]

### Forearm Level and Wrist Disarticulation

The transradial or forearm level amputation is the most common amputation performed in the civilian and military population. In the years leading up to published data from Operations Iraqi and Enduring Freedom, data compiled in 2015 from the Expeditionary Medical Encounter Database, Naval Health Research Center illustrated 50% of all UE amputations were transradial versus 10% wrist disarticulation. Limb length and soft tissue coverage must be balanced, as well as the considerations for prosthetic capabilities. Fractures should be stabilized to facilitate functional length. Rotational and free flaps should be entertained when necessary to provide optimal length. When prudent, the elbow should be preserved unless contraindicated by infection or necessary oncologic margin (**Fig. 2**).[8] A dorsal to volar flap is preferred for distal coverage to place the more resilient dorsal skin over the end of the residual. Forearm level amputations facilitate myoelectric control of hand and wrist function, whereas a wrist disarticulation preserves forearm rotation through the distal radioulnar joint and eliminates painful radioulnar convergence.[9] However, a wrist disarticulation can limit prosthetic options (ie, exclusion of wrist rotators because of added length) and can also be difficult to close in terms of soft tissue, often requiring a "fish mouth" closure but preferably the thick palmar skin is used to cover the disarticulation.

### Partial Hand Amputation

When prehensile grasp and sensation can be preserved, reconstruction through single ray, double ray, or partial hand is efficacious. Surgical reconstruction should focus on preserving power ulnar motor control or border digit apposition and, at all costs, preserve the thumb. Transposition of digits and toe-to-thumb reconstruction can facilitate success in thumb loss. Osseointegration for thumb preservation has been advocated as early as 1996.[10] Prosthetic fitting is cosmetic and functional in terms of providing a stable base to oppose residual grip. It is important for the surgeon to create a nonpainful, durable, osseous and soft tissue reconstruction to optimize this process.[11]

### Targeted Muscle Reinnervation

Traction neurectomy has been used historically to handle major peripheral nerves. However, this technique can result in painful end neuroma and residual proximal muscle deinnervation, which can cause atrophy and coverage issues. Based on the work of Kuiken, and colleagues,[12] terminal nerve branches can be non-anatomically transferred to provide control sites for intuitive myoelectric prostheses and decrease end

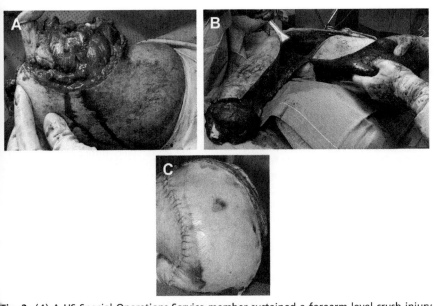

**Fig. 2.** (*A*) A US Special Operations Service member sustained a forearm level crush injury. Conventional surgical theory would have the patient amputated above the elbow for classic flaps. (*B*) A long latissimus dorsi rotational flap was selected to provide coverage of the elbow. An anterolateral thigh flap was entertained; however, with a previous leg injury this flap was not selected. The patient was counseled regarding a planned reduction given the bulk of the latissimus. (*C*) Latissimus flap inset to cover radius and ulna with myoplasty to posterior triceps, anterior flexor pronator, and brachioradialis. To prevent translation in healing, a fascial myodesis to radius and ulna is also performed.

neuroma by organized regeneration. In our experience with combat amputations, cancer amputations, and civilian trauma, this has become our center's preferred technique.

## Osseointegration

The marriage of prosthesis to skeleton through a viable skin interface has been one of the most significant advances in amputee science in the twenty-first century. Many patients do not wear UE prostheses because of difficulties with suspension. This is especially true in the transhumeral level and proximal where suspension often has to come from the contralateral shoulder girdle. Osseointegration affords the ability to obviate a socket and also allows for prosthetic rigidity to the skeleton, facilitating greater confidence and range of motion (ROM) to the amputee. This process is combined with TMR for improved precision and control. Risks include superficial and deep infection, and osteomyelitis and catastrophic failure. Despite these risks, this technique provides so much independence to the prosthetic wearer that the understanding of this process must continue to advance.[13]

## PROSTHETIC DESIGNS

The design of UE prostheses is broadly categorized by the power source: body powered; externally powered; hybrid; or passive, where the terminal device (TD) requires no power. Externally powered prostheses are further categorized by control input sources: traditional myoelectric, myoelectric pattern recognition, and switches. Oppositional prostheses and activity-specific prostheses are examples that may not use either body or external power to activate a TD.

Body-powered prostheses capture the user's own body movement through harnessing to produce the power required to activate a TD. Because there are no electronics involved, they are generally more durable and are used in a wider variety of environments, compared with externally powered prostheses. Body-powered prostheses most commonly capture the motion of biscapular abduction with a figure-of-eight or figure-of-nine harness, which is positioned to run over the inferior third of the scapulae, to capture maximum scapular movement. In the case of a transhumeral prosthesis, this motion pulls on a cable that first flexes the elbow, and then operates the TD device once the elbow is locked in position (**Fig. 3**). In a transradial prosthesis the cable operates the TD only. TDs for body-powered prostheses are either voluntary closing, where the device at rest is in the open position and the user actively closes it, or more commonly, voluntary opening, where the device is closed when at rest and the user actively opens it. The pinch force of voluntary closing TDs is determined by the user's strength, whereas voluntary opening devices rely on adjustable tension in the TDs.

Externally powered prostheses draw power from a battery and can obtain control input from a variety of sources to activate the prostheses. The rechargeable battery is usually incorporated within the forearm section of the prosthesis. The source of control for these prostheses may be input from electromyographic (EMG) surface electrodes and/or switches. EMG signals are used with either direct control or pattern recognition. For direct control, the signal from one electrode directly controls one motion at a time. The user switches between modes of operation using an EMG signal, such as simultaneous contraction of two muscles, or a switch, such as a bump switch on the side of the socket.

Another control strategy that uses EMG signals captured with surface electrodes is pattern recognition. In pattern recognition, input from an array of electrodes is captured as the user contracts their muscles as if they were performing the desired motion with their missing limb. The input from the array of electrodes is analyzed to enable the system to learn the EMG pattern for each motion. The pattern recognition system is then able to acquire input from multiple electrodes simultaneously and determine a user's intended motion. Electrodes within the socket do not have to be placed over specific muscle groups but, rather, over general areas of muscle activity. With pattern recognition there is no need to switch between modes to control elbow, wrist, and TD. Pattern recognition may be used with transradial prostheses, and when incorporated into

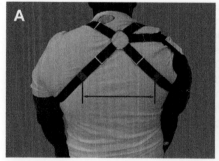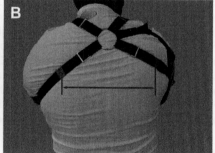

**Fig. 3.** A figure-of-eight harness on a body-powered transhumeral prosthesis. The inferior strap on the prosthetic side pulls on the cable to flex the elbow and activate the terminal device. Note the increase in distance between the reference lines at rest (*A*) (21 cm) and when performing biscapular abduction (*B*) (27 cm), producing the pull on the cable.

ranshumeral or shoulder disarticulation sockets of individuals who have had TMR, it can readily take advantage of the EMG signals of the reinnervated muscles.

Hybrid prostheses incorporate elements of body powered and externally powered prostheses to actuate all degrees of freedom of a prosthetic arm. They may be used when an individual cannot produce enough body motion necessary to operate both an elbow and a TD on a body powered prosthesis, or when the individual desires a lighter weight prosthesis than a fully electronic one. Therefore, they are particularly useful for individuals with higher levels of amputation.

Nonpowered prostheses, such as those for gross opposition or specific activities, remain common. This design may be used to restore an individual's body image and improve body symmetry to prevent postural issues, which may develop following the loss of a limb. These prostheses are often referred to as passive, although they are effective functionally in performing tasks requiring gross opposition. Activity-specific prostheses usually have a unique TD purposely designed to grip, lock on to, catch, push, or support a particular device/instrument. Examples include a TD that locks on to a weight lifting bar, one that can quick-disconnect from a bicycle handlebar, and a paddle-like device for swimming (**Fig. 4**).

Despite the existing range of options in UE prosthetic design, the Defense Advanced Research Projects Agency recognized the persistent need for better alternatives, and through the Revolutionizing Prosthetics program funded the development

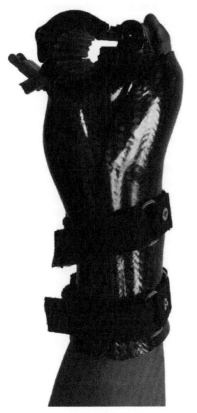

**Fig. 4.** A partial hand prosthesis for weight lifting. This activity-specific prosthesis includes a terminal device that can lock on to a weight lifting bar.

of two advanced prosthetic arms: the LUKE arm and the modular prosthetic limb. The LUKE arm was developed by DEKA Research and Development Corporation (Manchester, NH) and was commercialized by Mobius Bionics (Manchester, NH). The modular prosthetic limb was developed by the Johns Hopkins University Applied Physics Laboratory and is being used in research laboratories around the country.

## PREPROSTHETIC REHABILITATION

Over the course of the rehabilitation process, individuals with newly acquired amputations encounter a variety of health care professionals that work as an interdisciplinary team to address all aspects of care. This team includes physiatrists, surgeons, nurses, certified prosthetists, behavioral health specialists, social workers, physical and occupational therapists (OTs), recreation therapists, vocational rehabilitation specialists, driver rehabilitation therapists, and others.[14] OTs provide the tools, interventions, and education necessary to relearn the skills needed to complete basic ADLs and instrumental ADLs; manage residual limb deficits including edema control, shaping, and preprosthetic and post-prosthetic training; and facilitate community reintegration for successful resumption of life roles.[15]

Initial evaluation determines prior and current level of function, patient goals and background are assessed, and physical and emotional health are evaluated. Prior hand dominance, education level, vocation and recreational activities, living situation, and access to medical care are all important components of a holistic evaluation to establish a plan of care.[16] Change of dominance is addressed during this phase if needed to ensure independence with unilateral function when the prosthesis is not available and includes interventions directed at increasing fine motor coordination, reaction time, improving handwriting, and developing one handed typing skills. Ensuring independence with and without the prosthesis is an important component of overall function in variable situations throughout life.[16,17]

Prosthesis fitting and training rely on successful wound healing and limb shaping to ensure correct fit and functional use. Immediately postoperatively, medical interventions, such as provision of antibiotics, surgical site drains, and use of negative pressure wound therapy via vacuum-assisted closure systems, are implemented by physicians and wound care specialists.[16] In conjunction, the OT provides education regarding postoperative limb protection, initiation of edema management and limb shaping, and implementation desensitization activities.[14] Edema management and limb shaping begins with distal to proximal compression achieved with figure-of-eight wrapping using elastic bandages. A residual limb shrinker is introduced once wounds are sufficiently healed and are able to tolerate increased shearing forces. A silicon liner may also be used for the residual limb to provide constant concentric, distal to proximal compression, and can also assist with softening any scar tissue present. During this progressive volume reduction and shaping of the residual limb, size changes should be measured and monitored to ensure optimal residual limb shape for eventual prosthesis prescription, fitting, and use.[16]

Desensitization is another aspect that is addressed during this time. After amputation, it is common for the patient to report hypersensitivity in the residual limb. Compression, various texture exposure to the limb, massage, gradual loading, and tapping are all therapeutic interventions used to reduce hypersensitivity.[14,16] Addressing pain, in the phantom and residual limb, plays a large role in the management of hypersensitivity and is important for successful prosthetic integration and use.[16]

Overall strength and ROM are also addressed. Establishing a self-ROM stretching routine and low-load prolonged stretching of joints with ROM limitations during therapy helps increase effective gross motor movements and appropriate body mechanics. This helps reduce the use of compensation strategies that may lead to cumulative trauma or overuse injuries. Once ROM is addressed, overall strengthening and conditioning, postural exercises, and cardiovascular endurance are introduced to promote proximal stability for distal function without compensation.[14,16] Visual feedback is often used to help the patient identify and self-correct abnormal movement patterns. Introduction of isometric and isotonic strengthening can assist with improving core stability and strength, and improving symmetry of the contralateral extremity.[16]

The OT and prosthetist work with the patient to identify potential myosites, or muscles, which can be used to control electrodes that in turn control the prosthesis. Treatment focuses on individual activation of the targeted muscles, and progresses to learning proportional control of their activation. This allows graded movements of the TD attached to the prosthesis during functional activities.[14,16] Use of software programs specifically designed to provide biofeedback help the client to visualize their successes and improve proficiency and muscle endurance to maximize prosthesis wearing time and integration.

## PROSTHESIS FITTING

The fitting of a UE prosthesis should occur as early as possible so that the individual can begin training and performing bimanual tasks. The evaluation, design, and fitting of the prosthesis should involve a trained prosthetist working with the interdisciplinary team and includes: (1) a method to suspend the prosthesis from the residual limb, (2) an interface between the residual limb and the prosthesis, (3) a prosthetic socket, and (4) structural elements and a control system to connect the socket with the prosthetic joints and TD.

The prosthetic socket represents an important connection between the individual and prosthesis and provides the following principal functions. First, it should enable the user flexibility to maximize ROM of the remaining anatomic joints while serving to facilitate energy transfer between the user and the end point of the limb to interact with the environment. This means the socket design should incorporate methods to resist torques and forces that act to twist or move the socket relative to the residual limb. These two functions are often in conflict. Generally, the more the residual limb is encompassed by a prosthetic socket, the better it can resist torques and forces; however, this comes at the expense of limiting ROM of the remaining anatomic joints. Another function of a prosthetic socket is to protect the skin of the residual limb from damaging pressures. This is particularly important over boney prominences where skin breakdown can result in skin breakdown. The socket should also be a rigid platform for distal components, such as the forearm and TD. Optimization of prosthetic socket design should consider all of these functions, how that interacts with how the person intends to use their prosthesis, and how the prosthesis will be suspended and controlled.

Socket designs are constantly evolving as prosthetists continue to innovate through incorporating materials with different stiffness, development of new suspension methods, and superior techniques to shape the socket to distribute the within socket pressures over fragile tissue.[18] The primary interface between the residual limb and prosthetic socket is generally accomplished in one of the following methods: (1) skin-fit, (2) a prosthetic sock, or (3) a silicone liner. The skin may contact the inside of the socket directly (ie, "skin-fit"). This method offers the most direct control of the prosthetic limb and ways for an externally powered, myoelectrically controlled TD to receive the electrical signals from the underlying muscles. The limitation of this interface is potentially exposing the skin to areas of high pressures and sheering forces, and usually requires the use of a pull-sock. The second interface is through a prosthetic sock. These woven socks provide an easy method to don the socket and provide some cushioning between the skin and the socket. However, this method does require additional means to suspend the socket, normally through the harness of a body-powered control system. A third common interface is to use a silicone liner that is rolled onto the residual limb and inserted into the socket. Silicone liners may be pre-fabricated or custom made for the individual and offer a superior way to protect the skin (especially for those with skin grafts or fragile skin) while providing an intimate fit. **Fig. 5** provides a brief review of more traditional designs for partial hand amputations up to interscapulothoracic levels.

Prosthetic socket designs for partial hand amputations have benefited from recent advances in silicone interface technologies. These designs generally include a custom made silicone liner that is rolled on proximal to the wrist joint in which a small rigid socket is attached that provides a platform for the attachment of the missing digits.[19] Wrist disarticulation sockets may involve a method to suspend the prosthesis contouring the socket proximal to the styloid processes of the radius and ulna. A challenge with wrist disarticulation designs is that the distal end of the residual limb is wider than the portion of the limb just proximal to the styloid processes. Therefore, these design typically involve some method allow the styloid processes to push through the narrow section and provide suspension by the tightness of the socket proximal to the processes.[20,21] Transtibial prosthetic socket designs for a long residual limb may not require trim lines that extend far up the forearm section and therefore allow more pronation and supination of the forearm. A simple traditional design would be to have a prosthetic socket as the interface with the harness for body-powered control provide the suspension.[21,22] Short transradial residual limbs may require socket trim lines that extend proximal to the epicondyles of the humerus to provide a method for suspension and more control of the prosthesis but it is at the expense of limiting elbow ROM. The Muenster socket is a good example of this type of design.[23,24] Prosthetic design for transhumeral amputation is challenging because of the soft residual tissues around the humerus and because the shaft of the humerus does not provide skeletal contours that can resist torques developed at the TD. Therefore, these socket designs have traditionally included trim lines that extend proximally and medially to the humeral head to create deltopectoral and infraspinatus wings, a design described by McLaurin and coworkers[25] in the late 1960s. This type of design significantly limits ROM motion at the shoulder joint. Amputations through the shoulder joint or at the interscapulothoracic level typically require sockets that encompass large portions of the trunk to provide the biomechanical basis for supporting the prosthesis and resist the torques created by loads at the end of a long lever arm. Heat dissipation and comfort become major concerns and are addressed by removing large portions of the socket or using straps extending to the contralateral side.[26]

## POST-PROSTHESIS REHABILITATION

The transition to prosthetic training is a major milestone in the rehabilitative care of the UE amputee. The earlier phases lay a foundation for the actual training and use of a prosthesis. Focus of training shifts to mastery of prosthetic limb control, the integration of prosthesis into daily tasks, and complete independence with meaningful daily occupations.[27] Clinical evidence regarding UE prosthetic training is limited and relies on clinical judgment and expertise.[28] However, there is a belief that lack of training may be a significant contributing factor to device abandonment and rejection rates.[17] Studies

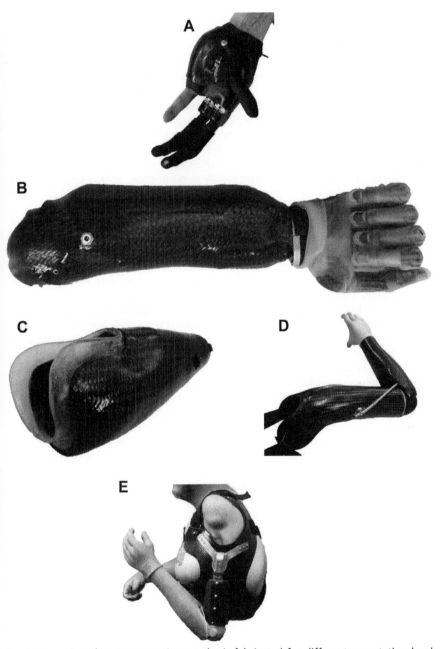

**Fig. 5.** Examples of upper extremity prosthesis fabricated for different amputation levels and using different technologies. (*A*) Myoelectric-operated partial hand prosthesis. (*B*) Myoelectric-operated wrist disarticulation prosthesis with a multiarticulated prosthetic hand. (*C*) Example of the Munster style transradial prosthetic socket where the trimlines extend around the condyles of the humerus to provide suspension. (*D*) Transhumeral prosthesis with a body-powered elbow joint and a myoelectric controlled prosthetic hand. (*E*) Shoulder disarticulation prosthesis with an X-frame-type prosthetic socket, passive shoulder joint, and myoelectrically operated elbow and prosthetic hand.

show that the sooner an amputee is fit and begins working with a prosthesis, the more successful functional outcomes. When patients are fit for an initial prosthesis within 30 days of amputation ("the golden window"), they show significantly higher rehabilitation success rates and likelihood for return to work within 4 months of injury.[16,17]

The patient, therapist, and prosthetist work together to select a prosthesis that best meets the needs of the patient. Myoelectric prostheses are tolerated much sooner than body-powered prosthesis because of lower shearing and end bearing forces, and are often the first prosthesis prescribed.[14] Regardless of the type of prosthesis, it is important that the patient develop a good understanding of component terminology and basic maintenance. This knowledge is important during training and when communicating mechanical difficulties or malfunctions with the treatment team. The patient should also be able to independently perform basic socket inspection and cleaning; battery changes (if myoelectric); and harness adjustment, rubber band replacement, and cable changes (if body powered).

The end goal is for the patient to tolerate wearing a prosthesis for 8 to 10 hours per day for use during functional activities. However, the basic tasks of wear, care, and operation must be accomplished first. The patient is first educated on limb inspection and donning and doffing the prosthesis with the establishment of a progressive wearing schedule. Frequent inspection (several times per day) of the residual limb for redness and/or irritation should be completed (especially after removing the prosthesis) and should become part of the daily routine. The patient is then taught the process of putting on and removing the prosthesis. The Reduced Friction Donning System (Advanced Arm Dynamics, Inc, Redondo Beach, CA) may be a helpful tool when donning the prosthesis. It is a low friction material that is placed on the residual limb and used to pull the arm into the socket and is especially helpful with a myoelectric prosthesis because the limb must fit securely into the socket for optimal skin-to-electrode contact. Smurr and colleagues[27] provides a step-by-step explanation on how to don a body-powered and myoelectric prosthesis. The methods for donning and doffing a prosthetic system for bilateral amputees can significantly vary depending on the level of amputation.[29] The end goal for all levels is to ensure the patient is able to perform the task independently.[29]

A recommended wear schedule is three 30-minute sessions per day with advancement of 30 minutes each day.[30] Special consideration is taken for a patient with decreased sensation or extensive scarring (eg, burns). The residual limb should be examined after removal and prosthetic wear should be discontinued should any redness persists for more than 20 minutes.[29]

Next, the focus shifts to accommodation of the weight of the prosthesis while standing and moving the extremities. The patient can be positioned in front of a mirror for increased body awareness during movement and learn to self-correct body asymmetry and awkward postures caused by the weight of the prosthesis.[27,31] After the patient becomes familiar with the weight of the prosthesis, the rehabilitation transitions to control and operation of the prosthetic limb.

Yancosek[29] recommends control training progress in the following way (regardless of the power source of the prosthesis): (1) standing to sitting, (2) prosthetic side to midline to across the body, and (3) table-top-height to overhead and floor levels. The tasks should be simple and repetitive during this phase and media used in training should include objects of various shapes, sizes, textures, density, and weight.[29] The focus of the controls training should include joint positioning to place the prosthesis in the proper position to access an intended target and proportion control (ie, force regulation) to control the accuracy of the TD to grasp different objects. Smurr and colleagues[16] provides a description of controls training by each amputation level for myoelectric and body-powered devices.

Once mastery over basic prosthetic limb control is reached the patient transitions to the intermediate phase of prosthetic rehabilitation where there is less focus on repetition of basic function and more emphasis on the completion ADLs and valued functional activities. The patient is trained to incorporate the prosthesis as the assisting limb in the case of a unilateral amputation.[30] There are checklists available that provide a comprehensive list of ADL tasks the patient should be able to complete with the use of the prosthesis.[32]

During the advanced prosthetic training phase the patient should be encouraged to select personally meaningful tasks and should select and become proficient at one type of prosthetic device (body-power, myoelectric).[14] The patient should trial various TDs and adaptive tools to decide what tools and techniques best meet his or her specific needs.[29] Training tasks should be multistep and challenging, and may include the completion of a tangible product or outcome.[16,29,33] Consultations with vocational rehabilitation for return-to-work, recreational therapy for adaptive sports and leisure tasks, and a driving rehabilitation specialist for vehicle modifications should also occur.

The importance of using standardized measurement instruments to assess UE function is well recognized[34] and is driven by the need for more cost-effective treatment from third party payers. Outcome assessment should be initiated at the beginning of treatment or in the case of performance measures, as soon as the patient receives the prosthetic limb. Some self-report and functional outcome measures that have been reported to be valid and reliable for UE amputation population in the literature include the shortened version of the Disabilities of the Shoulder Arm and Hand,[35] the Trinity Amputation and Prosthetics Experience Scale,[36] modified Box and Block Test,[36] and Modified Jebsen Taylor Hand Function Test. Additional measures to consider include: South Hampton Hand Assessment Procedure,[37] Assessment of Capacity for Myoelectric Control version 2.0,[38] and the Patient Specific Functional Scale.[39]

## SUMMARY

UE amputation rehabilitation continues to advance because of surgical, technologic, and rehabilitation advances. Barriers to acceptance of advanced UE prostheses continue to involve weight, battery life, function, and durability but research funding in this area continues to push the technology forward. Support (political, research funding, medical infrastructure, and emotional) for the combat injured continues to push innovations in UE amputation rehabilitation and these advances ultimately extend to the civilian health care sphere. Because of the complexity of this area, patients are best served by centers with interdisciplinary teams experienced in UE amputation rehabilitation.

## REFERENCES

1. Baumgartner R. Upper extremity amputation and prosthetics. J Rehabil Res Dev 2001;38(4):357.

2. Muller M. Transfemoral amputation: prosthetic management. In: Krajbich J, Pinzur M, Potter BK, et al, editors. Atlas of amputations and limb deficiencies: surgical, prosthetic and rehabilitation principles. 4th edition. Rosemont (IL): American Academy of Orthopaedic Surgeons; 2016. p. 537–54.

3. Alderete J. Amputations about the shoulder. In: Krajbich J, Pinzur M, Potter B, et al, editors. Atlas of amputations and limb deficiencies: surgical, prosthetic, and rehabilitation principles. 4th edition. Rosemont (IL): American Academy of Orthopaedic Surgeons; 2016. p. 271–86.

4. Cordeiro PG, Cohen S, Burt M, et al. The total volar forearm musculocutaneous free flap for reconstruction of extended forequarter amputations. Ann Plast Surg 1998;40(4):388–96.
5. Zachary LS, Gottlieb LJ, Simon M, et al. Forequarter amputation wound coverage with an ipsilateral, lymphedematous, circumferential forearm fasciocutaneous free flap in patients undergoing palliative shoulder-girdle tumor resection. J Reconstr Microsurg 1993;9(2):103–7.
6. Beltran MJ, Kirk KL, Hsu JR. Minimally invasive shortening humeral osteotomy to salvage a through-elbow amputation. Mil Med 2010;175(9):693–6.
7. Marquardt E, Neff G. The angulation osteotomy of above-elbow stumps. Clin Orthop Relat Res 1974;104:232–8.
8. Baccarani A, Follmar KE, De Santis G, et al. Free vascularized tissue transfer to preserve upper extremity amputation levels. Plast Reconstr Surg 2007;120(4):971–81.
9. Nanos GP. Wrist disarticulation and transradial amputation: surgical management. In: Krajbich J, Pinzur M, Potter BK, et al, editors. Atlas of amputation and limb deficiencies: surgical, prosthetic, and rehabilitation principles. 4th edition. Rosemont (IL): American Academy of Orthopaedic Surgeons; 2016. p. 221–323.
10. Lundborg G, Branemark PI, Rosen B. Osseointegrated thumb prostheses: a concept for fixation of digit prosthetic devices. J Hand Surg 1996;21(2):216–21.
11. Puhaindran ME, Steensma MR, Athanasian EA. Partial hand preservation for large soft tissue sarcomas of the hand. J Hand Surg 2010;35(2):291–5.
12. Souza JM, Cheesborough JE, Ko JH, et al. Targeted muscle reinnervation: a novel approach to postamputation neuroma pain. Clin Orthop Relat Res 2014;472(10):2984–90.
13. Branemark R, Branemark PI, Rydevik B, et al. Osseointegration in skeletal reconstruction and rehabilitation: a review. J Rehabil Res Dev 2001;38(2):175–81.
14. Management of Upper Extremity Amputation Rehabilitation Working Group. VA/DoD clinical practice guidelines for the management of upper extremity amputation rehabilitation. Washington, DC: Department of Veterans Affairs, Department of Defense; 2014.
15. Amputation Coalition of America. A team-based approach to amputee rehabilitation. Military in-Step. 2005. Available at: http://www.amputee-coalition.org/military-instep/amputee-rehab.html. Accessed April 15, 2018.
16. Smurr L, Gulick K, Yancosek K, et al. Managing the upper extremity amputee: a protocol for success. J Hand Ther 2008;21(2):160–75.
17. Resnik L, Meucci MR, Lieberman-Klinger S, et al. Advanced upper limb prosthetic devices: implications for upper limb prosthetic rehabilitation. Arch Phys Med Rehabil 2012;93(4):710–7.
18. Lake C. The evolution of upper limb prosthetic socket design. J Prosthetics Orthotics 2008;20(3):85–92.
19. Uellendahl J. Partial hand amputation: prosthetic management. In: Krajbich J, Pinzur M, Potter B, et al, editors. Atlas of amputations and limb deficiencies: surgical, prosthetic, and rehabilitation principles, Vol 2, 4th edition. Rosemont (IL): American Academy of Orthopaedic Surgeons; 2016. p. 213–20.
20. Uellendahl J, Mandacina S, Ramdial S. Custom silicone sockets for myoelectric prostheses. J Prosthetics Orthotics 2006;18(2):35–40.
21. Miguelez J, Conyers D, Lang M, et al. Transradial and wrist disarticulation socket considerations: case studies. J Prosthetics Orthotics 2008;20(3):118–25.
22. Fryer C, Michael J. Harnessing and controls for body powered devices. In: Smith D, Michael J, Bowker J, editors. Atlas of amputations and limb deficiencies:

surgical, prosthetic, and rehabilitation principles. 3rd edition. Rosemont (IL): American Academy of Orthopedic Surgeons; 2004. p. 131–44.

23. Fishman S, Kay H. The Munster-type-below-elbow socket: an evaluation. Artif Limbs 1964;8(2):4–14.

24. Miguelez J, Lake C, Conyers D, et al. The transradial anatomically contoured (TRAC) interface: design principles and methodology. J Prosthetics Orthotics 2003;15(4):148–57.

25. McLaurin CA, Sauter WF, Dolan CM, et al. Fabrication procedures for the open-shoulder above-elbow socket. Artif Limbs 1969;13(2):46–54.

26. Peterson B. Amputations about the shoulder: prosthetic management. In: Krajbich J, Pinzur M, Potter BK, et al, editors. Atlas of amputations and limb deficiencies: surgical, prosthetic, and rehabilitation principles. 4th edition. Rosemont (IL): American Academy of Orthopaedic Surgeons; 2016. p. 287–98.

27. Smurr LM, Yancosek K, Gulick K, et al. Occupational therapy for the polytrauma casualty with limb loss. In: Pasquina PF, Cooper RA, editors. Care of the combat amputee. Washington, DC: Dept. of the Army. Office of the Surgeon General., Borden Institute (U.S.); 2009. p. 493–533.

28. Dromerick AW, Schabowsky CN, Holley RJ, et al. Effect of training on upper-extremity prosthetic performance and motor learning: a single-case study. Arch Phys Med Rehabil 2008;89(6):1199–204.

29. Yancosek K. Amputations and prosthetics. In: Skirven T, Osterman AL, Fedorczyk JM, et al, editors. Rehabilitation of the hand and upper extremity. 6th edition. Philadelphia: Elsevier; 2011. p. 1293–305.

30. Atkins D, Edelstein J. Training patients with upper-limb amputations. In: Carroll K, Edelstein J, editors. Prosthetics and patient management: a comprehensive clinical approach. New York: SLACK; 2006. p. 167–80.

31. Yancosek K, Daugherty SE, Cancio L. Treatment for the service member: a description of innovative interventions. J Hand Ther 2008;21(2):189–95.

32. Atkins J, Meier R. Comprehensive management of the upper-limb amputee. New York: Springer-Verlag; 1989.

33. Oliver R, Schoonover C, Tu T, et al. Prosthesis thesis: a task-oriented approach to motor learning. OT Pract 2017;22(8):14–7.

34. Yancosek KE, Howell D. A narrative review of dexterity assessments. J Hand Ther 2009;22(3):258–70.

35. Resnik L, Borgia M. Reliability, validity, and responsiveness of the QuickDASH in patients with upper limb amputation. Arch Phys Med Rehabil 2015;96(9): 1676–83.

36. Resnik LPTP, Borgia MMS. Reliability and validity of outcome measures for upper limb amputation. J Prosthetics Orthotics 2012;24(4):192–201.

37. Light CM, Chappell PH, Kyberd PJ. Establishing a standardized clinical assessment tool of pathologic and prosthetic hand function: normative data, reliability, and validity. Arch Phys Med Rehabil 2002;83(6):776–83.

38. Lindner HY, Linacre JM, Norling Hermansson LM. Assessment of capacity for myoelectric control: evaluation of construct and rating scale. J Rehabil Med 2009;41(6):467–74.

39. Stratford P, Gill C, Westaway M, et al. Assessing disability and change on individual patents: a report of a patient specific measure. Physiother Can 1995;47(4): 258–63.

# Lower Limb Amputation Care Across the Active Duty Military and Veteran Populations

Joseph B. Webster, MD

## KEYWORDS

- Lower extremity • Amputation • Limb salvage • Rehabilitation • Prostheses
- Artificial limbs

## KEY POINTS

- Individuals with lower extremity amputations resulting from trauma have unique needs and require specialized expertise in order to facilitate optimal recovery.
- The wide-ranging needs of this population include issues related to the amputation itself, issues related to other traumatic injuries, and the management of longer-term secondary conditions.
- Successful management of individuals with trauma-related amputation involves an interdisciplinary team approach and care coordination across the continuum of care.
- Advances in surgical management, therapy techniques, and prosthetic limb technology have resulted in improved functional outcomes for individuals with trauma-related lower limb amputations.

## INTRODUCTION

Individuals with trauma-related amputations, whether from combat or noncombat activities, have unique needs and require specialized management expertise in order to facilitate optimal outcomes. These management considerations begin before the amputation and persistent throughout the lifetime of the individual. Successful management of individuals with trauma-related amputation requires an interdisciplinary team approach and care coordination across the continuum of care. This article covers the unique management considerations specifically related to the amputated residual limb and prosthetic restoration as well as management considerations related to comorbid injuries and to the commonly encountered longer-term consequences of traumatic amputation.

Disclosure: The author has nothing to disclose.
Department of Physical Medicine and Rehabilitation, Virginia Commonwealth University School of Medicine, Hunter Holmes McGuire VA Medical Center, Building 514, 1201 Broad Rock Boulevard, Richmond, VA 23249, USA
E-mail address: joseph.webster@va.gov

Phys Med Rehabil Clin N Am 30 (2019) 89–109
https://doi.org/10.1016/j.pmr.2018.08.008
1047-9651/19/© 2018 Elsevier Inc. All rights reserved.

## GENERAL CONSIDERATIONS

Individuals with trauma-related amputations have wide-ranging medical needs comprising issues with the amputation itself, issues related to traumatic injury of other body parts, and longer-term secondary conditions. Some of these issues are more prevalent and of greater severity in the early recovery period following the traumatic event, whereas others develop later and have the potential for progressive worsening over time.

In the acute care setting, management of the amputation may be a secondary consideration in the patients with polytrauma with a severe traumatic brain injury (TBI) or other life-threatening injuries. Once the patient is stabilized medically and begins showing improvements in their awareness and level of consciousness, management and rehabilitation of the amputation and/or salvaged limb become a greater priority and demand increased attention. As the patient emerges from posttraumatic amnesia, it is important to anticipate the psychological adjustment and support that will be required in understanding and accepting the longer-term implications of lower limb amputation.

## EPIDEMIOLOGY OF TRAUMATIC AMPUTATION

Traumatic amputation can result from injuries sustained both within and outside the military setting. Traumatic amputations that occur in military personnel can be directly related to combat operations or related to other, noncombat military activities. Data provided by the Extremity Trauma and Amputation Center of Excellence database show that 1718 United States service members sustained at least 1 amputation (excluding digit amputations) in conflict-related activities between January 1, 2001 and December 31, 2017.[1] Thirty-one percent of these individuals sustained 2 or more major limb amputations. Most of these amputations (73%) were a result of an improvised explosive device blast injury. Among the 1718 patients who underwent an amputation, 84% involved the lower limb (76% 1 lower limb, 8% both lower limbs). Among lower limb amputations, 56% were transtibial-level amputations and 38% were transfemoral-level amputations.[2]

Although combat-related traumatic amputations are frequently the result of a direct blast exposure, noncombat military and civilian traumatic amputations are most commonly the result of blunt trauma to the extremity. There are approximately 30,000 to 40,000 civilian injury-related amputations performed in the United States annually.[2,3] In civilians, traumatic amputations most commonly involve the lower limb compared with the upper limb (59% vs 41%). Motor vehicle accidents account for 51% of these amputations and 19% are the result of machinery accidents. Motor vehicle collisions and machinery accidents are more likely to involve upper limb amputation, whereas motorcycle and pedestrian accidents more commonly involve lower limb amputation.[2–4]

## MANAGEMENT IN THE MILITARY HEALTH SYSTEM

During the military conflicts in Iraq and Afghanistan since 2001, the sophisticated military trauma care system in conjunction with advances in personal protective equipment have led to high survival rates for those military personnel injured in combat. Despite these advances, the extremities remain susceptible to traumatic injury. The Department of Defense (DoD) has developed programs with specialized amputation surgical and rehabilitation care and these services are focused primarily at 3 DoD advanced rehabilitation centers. These centers provide highly advanced and nnovative care in all areas of amputation rehabilitation and prosthetic fabrication. Unique aspects of these programs include the use of a sports medicine rehabilitation approach, the incorporation of virtual care environments for advanced mobility raining, and an emphasis on community-based, adaptive sports and recreation nvolvement. The DoD amputation care programs operate in close collaboration with the Department of Veterans Affairs (VA) to ensure that care across the two systems is well coordinated.

## THE VETERANS HEALTH ADMINISTRATION APPROACH

The Veterans Health Administration (VHA) has long recognized that veterans with battle-related amputations epitomize the sacrifices of military service made on the nation's behalf. The wide-ranging and lifelong care considerations for these individuals were one of the driving forces behind implementation of VHA's Amputation System of Care (ASoC). The ASoC was implemented in 2008 in partnership with the VHA Polytrauma System of Care to ensure that veterans with both traumatic amputation and polytrauma can be provided comprehensive and coordinated services.

The VHA ASoC is an integrated health care delivery system that provides patient-centered, lifelong, holistic care and care coordination for veterans with amputations.[5] The ASoC provides care for veterans with extremity amputations related to disease processes such as diabetes and for veterans with amputations secondary to traumatic injuries. VHA outpatient amputation specialty clinics provide interdisciplinary and comprehensive services to meet the complex rehabilitation needs of veterans with traumatic amputations. Through care coordination and close collaboration with both primary care and other specialty care services, these amputation care teams ensure that all medical, rehabilitation, and prosthetic needs of veterans with traumatic amputations are met.[5]

## EXTREMITY TRAUMA
### Limb Salvage Versus Amputation

Extremity trauma is a term that encompasses a broad spectrum of injury severity with no consensus definition. When considered broadly, extremity trauma represents one of the most common combat-related injuries.[6,7] During the military operations in Iraq and Afghanistan since 2001, there have been an estimated 30,000 military personnel who have sustained some degree of extremity trauma with more than 19,000 having significant enough injuries to require hospitalization. Many of these injuries result in residual long-term impairments and associated functional limitations.[2,6–8]

The term limb salvage is defined as extremity trauma involving at least 3 of 4 systems (soft tissue, bone, nerves, and vascular supply) and requiring advanced surgical interventions in order to avoid amputation.[6,9] Early management of individuals who have undergone limb salvage may include the need for aggressive debridement and irrigation of remaining wounds, fasciotomies to reduce compartment pressures, delayed definitive closure of wounds, and additional reconstructive surgical procedures to salvage all viable tissue. Longer-term staged management may require additional fracture fixation or bone lengthening procedures and aggressive infection prevention and treatment. Soft tissue and skin management may involve negative pressure wound therapy, soft tissue expansion, skin grafting, or microvascular tissue transfer.[7,9,10]

Studies have been performed to evaluate outcomes following limb salvage compared with amputation of the lower extremity.[11,12] The Lower Extremity Assessment Project (LEAP) enrolled 569 patients with severe lower extremity injuries and this cohort was followed prospectively for 24 months. Functional outcomes were assessed with the Sickness Impact Profile (SIP). Although the rehospitalization rate was higher with limb reconstruction, there were no differences in functional outcomes between limb reconstruction and amputation.[11] A long-term follow-up study followed the same cohort for an average of 84 months postinjury. Most of the subjects reported that physical and psychosocial functioning had deteriorated since their 24-month follow-up, with 50% of the patients reporting severe disability. There was still no significant difference in SIP scores between treatment groups at long-term follow-up.[13] A meta-analysis of studies on complex limb salvage or early amputation for severe lower limb injury found similar outcomes between groups in the area of pain and no significant differences in functional outcome, including competitive employment.[14]

Additional studies have been performed looking more specifically at military personnel and comparing outcomes of limb salvage with amputation.[15,16] The Military Extremity Trauma Amputation/Limb Salvage (METALS) study is a retrospective cohort study of 324 Operation Enduring Freedom/Operation Iraqi Freedom service members with lower limb injuries requiring either amputation or limb salvage. The Short Musculoskeletal Function Assessment (SMFA) questionnaire was used to measure overall function. This study found that the amputation group had better scores in all SMFA domains as well as a lower likelihood of posttraumatic stress disorder (PTSD) and a higher likelihood of being engaged in vigorous sports. There were no significant differences between the groups with regard to depressive symptoms, pain interfering with daily activities, or work/school status.[16] Other studies have examined outcomes in individuals with lower limb reconstruction wearing a custom ankle-foot orthosis (intrepid dynamic exoskeletal orthosis – [IDEO]).[17,18] A systematic review of this research concluded that use of an IDEO combined with an intensive therapy program can enable return to duty, return to recreation and physical activity; improve agility, power, and speed; as well as decrease pain in some high-functioning patients.[18]

### Delayed Amputation

For those individuals with extremity trauma who are initially managed with limb salvage procedures, some later proceed to having a delayed amputation. As previously noted, limb salvage may result in the need for additional surgical procedures as well as chronic pain and persistent functional impairments.[9,10,19] The decision to proceed to amputation may occur in the first several months following the original injury, but, in other circumstances, the move toward amputation can occur years after the initial injury. In these circumstances, it is important for limb salvage patients who are considering amputation to be well informed about both the potential advantages and disadvantages of amputation. Those undergoing delayed amputation have been found to require a greater number of hospitalization days as well as significantly higher rates of many mental and physical health diagnoses.[20,21] Patients should also be fully educated that amputation may or may not improve their pain situation. Involvement of a peer or peer support visitor can be beneficial in these situations.

Whether performed at the time of initial injury or at a later period, the primary goal of the surgical amputation procedure is a well-healed residual limb that is free from pain and able to tolerate fitting of a prosthetic socket. A literature review completed as part of the VA-DoD Clinical Practice Guideline for Lower Limb Amputation Rehabilitation found that there was insufficient evidence to recommend one type of surgical amputation procedure rather than another. This finding highlights the importance of shared decision making between surgeons and the patients. Involvement of other members of the rehabilitation care team in the decision-making process can also be of benefit to provide additional input regarding longer-term rehabilitation outcome considerations.[2]

When more specifically considering the optimal surgical technique for performing a transtibial amputation in a young patient with traumatic lower limb injuries, the Ertl procedure, in which the cut ends of the tibia and fibula are joined with a bone bridge synostosis, has been proposed to result in a residual limb that is more stable with improved function, especially among high-performing individuals.[22] At the same time, the Ertl procedure has associated with longer operative and healing time and may be associated with a higher complication rate compared with the standard Burgess procedure.[23,24]

A literature review to determine the benefits of a bone bridge technique concluded that current evidence supports a bone bridge technique as an equivalent option (as safe and effective) to the non–bone bridge transtibial amputation technique.[24]

## RESIDUAL LIMB MANAGEMENT
### Acute Management Considerations

Successful healing of the residual limb is an important step in the recovery from amputation. The desired outcome of residual limb management is a stable platform to serve as the functional connection between the person with an amputation and the prosthesis[25] (**Box 1**). Individual with traumatic amputation may be healthy compared with individuals with amputations resulting from vascular disease. This good health can result in quicker healing of the residual limb and provide the opportunity to proceed more rapidly to prosthetic fitting and prosthetic ambulation. However, with amputations that are required for traumatic injuries, residual limb management may need to take into consideration the presence of soft tissue defects, skin grafts, healed burns, and adherent scar tissue. More proximal lower extremity fractures may also be present. In these circumstances, prosthetic limb fitting needs to proceed accordingly based on healing of these other injuries.

In addition to promoting healing and maintaining the integrity of the residual limb, effective postoperative dressing management can reduce residual limb pain, provide protection from injury, promote edema control and residual limb shaping, as well as maintain range of motion (ROM).[25] A variety of postoperative dressings are available to address these goals. These dressings vary from soft dressings such as elastic wraps or residual limb shrinkers to rigid or semirigid dressings that can be either prefabricated or custom made. Individuals with traumatic amputation are frequently well suited for use of a rigid or semirigid residual limb dressing either immediately following surgery or in the early acute care setting. The use of rigid or semirigid dressings has been suggested to promote healing and early prosthesis use following transtibial amputation through reducing acute postamputation edema volume as well as accelerating residual limb healing time and reducing hospitalization time. Rigid

---

**Box 1**
**Goals for acute residual limb management**

- Residual limb healing and primary wound closure
- Edema control and residual limb shaping
- Protection from injury or further trauma
- Maintaining and improving range of motion and strength
- Pain management
- Desensitization and preparation for prosthesis fitting

postoperative dressings are specifically preferred in situations in which limb protection is a high priority.[2,25,26]

### Longitudinal Residual Limb Management Considerations

Following amputation, the residual limb undergoes several changes over time that have the potential to result in difficulties wearing a prosthesis (**Box 2**). Thinning of the soft tissues along with muscle atrophy can result in diminished cushioning over the remaining bony structures of the residual limb (**Fig. 1**), which can make prosthetic fitting more challenging secondary to discomfort and increase the risk of skin irritation and breakdown. This situation may be especially challenging in residual limbs with adherent scar tissue, healed burns, or skin grafting (**Fig. 2**). These soft tissue considerations may require accommodation with the socket suspension system and with the type of interface material used.

### Dermatologic Conditions

Skin irritation and breakdown on the residual limb is a very common long-term concern for individuals with limb loss. For individuals who use socket-based suspension systems, these skin complications are frequently the result of combined pressure, shear, and increased temperatures inside the socket with hyperhidrosis and skin maceration. Dermatologic changes such as verrucous hyperplasia can be the result of negative pressures or a lack of contact between the residual limb and the socket (**Fig. 3**). In situations in which the traumatic injury resulted in a contaminated wound at the time of initial injury, infection treatment and prevention are essential in order to achieve and maintain wound healing. Other common residual limb skin issues include ingrown hairs, folliculitis, allergic reactions, irritant dermatitis, atopic dermatitis, and cutaneous fungal infections.[27,28] These conditions have been found to affect the health-related quality of life of military personnel with traumatic amputations, and improvements have been noted with the use of laser hair removal for issues related to the pilosebaceous unit.[29]

### Musculoskeletal Conditions

Musculoskeletal conditions are also fairly common in the amputated residual lower limb over time.[30] Although joint contracture is more likely to develop in the early stages of recovery, maintenance of ROM is also important to monitor and address in the long

---

**Box 2**
**Longitudinal residual limb considerations**

- Soft tissue and muscle atrophy
- Skin irritation and breakdown
- Folliculitis and other dermatologic conditions
- Joint contracture and pain
- Infection (soft tissue and bone)
- Osteoarthritis and overuse syndromes
- Heterotopic ossification
- Osteopenia and osteoporosis
- Residual limb and phantom limb pain

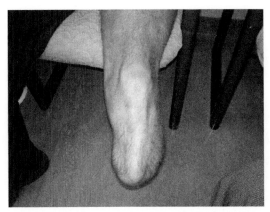

**Fig. 1.** Transtibial residual limb with atrophy of soft tissues and prominence of bony features.

term, especially when changes in health status occur. Other musculoskeletal complications, such as loss of bone mineral density, osteoarthritis, and overuse syndromes, are discussed in more detail later in this article. One of the goals of rehabilitation should be to address these issues early in the course of recovery and for patients to adopt prevention strategies that will help to maintain their long-term functional abilities.

Heterotopic ossification (HO) is the formation of bone tissue outside the normal bone structure. HO can develop in muscle tissue after trauma ranging from simple muscle sprains or contusions to open fractures of long bones[31] (**Fig. 4**). Although the precise cause of HO formation is unknown, development is considered to be triggered by inflammatory processes leading to proliferation of pluripotent mesenchymal cells and the inappropriate differentiation of these cells into osteoblasts.[31,32] Several proinflammatory mediators, such as platelet-derived growth factor, fibroblast-derived growth factor, transforming growth factor beta, and prostaglandins have been implicated in osteoblast DNA synthesis.[32–34]

The incidence of HO in military personnel who sustain combat-related amputations has been shown to be as high as 62%.[31] In 20% to 30%, the HO is severe enough to result in health and functional limitations. For individuals with HO involving the residual amputated limb, the HO can lead to numerous rehabilitation challenges, including

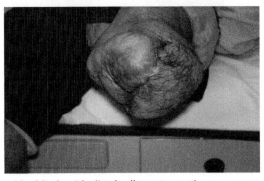

**Fig. 2.** Transtibial residual limb with distal adherent scar tissue.

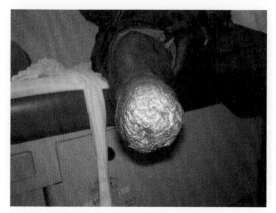

**Fig. 3.** Residual limb with verrucous hyperplasia secondary to a lack of distal contact.

wound healing difficulties and difficulties with prosthetic fitting. When the HO is mild, there can be circumstances where the HO has beneficial effects in promoting greater distal weight bearing or socket suspension. Treatment options for HO include the use of nonsteroidal antiinflammatory drugs and local radiation therapy to help prevent HO

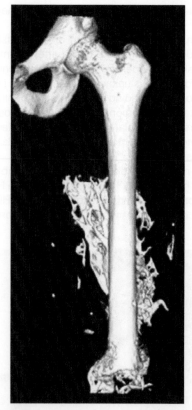

**Fig. 4.** Reconstruction of computed tomography scan with HO in a transfemoral residual limb.

ormation in high-risk patients.[31,35] Symptomatic HO may require pain management, physical therapy for improvement or maintenance of joint ROM, and prosthetic socket modifications. Surgical excision, if required, is best delayed until local inflammation has subsided and HO maturation can be shown on serial radiographs or triple phase bone scans.

## Pain Management

Pain may require longitudinal management following traumatic amputation. Amputation-related pain can generally be classified as residual limb pain or phantom limb pain. Residual limb pain typically improves with surgical healing following amputation but can be persistent and associated with prosthetic device fit and use. Phantom limb pain (pain that is perceived in the part of the body that is missing) can be chronic and severe enough to interfere with prosthetic use and functional mobility.

The VA and DoD clinical practice guidelines promote assessment of pain throughout the perioperative and rehabilitation periods in individuals with lower limb amputation. The guideline suggests that measurement of the intensity of pain and interference with function should be separately assessed for each pain type and location using standardized tools. Assessing the various pain characteristics, such as location, intensity, character, duration, timing, and aggravating factors or triggers, is important, and clinicians are also encouraged to consider the impact of the patient's pain on function.[2,36] Standardized tools such as the McGill Pain Scale and the Defense and Veterans Pain Rating Scale, when used with the supplemental questions that specifically measure the impact of pain on function, uniquely provide the ability to measure the pain intensity as well as pain's interference on function.[2,37]

Pain management is of great importance in promoting recovery and independence postamputation. Both pharmacologic and nonpharmacologic interventions should be considered and monitored for their effectiveness.[38,39] A multimodal, transdisciplinary approach to pain management including transition to a nonnarcotic pharmacologic regimen combined with physical, psychological, and mechanical modalities throughout the rehabilitation process has been suggested.[2] There are multiple pharmacologic and nonpharmacologic options for treating pain. Given the heterogeneity of patient characteristics, each pain management program should be individualized. Frequent adjustments to interventions should be considered on an individual basis. The need for an individualized approach is underscored by review articles that have determined that there is inconclusive evidence to support specific pharmacologic interventions in areas such as phantom limb pain.[38,39]

## OTHER TRAUMATIC INJURY CONSIDERATIONS
### General Considerations

Combat-related and other trauma-related amputations are commonly associated with moderate to severe injury severity scores and multiple other comorbid injuries (Box 3). These other injuries frequently have long-term consequences on both general health and amputation-specific outcomes. It is important to appreciate how commonly these associated injuries occur and the influence of these factors on outcomes such as functional independence, satisfaction, and quality of life. Management of these associated injuries is covered in detail elsewhere in this article, so only a few issues are mentioned here that relate specifically to individuals with traumatic amputation.

---

**Box 3**
**Common injuries associated with traumatic amputation**

- TBI
- Extremity fractures and other musculoskeletal injuries
- Soft tissue injuries and burns
- Peripheral nerve injuries
- Abdominal and genitourinary injuries
- Hearing loss and tinnitus
- Vision impairment or loss
- Mental health conditions such as PTSD, Depression, and Adjustment Disorder

---

### Traumatic Brain Injury Considerations

When TBI occurs in conjunction with traumatic amputation, the associated residual cognitive, emotional, and behavioral effects have to be taken into consideration when it comes to the selection of prosthetic limb componentry and rehabilitation interventions. One study found that, of military personnel with combat-related amputations, 23% also had a TBI diagnosis and those with TBI were more likely to have postinjury complications requiring increased medical and rehabilitative care.[40] Persistent cognitive impairments may affect the sequencing required during donning of the prosthesis and appropriate maintenance of the prosthesis. These individuals may also show impulsivity or a lower frustration tolerance, and these factors should be considered when advanced prosthetic technology is being prescribed that requires greater attention to detail and maintenance.

### Psychological Health/Mental Health Considerations

Loss of a limb is a life-changing event that can have an impact on every aspect of a person's life from basic walking to social roles in the family and broader society. Amputation frequently also has an effect of the person's ability to work and pursue vocational goals. Amputation requires psychological adjustments to new-onset physical limitations, body-image changes, confidence, self-esteem, and self-worth,[41] especially for young, previously healthy individuals who require unanticipated traumatic amputation. Amputations involving the upper limb are more visible and frequently have a greater impact on body image and concept of self. Peer support and peer visitation are recommended as soon as feasible following amputation to assist with limb loss adjustment, and this type of support can be useful long term as well.[2,42,43] Although many of these adjustment issues can be addressed by rehabilitation team members, more formal mental health services are often required.

In addition to these adjustment issues, individuals who have sustained a traumatic amputation frequently struggle with serious mental health conditions such as anxiety, depression, PTSD, and substance abuse. In a study examining VA outpatient costs for combat veterans, PTSD was associated with increased prosthetic cost by amputation status and increased psychiatric and pharmacy costs.[44] Psychological adjustment and lifestyle adaptation are important to address during all stages of rehabilitation following amputation. PTSD symptoms and other mental health conditions can be long lasting and do not necessarily change in response to improvements in physical functioning.[45] Substance abuse issues can arise out of a need or desire for improved pain control but are also commonly seen as a coping strategy for symptoms of PTSD, depression, and anxiety. An awareness and recognition of potential substance abuse issues can lead to appropriate interventions if the individual is open to support and treatment.

## SECONDARY COMPLICATIONS

Amputation of 1 or more limbs has a longitudinal impact on many areas outside the residual limb (**Box 4**). These secondary conditions are of high importance for individuals with traumatic amputations because of their long life expectancy. Many of these conditions gradually progress or worsen over time, whereas others are more episodic. The 2 areas most commonly affected are the musculoskeletal and the cardiovascular systems, and these conditions highlight the importance of comprehensive prevention strategies including proper nutrition, exercise, avoidance of tobacco products, and wellness counseling. The potential to prevent or reduce the impact of these conditions also emphasizes the need for routine follow-up including medical monitoring and education.

### Osteoarthritis

Longitudinal musculoskeletal considerations include the increased potential for the development of osteoarthritis in the nonamputated extremity as well as in the proximal joints of the amputated limb. Symptomatic osteoarthritis of the nonamputated knee is greater in amputees compared with age-matched, uninjured individuals with a 65% greater incidence of osteoarthritis and pain.[46] Proposed factors include obesity, abnormal knee joint mechanics with greater loading forces during gait, muscle weakness, previous knee trauma, and altered physical activity level.[46,47] The risk of osteoarthritis development is also related to the level of amputation, with the incidence of hip osteoarthritis being increased 3-fold in individuals with a transfemoral compared with transtibial amputation.[48] Further research is needed to determine whether early identification and modification of risk factors for knee osteoarthritis, including advanced prosthetic technologies, can optimize long-term function and quality of life after traumatic amputation.[30,49]

### Overuse Syndromes

Overuse syndromes in both the remaining upper and lower extremities frequently develop in those with traumatic lower limb amputation. A study of 791 service members with deployment-related lower limb injury found the overall incidence of developing at least 1 musculoskeletal overuse injury within the first year after lower limb amputation was between 59% and 68%. Military personnel with unilateral lower

---

**Box 4**
**Common secondary conditions associated with traumatic amputation**

- Musculoskeletal conditions
  - Osteoarthritis in the nonamputated extremity
  - Overuse syndromes; nonamputated limb and upper body
  - Low back pain
- Weight gain and obesity
- Cardiovascular disease
- Aortic aneurysm

limb amputation were almost twice as likely to develop an overuse injury compared with those with a mild combat-related injury, and the risk of overuse injury was even greater in those with bilateral lower limb amputation.[50] Management strategies should include short-term interventions directed at the reduction of inflammation, swelling, and pain, including a period of relative rest or change in activity level. Longer-term strategies should target correction of the underlying biomechanical factors contributing to the condition.

## Low Back Pain

Low back pain (LBP) is a common secondary condition in patients with lower limb amputation, occurring in up to 70% of this population.[51–54] Patients with transfemoral amputations tend to have a greater incidence and severity of LBP than those with transtibial amputations.[52] This condition is not only highly prevalent but it can also be chronic and more bothersome than residual limb pain or phantom limb pain. LBP has been shown to have a significant impact on both function and quality of life.[54,55] The cause of LBP in people with lower limb amputation is commonly multifactorial, with research suggesting that limb length differences, altered lumbopelvic biomechanical forces with excessive trunk motion, and muscle imbalance all play a role.[30,53,54] Fit and alignment of the prosthesis can also be contributors. Management of LBP in this population needs to take into consideration all of these variables that are unique to the person with an amputation as well as the factors that contribute to back pain in those without amputations. An emphasis on maintaining core strength and avoiding excessive weight gain are especially important for those with traumatic lower limb amputations.

## Bone Density Loss (Osteoporosis and Osteopenia)

Loss of bone mineral density in the residual limb following amputation is well documented. In individuals with trauma-related amputation, this bone mineral density loss can lead to the development of both osteopenia and osteoporosis in the residual limb and spine.[56] Studies have also documented that bone mineral density loss is more severe with more proximal amputation at the transfemoral level and with reduced prosthesis fit and use.[57] Because these changes can occur rapidly in the early period following amputation, mobilization and weight bearing should be encouraged as soon as possible[58,59]; this is vital because bone health may affect longer-term prosthesis use and activity levels. It is commonly recommended that a dual energy x-ray absorptiometry studies be performed on patients with lower limb amputations before engaging in high-impact activities, including running.

## Weight Gain/Obesity/Cardiovascular Disease

Decreased activity levels and metabolic changes can result in weight gain and obesity development following lower limb amputation. This weight gain can contribute to additional problems, such as LBP and cardiovascular disease.[30] It can also lead to a vicious cycle in which weight gain makes prosthetic fitting and use more difficult, thus resulting in even greater declines in activity. These considerations highlight the importance of engaging in preventive treatment strategies and adopting an active lifestyle for those individuals who require an amputation secondary to trauma at a young age.

Patients aging with a traumatic amputation have significantly worse cardiovascular and metabolic issues, which appear to be directly related to their traumatic amputations and not accounted for by obesity, sedentary lifestyle, or tobacco use.[30,60] This population has been identified as having increased hypertension, ischemic heart disease, and diabetes mellitus. A 30-year follow-up of World War II veterans with lower limb amputation along with other research studies found that the relative risk of cardiovascular disease mortality is increased 2.4 to 4 times that of persons with limb salvage.[30,60–62] The increased mortality may be partly related to modifiable risk factors and increased insulin resistance, but the exact cause remains unclear.[61] Lower extremity amputees should also be monitored for aortic aneurysms, which occur at a reported rate of 6% versus 1% in the nonamputee population.[30]

## REHABILITATION CONSIDERATIONS

As mentioned previously, military rehabilitation programs have adopted a sports medicine approach to treating individuals with traumatic limb loss. This model places an emphasis on core strengthening, aerobic conditioning, and activity-specific training in addition to formal prosthetic gait training (**Fig. 5**). Because these individuals often use prosthetic components with advanced technology, it is essential that the rehabilitation disciplines working with these patients have a good understanding of the componentry capabilities. Close collaboration with the individual's prosthetist leads to optimal outcomes because the prosthesis can be modified or reprogrammed as the individual advances through rehabilitation. Clear communication regarding goal setting and establishing realistic expectations for rehabilitation are also central. The promotion of physical activity and participation in sport has been recommended for veterans with lower limb amputation because of their correlation to health-related quality of life.[63]

In addition to physical therapy and occupational therapy services for initial prosthetic gait and activities of daily living training, a course of therapy services should be considered when there are significant changes in prosthetic componentry, when there is a desire to learn skills, or if there has been a change in health status. Additional rehabilitation disciplines should be incorporated into the treatment program in the early phases of care and continued or reinstituted as needed.[64–66] This includes recreation therapy for participation in leisure activities, recreational pursuits, and adaptive sports. Adaptive sports can involve learning new ways to participate in previously enjoyed sports as well as introduction to new activities. For military and prior military personnel, returning to firearms training can be an important goal. Vocational rehabilitation services should also be provided for those who are likely to need to transition to a new career or line of work following their amputations.

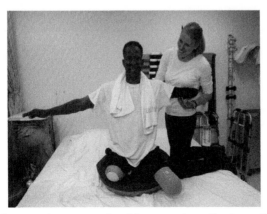

**Fig. 5.** Rehabilitation exercise program involving core strengthening activity.

## PROSTHESIS FABRICATION AND FITTING

Individuals with traumatic amputations have specialized and lifelong needs in the area of prostheses, orthoses, and equipment (**Box 5**). With regard to artificial limbs, these needs include the initial prosthesis prescription, fabrication, and fitting. It is important to proceed with the initial fitting as soon as possible, but, in individuals with polytraumatic injuries, prosthesis fitting may be delayed by other issues outside residual limb healing, such as the severity of the TBI or weight bearing that is restricted by other orthopedic injuries or complications. In these circumstances, it is imperative to continue aggressive preprosthetic therapy interventions and residual limb shrinkage and shaping.

Many factors need to be considered with the initial prosthesis prescription. One of the most important is to establish the person's premorbid functional abilities and their specific functional goals for use of the prosthesis. In most circumstances, individuals who sustain traumatic amputations were active and healthy before their traumatic events and have goals to return to the highest level possible of social, leisure, sport, and vocational activity. Potential long-term functional limitations related to the person's other traumatic injuries also need to be taken into consideration. In this population, it is common for individuals to have a desire to use their prostheses in various environments in which access to repairs and servicing of the prosthesis may be difficult. In these cases, the durability and reliability of the prosthetic components need to be evaluated. These factors can also affect the cosmetic appearance of the prosthesis and whether or not a cover is recommended.

Specific prosthetic componentry considerations include sockets with flexible inner liners and hard outer sockets with windows to accommodate muscular contraction and movement during higher-level activities (**Fig. 6**). Interface materials may need to provide additional cushioning and possess flow properties that reduce residual limb shear forces in individuals with limited soft tissue coverage, adherent scar tissue, or bony prominences. In contrast, patients with adequate residual limb soft tissues and a desire to participate in high-level activities, such as running, may benefit from interface materials that are thinner and provide an internal matrix for additional soft tissue support and stability.[26]

Microprocessor knee components (**Fig. 7**) are generally appropriate for everyday use for individuals with traumatic amputations at the knee disarticulation level and more proximal.[2,67,68] Nonmicroprocessor knees may be required for activity-specific prostheses such as a prosthesis used for running. Dynamic elastic response foot

---

**Box 5**
**Prosthetic device and equipment considerations**

Artificial limbs
- Initial limb prescription, fabrication, and fitting
- Routine repairs and replacement
- Need for new prostheses as needs and functional abilities change
- Need for new prostheses as new technology becomes available

Mobility assistive devices
- Standard devices, such as crutches, canes, and walkers
- Wheelchairs: manual and/or power

Durable medical equipment
- Bath benches, shower chairs, grab bars, hand-held showers
- Other durable medical equipment

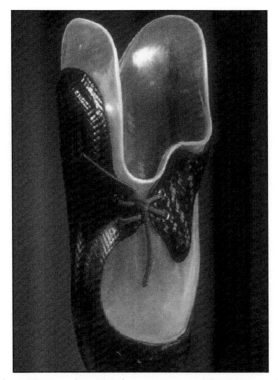

**Fig. 6.** Transtibial prosthetic socket with fenestrations and flexible inner liner to allow for residual limb volume changes.

and ankle components that provide energy storage and return properties as well as the ability to accommodate over uneven surfaces are commonly appropriate for this population (**Fig. 8**). Additional torque absorbers can be used to help absorb ground reaction forces and reduce shearing stress on the residual limb.

Once the initial fitting and prosthetic gait training have taken place, these individuals typically develop into active prosthetic users. For those with unilateral amputations at the transtibial and transfemoral levels, the expectation is that these individuals will be independent with prosthetic ambulation over all types of terrain and for long distances in the community. This functional outcome is also expected for individuals with bilateral transtibial-level involvement. Because of the high activity level in this population, their need for prosthesis repairs and servicing may be greater than that of less active prosthetic users. This consideration also places greater importance on the need for spare prostheses in case the primary prosthesis becomes broken and nonusable. In addition, because of the need and desire to participate in various activities, this population is more likely to benefit from the provision of specialty prostheses that can be used for specific activities such as running and water-based interests (**Fig. 9**). Dependability and reliability issues are also important to consider if the individual is going to be living or performing activities in more remote locations without ready access to prosthetic services.

Ongoing, routine follow-up for individuals with traumatic amputation needs to address their changing needs with regard to prosthetic fitting and componentry. It

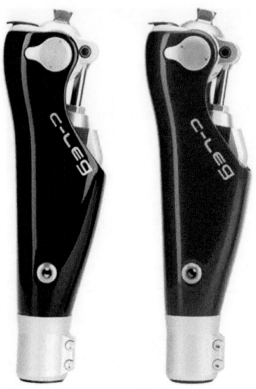

**Fig. 7.** Example of microprocessor knee unit. (*Courtesy of* Ottobock, Minneapolis, MN; with permission.)

is anticipated that functional abilities and goals will change over time, necessitating reevaluation of prosthetic restoration to best meet these functional goals. In addition, the desire for participation in various sport and recreation activities may change or decline over time. Routine follow-up is also a means by which routine health issues can be addressed along with providing reassessment of prosthetic needs as new technology becomes available. Routine follow-up should also include evaluation of needs in the area of mobility assistive devices and durable medical equipment.[2]

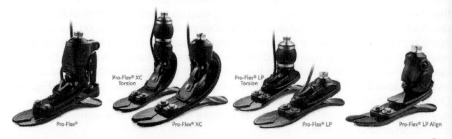

**Fig. 8.** Example of a dynamic elastic response foot with multiaxial features. (*Courtesy of* Össur, Reykjavik, Iceland; with permission.)

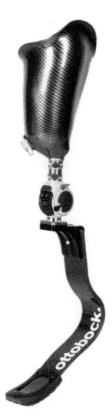

**Fig. 9.** Example of a specialty prosthesis used for running. (*Courtesy of* Ottobock, Minneapolis, MN; with permission.)

## SUMMARY

Greater sophistication in both military and civilian trauma care systems in conjunction with improved safety equipment has led to high survival rates for individuals with polytraumatic injuries, including those with trauma-related amputations. Management of individuals with trauma-related amputation must take into consideration issues directly related to the amputation as well as issues related to injury of other body parts and the management of longer-term secondary conditions. These management considerations begin before the amputation and persist throughout the lifetime of the individual.

Optimal outcomes are achieved with the use of an interdisciplinary team approach and coordination of services across the continuum of care. Advances in rehabilitation interventions and prosthetic technology have assisted individuals with trauma-related amputations to return to functional independence and attain great success in leisure activities, recreational pursuits, and competitive sports. Emerging advances in the areas of bioengineering, bionics, transplantation science, and regenerative medicine will undoubtedly lead to even greater achievements in the future.

## REFERENCES

1. Extremity trauma and amputation center of excellence. EACE-R amputee database. Accessed October 01, 2017.

2. VA/DoD clinical practice guideline for rehabilitation of individuals with lower limb amputation. 2017. Available at: https://www.healthquality.va.gov/guidelines/rehab/amp/index.asp. Accessed September 20, 2018.

3. Ziegler-Graham K, MacKenzie EJ, Ephraim PL, et al. Estimating the prevalence of limb loss in the United States: 2005 to 2050. Arch Phys Med Rehabil 2008;89(3): 422–9.

4. Barmparas G, Inaba K, Teixeira PG, et al. Epidemiology of post-traumatic limb amputation: a National Trauma Databank analysis. Am Surg 2010;76(11): 1214–22.

5. Webster JB, Poorman CE, Cifu DX. Guest editorial: department of Veterans Affairs amputations system of care: 5 years of accomplishments and outcomes. J Rehabil Res Dev 2014;51(4). vii–xvi.

6. Owens BD, Kragh JF Jr, Wenke JC, et al. Combat wounds in operation Iraqi Freedom and operation Enduring Freedom. J Trauma 2008;64(2):295–9.

7. Andersen RC, Fleming M, Forsberg JA, et al. Dismounted complex blast injury. J Surg Orthop Adv 2012;21(1):2–7.

8. Department of Defense Dismounted Complex Blast Injury (DCBI) task force report. 2011.

9. Pinzur MS, Gottschalk FA, Pinto MA, et al, American Academy of Orthopaedic Surgeons. Controversies in lower-extremity amputation. J Bone Joint Surg Am 2007;89(5):1118–27.

10. Fleming ME, Watson JT, Gaines RJ, et al. Extremity war injuries VII reconstruction panel. Evolution of orthopaedic reconstructive care. J Am Acad Orthop Surg 2012;20(Suppl 1):S74–9.

11. Bosse MJ, MacKenzie EJ, Kellam JF, et al. An analysis of outcomes of reconstruction or amputation after leg-threatening injuries. N Engl J Med 2002;347(24): 1924–31.

12. Prasarn ML, Helfet DL, Kloen P. Management of the mangled extremity. Strategies Trauma Limb Reconstr 2012;7(2):57–66.

13. MacKenzie EJ, Bosse MJ, Pollak AN, et al. Long-term persistence of disability following severe lower-limb trauma. Results of a seven-year follow-up. J Bone Joint Surg Am 2005;87(8):1801–9.

14. Busse JW, Jacobs CL, Swiontkowski MF, et al, Evidence-Based Orthopaedic Trauma Working Group. Complex limb salvage or early amputation for severe lower-limb injury: a meta-analysis of observational studies. J Orthop Trauma 2007;21(1):70–6.

15. Melcer T, Walker GJ, Sechriest VF 2nd, et al. Short-term physical and mental health outcomes for combat amputee and nonamputee extremity injury patients. J Orthop Trauma 2013;27(2):e31–7.

16. Doukas WC, Hayda RA, Frisch HM, et al. The Military Extremity Trauma Amputation/Limb Salvage (METALS) study: outcomes of amputation versus limb salvage following major lower-extremity trauma. J Bone Joint Surg Am 2013;95(2):138–45.

17. Russell Esposito E, Stinner DJ, Fergason JR, et al. Gait biomechanics following lower extremity trauma: Amputation vs. reconstruction. Gait Posture 2017;54: 167–73.

18. Highsmith MJ, Nelson LM, Carbone NT, et al. Outcomes Associated With the Intrepid Dynamic Exoskeletal Orthosis (IDEO): a systematic review of the literature. Mil Med 2016;181(S4):69–76.

19. Bjerke H, Stuhlmiller D. Extremity vascular trauma. Medscape 2015.

20. Clarke P, Mollan RA. The criteria for amputation in severe lower limb injury. Injury 1994;25(3):139–43.

21. Melcer T, Sechriest VF, Walker J, et al. A comparison of health outcomes for combat amputee and limb salvage patients injured in Iraq and Afghanistan wars. J Trauma Acute Care Surg 2013;75(2 Suppl 2):S247–54.

22. Plucknette BF, Krueger CA, Rivera JC, et al. Combat-related bridge synostosis versus traditional transtibial amputation: comparison of military-specific outcomes. Strategies Trauma Limb Reconstr 2016;11(1):5–11.

23. Keeling JJ, Shawen SB, Forsberg JA, et al. Comparison of functional outcomes following bridge synostosis with non-bone-bridging transtibial combat-related amputations. J Bone Joint Surg Am 2013;95(10):888–93.

24. Kahle JT, Highsmith MJ, Kenney J, et al. The effectiveness of the bone bridge transtibial amputation technique: a systematic review of high-quality evidence. Prosthet Orthot Int 2017;41(3):219–26.

25. Smith DG, McFarland LV, Sangeorzan BJ, et al. Postoperative dressing and management strategies for transtibial amputations: a critical review. J Rehabil Res Dev 2003;40(3):213–24.

26. Highsmith MJ, Kahle JT, Miro RM, et al. Prosthetic interventions for people with transtibial amputation: systematic review and meta-analysis of high-quality prospective literature and systematic reviews. J Rehabil Res Dev 2016;53(2):157–84.

27. Highsmith JT, Highsmith MJ. Common skin pathology in LE prosthesis users. JAAPA 2007;20(11):33–6, 47.

28. Highsmith MJ, Kahle JT, Klenow TD, et al. Interventions to manage residual limb ulceration due to prosthetic use in individuals with lower extremity amputation: a systematic review of the literature. Technol Innov 2016;18(2–3):115–23.

29. Miletta NR, Kim S, Lezanski-Gujda A, et al. Improving health-related quality of life in wounded warriors: the promising benefits of laser hair removal to the residual limb-prosthetic interface. Dermatol Surg 2016;42(10):1182–7.

30. Butowicz CM, Dearth CL, Hendershot BD. Impact of traumatic lower extremity injuries beyond acute care: movement-based considerations for resultant longer term secondary health conditions. Adv Wound Care (New Rochelle) 2017;6(8):269–78.

31. Edwards DS, Kuhn KM, Potter BK, et al. Heterotopic ossification: a review of current understanding, treatment, and future. J Orthop Trauma 2016;30(Suppl 3):S27–30.

32. Balboni TA, Gobezie R, Mamon HJ. Heterotopic ossification: pathophysiology, clinical features, and the role of radiotherapy for prophylaxis. Int J Radiat Oncol Biol Phys 2006;65:1289–99.

33. Centrella M, McCarthy TL, Canalis E. Transforming growth factor beta is a bifunctional regulator of replication and collagen synthesis in osteoblast-enriched cell cultures from fetal rat bone. J Biol Chem 1987;262:2869–74.

34. Schurch B, Capaul M, Vallotton MB, et al. Prostaglandin E2 measurements: their value in the early diagnosis of heterotopic ossification in spinal cord injury patients. Arch Phys Med Rehabil 1997;78:687–91.

35. Pakos EE, Ioannidis JP. Radiotherapy vs. nonsteroidal anti-inflammatory drugs for the prevention of heterotopic ossification after major hip procedures: a meta-analysis of randomized trials. Int J Radiat Oncol Biol Phys 2004;60:888–95.

36. Jensen MP, Smith DG, Ehde DM, et al. Pain site and the effects of amputation pain: Further clarification of the meaning of mild, moderate, and severe pain. Pain 2001;91(3):317–22.

37. Melzack R. The short-form McGill pain questionnaire. Pain 1987;30(2):191–7.

38. Brunelli S, Morone G, Iosa M, et al. Efficacy of progressive muscle relaxation, mental imagery, and phantom exercise training on phantom limb: a randomized controlled trial. Arch Phys Med Rehabil 2015;96(2):181–7.
39. Alviar MJM, Hale T, Dungca M. Pharmacologic interventions for treating phantom limb pain. Cochrane Database Syst Rev 2016;(10):CD006380.
40. Rauh MJ, Aralis HJ, Melcer T, et al. Effect of traumatic brain injury among U.S. servicemembers with amputation. J Rehabil Res Dev 2013;50(2):161–72.
41. Kratz AL, Williams RM, Turner AP, et al. To lump or to split? Comparing individuals with traumatic and nontraumatic limb loss in the first year after amputation. Rehabil Psychol 2010;55(2):126–38.
42. Purk JK. Support groups: why do people attend? Rehabil Nurs 2004;29(2):62–7.
43. Wegener ST, Mackenzie EJ, Ephraim P, et al. Self-management improves outcomes in persons with limb loss. Arch Phys Med Rehabil 2009;90(3):373–80.
44. Bhatnagar V, Richard E, Melcer T, et al. Lower-limb amputation and effect of posttraumatic stress disorder on Department of Veterans Affairs outpatient cost trends. J Rehabil Res Dev 2015;52(7):827–38.
45. Talbot LA, Brede E, Metter EJ. Psychological and physical health in military amputees during rehabilitation: secondary analysis of a randomized controlled trial. Mil Med 2017;182(5):e1619–24.
46. Norvell DC, Czerniecki JM, Reiber GE, et al. The prevalence of knee pain and symptomatic knee osteoarthritic among veteran traumatic amputees and non-amputees. Arch Phys Med Rehabil 2005;86:487–93.
47. Kulkarni J, Adams J, Thomas E, et al. Association between amputation, arthritis, and osteopenia in British male war veterans with major lower limb amputation. Clin Rehabil 1998;12:348–53.
48. Davies P. Between health and illness. Perspect Biol Med 2007;50:444–52.
49. Farrokhi S, Mazzone B, Yoder A, et al. A narrative review of the prevalence and risk factors associated with development of knee osteoarthritis after traumatic unilateral lower limb amputation. Mil Med 2016;181(S4):38–44.
50. Farrokhi S, Mazzone B, Eskridge S, et al. Incidence of overuse musculoskeletal injuries in military service members with traumatic lower limb amputation. Arch Phys Med Rehabil 2018;99(2):348–54.e1.
51. Ehde DM, Smith DG, Czerniecki JM, et al. Back pain as a secondary disability in persons with lower limb amputations. Arch Phys Med Rehabil 2001;82:731–4.
52. Ehde DM, Czerniecki JM, Smith DG, et al. Chronic phantom sensations, phantom pain, residual limb pain, and other regional pain after lower limb amputation. Arch Phys Med Rehabil 2000;81:1039–44.
53. Friberg O. Leg length inequality and low back pain. Lancet 1984;2:1039.
54. Friel K, Domholdt E, Smith DG. Physical and functional measures related to low back pain in individuals with lower-limb amputation: an exploratory pilot study. J Rehabil Res Dev 2005;2:155–66.
55. Foote CE, Mac Kinnon J, Robbins C, et al. Long-term health and quality of life experiences of Vietnam veterans with combat-related limb loss. Qual Life Res 2015;24:2853–61.
56. Rush PJ, Wong JS, Kirsh J, et al. Osteopenia in patients with above knee amputation. Arch Phys Med Rehabil 1994;75:112–5.
57. Leclercq MM, Bonidan O, Haaby E, et al. Study of bone mass with dual energy x-ray absorptiometry in a population of 99 lower limb amputees. Ann Readapt Med Phys 2003;46:24–30.

58. Stocker D, Stack A, Goff B, et al. Patients experience rapid, substantial bone loss following a trauma-related amputation: the Walter Reed experience. J Nucl Med 2007;48(Suppl 2):286P.

59. Bemben DA, Sherk VD, Ertl WJJ, et al. Acute bone changes after lower limb amputation resulting from traumatic injury. Osteoporos Int 2017;28(7):2177–86.

60. Rose HG, Schweitzer P, Charoenkul V, et al. Cardiovascular disease risk factors in combat veterans after traumatic leg amputations. Arch Phys Med Rehabil 1987; 68:20–3.

61. Peles E, Akselrod S, Goldstein DS, et al. Insulin resistance and autonomic function in traumatic lower limb amputees. Clin Auton Res 1995;5:279–88.

62. Modan M, Peles E, Halkin H, et al. Increased cardiovascular disease mortality rates in traumatic lower limb amputees. Am J Cardiol 1998;82:1242–7.

63. Christensen J, Ipsen T, Doherty P, et al. Physical and social factors determining quality of life for veterans with lower-limb amputation(s): a systematic review. Disabil Rehabil 2016;38(24):2345–53.

64. Jelić M, Eldar R. Rehabilitation following major traumatic amputation of the lower limbs. A review. Phys Rehab Med 2003;15(3&4):235–52.

65. Penn-Barwell JG. Outcomes in lower limb amputation following trauma: a systematic review and meta-analysis. Injury 2011;42(12):1474–9.

66. Rau B, Bonvin F, de Bie R. Short-term effect of physiotherapy rehabilitation on functional performance of lower limb amputees. Prosthet Orthot Int 2007;31(3): 258–70.

67. Sawers AB, Hafner BJ. Outcomes associated with the use of microprocessor-controlled prosthetic knees among individuals with unilateral transfemoral limb loss: a systematic review. J Rehabil Res Dev 2013;50(3):273–314.

68. Kahle JT, Highsmith MJ, Hubbard SL. Comparison of nonmicroprocessor knee mechanism versus C-leg on prosthesis evaluation questionnaire, stumbles, falls, walking tests, stair descent, and knee preference. J Rehabil Res Dev 2008;45(1): 1–14.

# Rehabilitation of Burn Injuries: An Update

Alan W. Young, DO[a,b,*], William Scott Dewey, PT[c],
Booker T. King, MD[d]

## KEYWORDS

- Burns • Burn rehabilitation • Burn scar • Pain management
- Cutaneous functional unit • Burn contracture

## KEY POINTS

- Understanding burn injuries and the requirements for treatment of various burn causes.
- Understanding wound care because it is an important part of the practice of all providers that work with burn survivors.
- Understanding how to evaluate burn scar contracture and the best therapeutic treatments to decrease the functional disability and cosmetic impairments of burn scars and contractures.
- Understanding the need for aggressive treatment of all causes of burn pain keeping in mind the need to taper pharmacologic interventions as functional improvements and wound closure progresses.
- Remain mindful of the psychological impact short and long term from burn injuries.

A major burn is a severe injury with a global impact. It affects survivors and their families physically, psychologically, emotionally, and spiritually.[1] If this injury occurs with other trauma, such as brain injury, massive soft tissue loss, multiple orthopedic

Disclosure Statement: The views expressed in this paper are those of the authors and do not reflect the official policy or position of Brooke Army Medical Center/Joint Base San Antonio, the Army Institute of Surgical Research, or the Department of the Army or the Department of Defense. The authors declare that there is no conflict of interest regarding the publication of this article.
[a] Complementary and Integrative Medicine Service, Department of Pain Management, Brooke Army Medical Center, JBSA, 3551 Roger Brooke Drive, Fort Sam Houston, TX 78234, USA; [b] Rehabilitation Medicine, UT Health San Antonio, 7703 Floyd Curl Drive, San Antonio, TX 78229, USA; [c] Rehabilitation Services, Army Burn Center, U.S. Army Institute of Surgical Research, JBSA, 3698 Chambers Pass Suite B, Fort Sam Houston, TX 78234-7767, USA; [d] Medical Corps US Army, Army Burn Center, U.S. Army Institute of Surgical Research, JBSA, 3698 Chambers Pass Suite B, Fort Sam Houston, TX 78234-7767, USA
* Corresponding author. Department of Pain Management, Brooke Army Medical Center, JBSA, 3551 Roger Brooke Drive, Fort Sam Houston, TX 78234.
E-mail address: alan.w.young4.civ@mail.mil

Phys Med Rehabil Clin N Am 30 (2019) 111–132
https://doi.org/10.1016/j.pmr.2018.08.004
1047-9651/19/Published by Elsevier Inc.

injuries, amputations, or spinal cord injuries, the impact is magnified. These combinations, unfortunately, were seen with increasing frequency among our combat casualties as our most recent conflict progressed. Our system of medical evacuation and treatment led to the survival of many of these severely injured service members. Their ultimate recovery requires a comprehensive, interdisciplinary, team-based approach, individually designed to maximize function, minimize disability, promote self-acceptance, and facilitate survivor and family reintegration into the community.[2] The purpose of this article is to discuss the rehabilitation management of military burn casualties.

Because of air superiority in theater during Operation Iraqi Freedom and Operation Enduring Freedom, casualties were airlifted directly from the battlefield to a Forward Surgical Team or a Combat Support Hospital. More severely injured were transferred directly to the Air Force Theater Hospital such as Bagram. Once stabilized, they were transferred by Critical Care Air Transport teams to Landstuhl Regional Medical Center in Germany for treatment. From there they were air lifted again to US military treatment facilities for definitive treatment and rehabilitation. These military treatment facilities were primarily Walter Reed National Medical Center and Brooke Army Medical Center, Joint Base San Antonio (BAMC, JBSA). From there, they progressed to Veterans Administration care, including the Polytrauma System.[1] The potential for lack of air superiority and the generation of large numbers of casualties in a peer or near peer engagement may jeopardize this strategy. A review of this process is ongoing.

The US Army Institute of Surgical Research, at BAMC, JBSA has the only dedicated Burn Center in the Department of Defense and as such takes care of all the military beneficiaries who receive serious burns wherever they are stationed or deployed. In addition, it is verified by the American Burn Association as the regional burn center for most of South Texas. It is also a primary research center for combat casualty care.

As noted, a multidisciplinary approach is needed to care for these patients. The disciplines include general surgery, trauma surgery, plastic surgery, physical medicine and rehabilitation, critical care, infectious disease, and behavioral medicine. Other professionals include nursing, physical therapy, occupational therapy, respiratory therapy, psychology, orthotics and prosthetics, licensed clinical social workers, case management, recreational therapy, and vocational counselors. Other ancillary personnel, such as peer counselors, have a role as well.[2]

## GENERAL INFORMATION

The skin is body's largest organ system (**Fig. 1**). It functions to maintain homeostasis, including fluid balance, and thermoregulation and provides an immune barrier. In addition, it has a cosmetic function that is particularly important in our culture.

In 2016, 486,000 people sustained burn injuries in the United States that required treatment, and 40,000 required hospitalization. Survival rate was 93%. A total of 3275 people died prehospitalization and posthospitalization.[3]

## CLASSIFICATION

Burn classification is shown in **Box 1** and discussed in further detail later.

## CAUSES
### Thermal

Excessive heat or cold applied to the skin causes injury by direct tissue destruction and generating a surrounding zone of stasis or vasoconstriction causing ischemia.

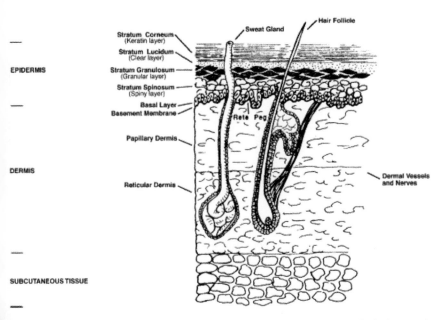

**Fig. 1.** Anatomy of the skin. Normal skin has an epidermis that is composed of 5 layers. The basement membrane separates the dermis from the epidermis. The cells of the epidermal basal layer continue into the dermis as they line the hair follicles and other skin appendages. (*From* Young A. Rehabilitation of burn injuries. Phys Med Rehabil Clin 2002;13(1):86; with permission.)

This area may improve or deteriorate depending on treatment. Severity of either injury is related to the duration and the intensity of exposure. Eighty-five percent to 95% of burns are secondary to heat.[1]

## Chemical

Chemical burns can result from acid, alkali, or vesicant exposure. Acid causes coagulation necrosis and alkaline liquefaction necrosis. It is easy to underestimate the severity of these burns. They may initially appear superficial, but some chemical agents will continue to cause damage despite topical treatment. White phosphorus, for example, ignites on contact with the air and must be physically removed to stop ongoing injury.[4]

## Radiation

The degree of injury will depend on the duration, location, total surface area of involvement, and intensity of exposure. Damage results from the excitation of molecules causing breakdown of chemical bonds, damage to DNA and RNA, loss of continuity of other molecular cross-linkages, and the production of virulent-free radicals. Cells that are undifferentiated, divide quickly, and have a high rate of metabolic activity, such as hematopoietic, reproductive, and gastrointestinal tissue, are most susceptible. The dose at which 50% of the population will die in 30 days (lethal dose 50/30) after whole-body exposure is 4 to 5 Sieverts (400–450 rad).[5] The most common radiation injury is sunburn. The next most common is from radiation therapy with 95% of treated patients developing some degree of radiodermatitis.[6]

---

**Box 1**
**Burn classification**

*Causative agent*

Thermal
  Heat
  Cold

Electrical

Chemical

Radiation

*Depth of burn*

Older terminology
  First degree: epidermis injured
  Second degree: dermis partially damaged
  Third degree: all dermis destroyed
  Fourth degree: muscle, nerve, and bone damaged

Newer terminology
  Superficial partial thickness: epidermis and upper part of dermis injured
  Deep partial thickness: epidermis and large upper portion of dermis injured
  Full thickness: all skin destroyed

*Size of burn: rule of nines*

Head = 9% BSA

Each upper extremity = 9% BSA

Each lower extremity = 18% BSA

Anterior trunk = 18% BSA

Posterior trunk = 18% BSA

Perineum = 1% BSA

*American Burn Association classification*

Minor
  <15% BSA partial thickness (10% in child)
  <2% BSA full thickness (not involving eyes, ears, face, or perineum)

Moderate[a]
  All 15%–25% BSA (10%–20% in child)
  2%–10% BSA full thickness (not involving eyes, ears, face, or perineum)

Major
  All >25% BSA partial thickness (20% in child); ≥10% BSA full thickness
  All burns to face, eyes, ears, feet, perineum
  All electrical
  All inhalation
  All burns with fracture or major tissue trauma
  All with poor risk secondary to age or illness

*Abbreviation:* BSA, body surface area.
[a] Most moderate and all major burns should be hospitalized.

---

## Electrical

Injuries from electrocution result from the conduction of electrical energy through tissue. Contact is not required because current can arc through the air. Electrical burns are difficult to assess. Superficially, damage may appear minimal, but the current ollows the path of least resistance, that is, nerves, arteries, veins, and bones, and all must be evaluated for injury. Low voltage, less than 1000 V, may cause ventricular fibrillation and arrhythmia but rarely significant tissue damage. Injury from greater than 1000 V can be extensive. Exit wounds are worse than entrance wounds because energy is slowed as it is conducted through the body. When it reaches an exit point, improved conduction generates an explosive release.[7] Creatine kinase (CK) is a sensitive indicator of total muscle damage. Total CKs of less than 2500 IU are associated with few skin grafts or amputations. Greater than 2500 IU has a risk of major amputation.[8] Specific complications from electrocution that have an impact on rehabilitation include: hyperextension caused by tonic/clonic contractions, peripheral neuropathy, cognitive impairment, long bone fractures, spinal cord injury, formation of heterotopic bone around joints and residual limbs, cardiopulmonary arrest, amputation, early development of cataracts, and hearing loss.[7]

## DEPTH OF BURN

For many years, burns were classified by degree: first, second, and third (**Fig. 2**). This terminology, however, does not give an accurate description of clinical findings or decision making. Currently, the term superficial partial thickness is used to describe any burn of the epidermis. This term may also be used to describe burns that involve the very upper layers of the dermis as well. These burns usually heal without surgery. Deep partial thickness burns involve the entire epidermis and a large part of the dermis. This distinction is important because some deep partial thickness burns will require skin grafting. Full-thickness burns involve the epidermis and dermis and extend into the subcutaneous tissue. Skin grafting is required.[9]

## AREA OF INVOLVEMENT

Burn size is determined using the rule of 9s (**Fig. 3**). The body is divided into 11 areas each assigned a value of 9. For example, the head is 9% (4.5 front and 4.5 back); the chest is 18%, and so on. This calculation works well except with children, particularly infants, because of the disproportionately large relationship of the head to the rest of the body. The Lund and Browder method accounts for this difference by assigning a larger value to the head of the infant and decreasing all other values. For example, at age one, the head is 17%.[9] It progressively returns to the adult norm as the child ages (**Fig. 4**).

In general, injuries are described as the sum of all body parts involved, stated as total body surface area (TBSA) of involvement. Minor burns, defined as less than 15% partial-thickness TBSA (10% in children), or no more than 2% full thickness, can be treated as an outpatient. Any burn that is greater than 25% partial-thickness TBSA (20% in children), or 10% full thickness, or involve the eyes, ears, face, perineum, electrical, or inhalational injuries, occurred with fractures or other major injuries, or occurred in patients at risk because of age or concurrent illness, is considered major and should be hospitalized in specialty burn units. Moderate burns fall in between these parameters, and hospitalization is judged on a case-by-case basis.[9]

## INITIAL CARE

Although this review is not intended to be a comprehensive guide to initial burn management, it is important to have a basic understanding of burn care.

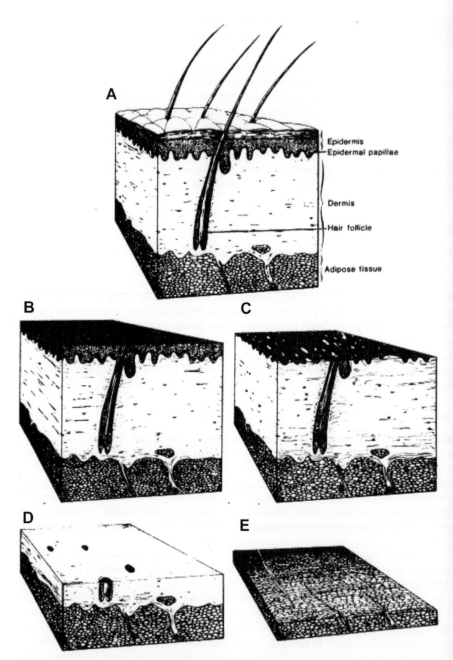

**Fig. 2.** Depth of burns: (A) normal skin; (B) superficial partial thickness (first degree); (C) superficial partial thickness (second degree); (D) deep partial thickness (second degree); and (E) full thickness (third degree). (*From* Young A. Rehabilitation of burn injuries. Phys Med Rehabil Clin 2002;13(1):91; with permission.)

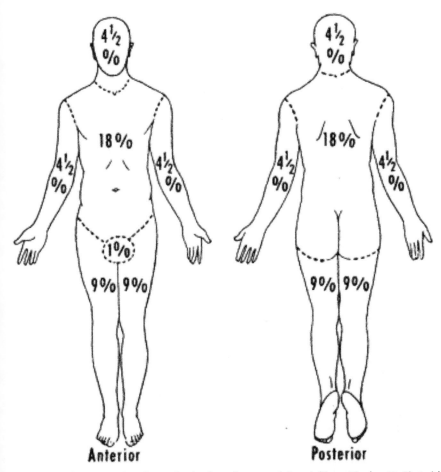

**Fig. 3.** Rule of nines used to determine body surface area injured. (*From* Moylan JA. First aid and transportation of burned patients. In: Artz CP, Moncrief JA, Pruitt BA, editors. Burns: a team approach. Philadelphia: WB Saunders; 1979. p. 153; with permission; and Young A. Rehabilitation of burn injuries. Phys Med Rehabil Clin 2002;13(1):85–108.)

The treatment of the burn survivor is not a strict progression from one step to another, but an ongoing dynamic process. It is adjusted based on the survivor's response to interventions as they advance from initial insult to medical stability. The process may be completed within a few days or may take months depending on the age, severity, depth, TBSA involved, and other concurrent injuries.

The initial evaluation of the burn patient begins with the evaluation of the airway, breathing, and circulation. Once the airway is stabilized, all other life-threatening processes, such as pneumothorax and hemorrhage, are addressed. Inhalational injury is evaluated by history, presenting symptoms, physical examination, and bronchoscopy. The extent of the burn injury is assessed, and the patient is taken to the shower for debridement and cleaning, and then dressed with topical antimicrobials. A deep circumferential burn of an extremity or around the upper torso may require an escharotomy. The patient is evaluated, and treatment is initiated for all other non-life-threatening injuries.[9]

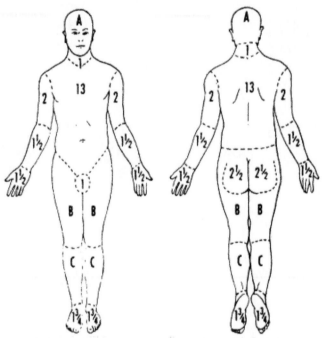

*Relative Percentage of Areas Affected by Growth*

| Age in Years | 0 | 1 | 5 | 10 | 15 | Adult |
|---|---|---|---|---|---|---|
| A—½ of head | 9½ | 8½ | 6½ | 5½ | 4½ | 3½ |
| B—½ of one thigh | 2¾ | 3¼ | 4 | 4¼ | 4½ | 4¾ |
| C—½ of one leg | 2½ | 2½ | 2¾ | 3 | 3¼ | 3½ |

**Fig. 4.** Lund and Browder method of determining skin surface area; method corrects for differences in percentage of body surface areas by age. (*From* McManus WF. Immediate emergency department care. In: Artz CP, Moncrief JA, Pruitt BA, editors. Burns: a team approach. Philadelphia: WB Saunders; 1979. p. 154; with permission; and Young A. Rehabilitation of burn injuries. Phys Med Rehabil Clin 2002;13(1):85–108.)

While all these other evaluations are occurring, fluid resuscitation begins. The replacement of fluid loss from the burn wound is critical, especially in the first 24 hours. The requirement can be calculated from a variety of formulas. The Modified Brooke and Parkland formulas are commonly used and rely on hourly measurement of the patient's urine output to adjust the rate of intravenous fluid replacement.[10]

Early burn wound excision followed by definitive wound coverage in patients with large surface area burns improves survival.[11] Even coverage with temporary dressing such as allograft and xenograft will help decrease fluid loss, provide protection from infection, help with thermal regulation, and decrease perceived pain.[11]

The care of the burn survivor is complex and dynamic. Many processes are operating concurrently to achieve the goal of medical stabilization. Rehabilitation, reconstruction, and restoration occur simultaneously, often with conflicting goals. At the same time that a free muscle transfer may require immobilization, a proximal joint may need mobilization. When a wound is most friable may also be the time that compression on surrounding scar is most required. The art of rehabilitation of the burn survivor is maintaining the balance of continuous conflicting treatments to optimize outcome. It demands close cooperation and communication between team members so the goals of one discipline do not overwhelm the goals of others.

## WOUNDS

Wound care is continuous throughout all phases of treatment. Physicians, physician assistants, nurses, physical and occupational therapists, will all be involved. A good understanding of wound care is important for the rehabilitation and occupational therapist.

Healing begins at the moment of injury. The body's first response is inflammation with an influx of neutrophils, lymphocytes, and macrophages to remove damaged cells. A new matrix is formed of fibroblasts and angiogenesis begins. Collagen is laid down into the matrix, and the typical appearance of granulation tissue develops. This tissue has a greater than normal percentage of calcium with more crosslinks that add rigidity to the granulation tissue resulting in eschar. Wound remodeling begins to shape the eschar over the burned areas. As time passes, it begins to contract and form scars that can be painful, can be prone to infection, and can convert a semi-closed wound into a deeper injury. Because of scar formation, burn survivors may require surgical procedures for months to years to improve function.[12]

The first step in wound care is the debridement and/or excision of eschar/devitalized tissue to prepare the wound bed for coverage. Initially patients are taken to the shower for superficial mechanical debridement. Superficial debridement involves the use of wet-to-moist (never dry in burn patients) dressings, liquid aseptic cleansers, and hydrotherapy to clean wounds and remove loose tissue and debris. Hydrotherapy, at the authors' institution, no longer involves immersing or tanking because this is thought to spread infection to unaffected areas. Instead, mechanical removal of the devitalized tissue and cleansing is achieved by placing the patient on an appropriate lifting device and going to the shower where low-pressure water can flow over and around the affected areas.[12]

Surgical debridement is often required to expose viable tissue and is accomplished by the use of tangential, or for very deep burns, fascial excision. The amount of burn wound excision and grafting that can be performed at any one time is limited by 2 factors: (1) the amount of unburned skin available to become donor sites for coverage, and (2) the amount of bleeding that occurs during surgery. Massive blood loss can quickly occur during burn surgery. As noted, however, early burn wound excision and definitive coverage will decrease mortality, morbidity, and hospital length of stay.[12]

## GRAFTS

Once a wound has been excised, it must be grafted or covered with a temporary dressing or biologic tissue. Autograft is tissue taken from donor sites on the patient. Grafts are usually harvested from the anterior thigh, but almost any area, including the scalp and the soles of the feet, can be used. The grafts are usually split thickness skin grafts (STSG), that is, skin harvested at a depth to include only the epidermis and a portion of the dermis. The STSG can be meshed to expand it and achieve greater surface of wound coverage and allow fluid and blood to pass through the graft. The major disadvantage is that STSG will contract as it heals. Contraction may result in functional limitations depending on the site. Full-thickness skin grafts include all the dermal layers and will not contract. However, it creates a very deep wound at the donor site and limits the amount of available tissue because it takes a very long time to heal sufficiently to be harvested again. Obviously there is no problem with rejection of autograft.[12]

When the TBSA is too large to obtain complete coverage with autografts, other temporary biological dressings can be used. Allograft is human cadaver skin. Xenograft is skin taken from another animal species such as pigs.[13] These coverings are temporary and will eventually slough off as the body rejects the foreign tissue. In the interim, they provide most of the benefits of STSG until the patient's donor sites are ready to be reharvested.

A very interesting biological dressing is cultured epithelial autograft. An unburned skin sample, approximately 2.5 square cm, is biopsied and sent to an outside laboratory for processing. From this biopsy, an unlimited amount of skin can be grown. Because the tissue is genetically identical to the patient's skin, there is no risk of rejection. Unfortunately, other problems exist. The final product is only a few cell layers thick and is very friable, making application technically challenging. Also, only superficial epithelial cells can be grown. The lack of deeper elements makes it difficult to cover irregular surfaces such as the face or joints because the product does not adhere as well. The final and not insignificant problem is the cost of hundreds of dollars for every few square centimeter of product delivered.[12]

Much effort is being expended in the development of synthetic dressings. An example is PermeaDerm, a bilaminar dressing with a pattern of slits in the surface. It produces less inflammation and fluid collection beneath the matrix, resulting in a greater surface area and more uniform depth of wound coverage than older synthetic dressings.[14]

Superficial and some deep partial-thickness wounds can heal without surgical intervention and can be treated with topical creams and dressings. Any wound that fails to close within 18 to 21 days should be reevaluated for possible grafting.[12]

There are many types of dressing materials that can be used. Every wound should be evaluated for depth, size, and location to determine which dressing will be the most appropriate. In general, open areas should have a topical antimicrobial applied as the initial layer. Historically mafenide acetate (Sulfamylon) and silver sulfadiazine (Silvadene) have been standard treatments, with the latter being most effective against pseudomonas. Bacitracin is frequently used as well. Many new dressings have been impregnated with silver, which has antimicrobial properties. For weeping wounds, products are available that are nonadherent and absorbent. Finally, everything is held in place with gauze bandages or other wraps. Whatever dressing is chosen, it is important that it is reapplied as often as necessary to remove old wound debris and prevent dessiccation.[12]

## Physical Rehabilitation

As noted, burn rehabilitation is an extremely complex and difficult process, and when combined with other injuries, is extremely challenging.

Burn rehabilitation has 2 primary functional goals: maintain mobility and prevent/mitigate scars and contractures. These goals are addressed concurrently and should begin as soon as medically and surgically possible. As survivability of major burns has increased, mobility and contracture management have become more challenging.

Although specific rehabilitation priorities change daily, these primary goals must be the foundation of all treatment plans.

## Mobility in the Intensive Care Unit

Patients with a large percentage of TBSA burn are critically ill and are typically admitted to an intensive care setting. Because the priority is intensive medical management in order to optimize survival,[15] there are many barriers to performing mobility. Despite these barriers, there is recent evidence that mobility in this setting can be done safely and reduces respiratory and vascular comorbidities associated with prolonged immobilization.[16–26] Because of the complex nature of patient mobilization in the intensive care setting, it is important to have the entire intensive care unit team participate in treatment planning and implementation,[21,22] including ambulating patients receiving extracorporeal membrane oxygenation.[27]

## Ambulation Following Skin Grafting

The lower extremity has fewer areas at risk for contracture compared with the upper extremity,[28] but still has potential problems. Grafting here can have a direct effect on patients' mobility due to traditional restrictions on motion thought to prevent graft loss in the acute setting. However, Nedelac and colleagues[29] found no evidence in the literature showing that early ambulation jeopardizes graft take. A retrospective review by Gawaziuk and colleagues[30] on the effect of early ambulation following lower extremity skin grafting with less than 30% TBSA burns found a 98% graft take rate with no repeat grafting required after waiting no more than 1 day to ambulate after surgery. In a prospective randomized controlled trial, Lorello and colleagues[31] observed no significant difference with graft loss between 2 groups of patients who underwent lower extremity grafting. One group ambulated on postoperative day 1 and the other group ambulated on postoperative day 5. Interestingly, the group that ambulated on postoperative day 5 actually had a significantly greater graft loss when the average loss percentage of the 2 groups was compared. Neither group required repeat grafting. It is important to note patients in this study were immobilized if the graft crossed a joint and kept non-weight-bearing if the graft crossed the ankle. Using these criteria, early ambulation after lower extremity skin grafting, particularly with larger TBSA burns, should be pursued.

## Contracture Risk Identification

A burn scar contracture has been defined as a loss of motion due to the replacement of skin with nonelastic tissue as a result of the wound healing process.[32] Contractures can have a profound impact on a burn survivor's outcome because of the loss of functional motion.[33,34] As discussed, consideration for contracture prevention must be included in every phase of treatment. In order to meet this challenge, the therapist must identify areas at risk for contracture.

Burn depth and location are key factors to predict contracture risk and establish treatment priorities. Range of motion (ROM) progression or regression must be tracked with objective, standardized techniques.[35] Goniometry provides objective measurements that can be tracked over time. Edgar and colleagues[36] demonstrated high intrarater and interrater reliability during goniometric measurement sessions for burn patients. To ensure this, measurement techniques must be standardized throughout a department. Goniometry should consider the location and relative tension of adjacent joints, and skin or scar tissue, identifying areas causing the impairment and monitoring the effectiveness of treatment.[37]

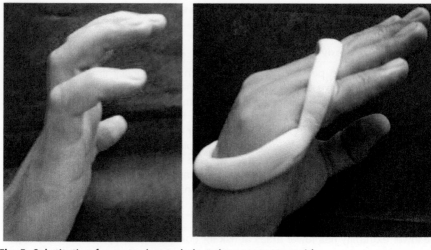

**Fig. 5.** Substituting for motor loss to help reduce contracture risk.

An additional determinant of contracture risk is the presence of any muscle loss or weakness combined with burns. Any motor deficit must be identified early, and splints that can substitute for this active ROM deficiency promptly used (**Fig. 5**). As shown in **Fig. 5**, a claw position is noted following an ulnar nerve injury putting the metacarpophalangeal (MCP) joints in extension and the interphalangeal (IP) joints in flexion. This position can increase the risk for an MCP joint extension contracture if the dorsal hand is burned or an IP joint flexion contracture if palmar burns are present. An anticlaw splint places the MCP joints into flexion and also blocks relative MCP extension during finger extension attempts, thus increasing active extension of the IP joints of the involved digits.[38–40]

It is important to use standardized nomenclature to ensure a universal understanding of contractures.[32–35] Richard and colleagues[32] suggest that contractures should be listed by the position that is opposite the direction of the desired motion. For example, a patient who lacks elbow extension would be considered to have an elbow flexion contracture.

Another nomenclature issue is that the term TBSA does not covey what the risk may be for contracture. A 2% burn to the hand is much more problematic than the same TBSA on the chest wall. Richard and colleagues[41] identified cutaneous functional units (CFU) as a solution for this issue. A CFU is defined as an area of skin that is serially recruited to permit ROM. This area of skin is proximal to the joint and is bordered by a skin crease.[41] By identifying the relationship between the burn location and the respective skin creases, risk can be assessed. The number and location of the CFU add to contracture risk particularly when sequential CFU are involved.[42] Schneider and colleagues[43] found that burn patients with a hand contracture averaged 10 involved CFU per subject. In the military setting, it has been shown that the finding of a hand contracture frequently results in an inability to return to duty.[44]

A correlation has been demonstrated between the CFU quantity and the total rehabilitation time required to treat contracture occurrence. Patients who received more therapy for each CFU involved were less likely to develop a contracture.[44–46] When compared with TBSA, CFU has been shown to be more relevant in determining how much therapy was required to prevent a contracture.[47] This information has a profound impact for treatment planning. Counting dorsal and palmar surfaces, there are more than 30 CFU or contracture risk areas per hand.[28] The treatment requirements of a patient with a hand burn are more accurately assessed using CFU than TBSA alone.

### Contracture Treatment

Preventing and treating burn scar contracture require prolonged stretch and optimal positioning. There are commonly recommended positions for regions that frequently contract[38,39] (**Fig. 6**). Unfortunately, no position is guaranteed to always prevent contractures of involved areas.[40]

Treating scar contractures is a primary mission for burn rehabilitation providers. Treatment interventions include, but are not limited to, exercise, positioning devices, splints, and casts.[32,38] These interventions use biomechanical principles, such as successive length induction, stress relaxation, and tissue creep.[38,48] Jacobson and colleagues[49] notes that it is important for providers to consider cutaneokinematic principles described in the CFU concept. The location, number of joints involved, and position of joints adjacent to involved areas are important considerations when determining an effective treatment strategy.

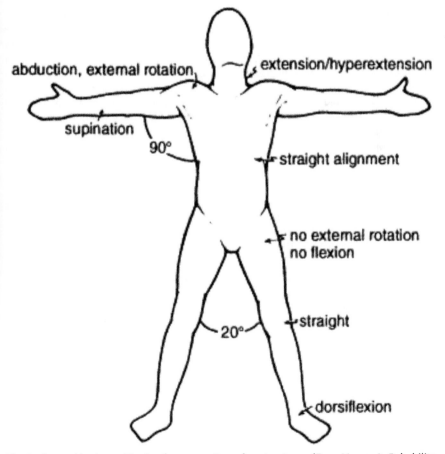

abduction, external rotation

extension/hyperextension

supination

90°

straight alignment

no external rotation
no flexion

20°    straight

dorsiflexion

**Fig. 6.** General body positioning for prevention of contractures. (*From* Young A. Rehabilitation of burn injuries. Phys Med Rehabil Clin 2002;13(1):99; with permission.)

Interventions for lengthening tissue depend on the duration and amount of force applied to the skin or scar during exercise and positioning. It should be a low-load force over a long duration.[50] In a retrospective evaluation of the effect of passive ROM on skin-grafted areas, Godleski and colleagues[51] found that a period of at least 3 minutes of end range stress to each involved area had a significant impact on increasing ROM. Although the investigators acknowledge some weaknesses in their findings, it does support the concept that calculated exercise can be beneficial for increasing ROM of affected areas after undergoing a skin graft.

Splinting and positioning devices are very helpful for treating burn scar contractures because they allow the clinician to extend the time of treatment beyond the active session. There are 3 classifications of splints commonly used for burn patients: static, dynamic, and static progressive splints.[32] Static splints keep the tissue at a constant length by maintaining one position (**Fig. 7**). They must be replaced as tissue lengthens.[38,40] Dynamic splints provide variable tension to involved areas, usually by using elastic or spring-loaded mechanisms.[38] Static progressive splints apply inelastic tension to soft tissue, and at end ROM, force adjusted as length gains are made (**Fig. 8**).[32,38,52] There are no specific best practice guidelines as to when or which type of splint to use. A tiered approach with dynamic splints followed by static-progressive splints if progress is inadequate with static splints is one strategy.[38,53] Dynamic and static progressive splints are technically challenging to fabricate and require adjustment at regular intervals to maintain optimal tissue stress. Richard and colleagues[54] found that treatment plans that included dynamic and static progressive splints for burn patients corrected contractures in less than half of the amount of days compared with treatments that did not include these splint types. Huang and colleagues[55] observed that treatments that included splinting for at least a 6-month period decreased the frequency of burn scar contractures in several body regions. Data show effectiveness of splinting in burn patients, but more study is required to provide clinicians with the answers as to the specific type, duration, and timing of splint application.[32]

## TREATMENT OF HYPERTROPHIC SCARRING

There is no way to predict how an individual's skin will respond to the burn injury (**Fig. 9**). All will have some scars, but there is no way to tell who will develop the most severe hypertrophic scarring. Therefore, attempts at prevention and mitigation must be applied universally. The international standard of treatment of burn scars is

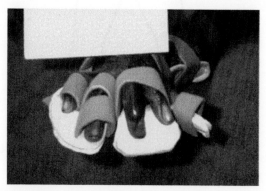

**Fig. 7.** Resting hand orthosis to correct deformity. (*From* Young A. Rehabilitation of burn injuries. Phys Med Rehabil Clin 2002;13(1):104; with permission.)

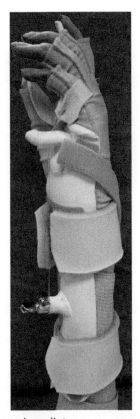

**Fig. 8.** Example of a static progressive splint.

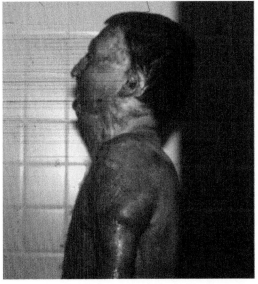

**Fig. 9.** Hypertrophic scarring on the face and upper body. (*From* Young A. Rehabilitation of burn injuries. Phys Med Rehabil Clin 2002;13(1):98; with permission.)

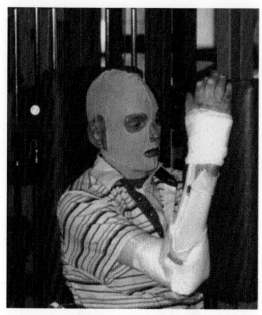

**Fig. 10.** Compression garment: fabric face mask. (*From* Young A. Rehabilitation of burn injuries. Phys Med Rehabil Clin 2002;13(1):101; with permission.)

the application of 25 mm Hg of pressure to the scar.[32] It is accomplished by wearing custom compression garments, gloves, and masks. Masks can be composed of either fabric or acrylic material. Everything used for compression should be worn 23 h/d. This requires multiple sets of garments, so one can be laundered as the other is worn. Treatment may begin even if there is still open area by wrapping with Kerlex and ace wraps, progressing to Coban and Tubigrip as skin heals. Finally, when only minimal scattered open areas remain, compression garments may be used. Custom measured garments are best because off the shelf cannot conform directly to the contours of the skin and scar and will fail to provide sufficient compression (**Fig. 10**). There are other treatments available that complement, but do not replace, compression garments for hypertrophic scar treatment. Although the mechanism is not clear, the application of Silastic/silicone gel to scars has been found to decrease height and erythema even without other sources of pressure. It is frequently used to line the surface of acrylic masks, any compression garment, and as sheets directly on scars. Evidence is statistically significant but considered susceptible to bias.[56] Laser treatments have been shown to help reduce both erythema and hypertrophy. Early application seems to be most beneficial. In particular, the pulse dye laser is helpful to decrease erythema. It takes the greater power of the $CO_2$ laser to reduce the height of scars.[57] Their use will undoubtedly increase.

## PAIN MANAGEMENT

Burns have been described as one of the most painful injuries that can occur. Pain management must address 3 different components of pain. Background or baseline pain is best treated by long-acting opioids. Breakthrough pain occurs with therapy treatments, general movement, and dressing changes and is addressed with short-acting narcotics. Procedural pain occurs with debridement, large dressing changes, bronchoscopy, line changes, skin grafting, and similar treatments. Procedures may require anything from conscious sedation to general anesthesia. There is discussion supporting requirements for as much as 70 mg of morphine equivalence daily to treat up to 20% TBSA and 150 mg to treat 30% or higher TBSA burns.[58] Currently, there is reticence and some legislative restriction to prescribing opiates. However, it is vital that pain is initially treated aggressively and adequately. It can subsequently be tapered as quickly as is reasonable for each individual. Other acute and chronic comorbidities will generate pain. Neuropathic pain is caused by damage to nerve endings. This occurs with deep partial and full-thickness burns. The use of gabapentin for neuropathic pain has additional positive effects on patients perception of pain from all causes decreasing overall narcotic requirements.[59] It should be started early. Phantom pain, myofascial pain, psychological distress, and sleep hygiene all contribute to pain and appropriate non–opioid treatment should be added as indicated.[58] Successful management requires an ongoing holistic evaluation of these comorbidities, the wound burden, and progress in the rehabilitation to optimize medication levels. In general, as wounds close, scars diminish, and as mobility improves, pain decreases. On a chronic basis, many burn survivors use little to no routine narcotic medication.[9]

## PSYCHOLOGICAL ISSUES

Many catastrophic changes occur in the moment of trauma, particularly burn trauma. One of the worst is a change in physical appearance. A core tenant of our self-esteem is based on how we perceive people respond to our appearance. Many burn survivors will not look in a mirror for months. In addition to the change in appearance, burn survivors also experience a loss of control over their lives. They are delivered into the medical system and subjected to the apparent whims of others for an unknowable period of time. They are acutely relegated to a position of dependence in their family and society at large. This dependence generates financial and social stress.[60] Additional stress comes from constant pain, and depending upon circumstances, survivor's guilt. Preexisting psychological disorders will complicate treatment, frequently during rehabilitation. Depression, even in patients without prior history, should be anticipated and can occur late. Posttraumatic stress disorder (PTSD) without other psychological diagnosis occurs in 45% of burns survivors within the first year.[61] Psychiatric and psychological intervention, counseling, treatment of sleep issues, antidepressants, antianxiety medication, and peer support groups such as the Phoenix Society all have a place in treatment. Early and aggressive reintegration into the community for vocational and avocational activity is very helpful.[60]

## NUTRITION

A major burn is accompanied by a hypermetabolic state. Adequate caloric intake and a positive nitrogen balance promote skin and muscle growth and repair. Healing cannot occur if the body is in a catabolic state. Required are 2000 to 2200 calories/$m^2$ TBSA with 1.5 to 2.0 g of protein per kilogram per day. A general multivitamin supplemented with vitamin C, A, zinc, copper, and manganese are essential for wound healing.[62]

## OTHER PROBLEMS

Neuropathy occurs in up to 9% of burns survivors regardless of burn size or cause. The incidence is higher in electrical burns.[63] The cause is not clear. Symptoms occur in burned and unburned areas. It can present as a mononeuropathy, multiple mononeuropathies, or a generalized sensorimotor polyneuropathy.[64] Treatment usually involves the use of oral medication indicated for neuropathy, that is, Lyrica, Neurontin, amitriptyline, Cymbalta, and occasionally, tramadol.

Pruritus is a common problem. Some burn survivors describe it as more uncomfortable than their pain. For many years, it was thought that histamine release was the cause but now seems that this is another example of neuropathic pain. Medications for neuropathy have been found to be more helpful for pruritus than antihistamines.[65]

Bone and joint changes can cause impairment with osteoporosis the most common finding. Osteophytes may form around joints, particularly the olecranon and coracoid process after burn injury.[66] Bones may be deformed by traction from burn scar contraction and by the application of compression garments, particularly in the face over the mandible and nose.[67] Subluxations or dislocations particularly the MCP and metatarsal phalangeal can occur with burns to the dorsal surface of the hand and foot. Splints and daily stretching are required if this occurs. Pediatric patients are very susceptible to pressure changes from scar and compression garments and must be monitored diligently until they stop growing.

Heterotopic ossification is the deposition of ectopic bone around joints and tendons. It most frequently occurs at the elbow, hip, shoulder, and to a lesser degree at the temporomandibular joint, wrist, hand, knee, and ankle. Occurrence seems to be related to metabolic factors released early in the hypermetabolic state.[68] Historically the incidence has been 3%. In our last conflict, the incidence was 17% for burns. Burns combined with amputation and traumatic brain injury as comorbidities push the percentage of patients requiring surgical revision to 74%.[69] The practice had been to wait at least a year until the bone matured before trying to excise it because of the risk of recurrence if it was still active. However, it has been shown that early excision does not significantly increase recurrence.[70] There is also some evidence that the use of IV bisphosphonates may be effective in decreasing/reversing effects of heterotopic ossification.[71]

## LONG-TERM CARE

It is very important for the burn survivor and their support group to have a clear understanding of the long-term problems they will have to manage to successfully reintegrate in the family and community. There must be education on any medications required long term. As discussed, it is important for pain medication to be tapered throughout the treatment process, and by this time the patient should be on little to no opioids for pain. If pain persists, other causes should be evaluated, such as painful contractures, subluxations, heterotopic ossification, nerve injuries, infection, and addiction. The skin must be well maintained. It will be sensitive to mechanical shearing and topical irritants. It is necessary to lubricate all affected areas at least twice a day. Burn skin is more susceptible to repeated thermal injury, particularly from sun exposure, which can lead to melanoma. Compression garments do not provide protection from UV rays. Sunscreen at least SPF 30 or more needs to be applied to the skin whenever the survivor goes outside. Long sleeve shirts and hats should be used even in cloudy weather. Areas of full-thickness burn cannot participate in thermal regulation secondary to loss of sweat glands. Extremes of hot or cold temperatures should be avoided. Compression garments should be worn 23 hours a day until scars have matured, that is, are no longer hyperemic and do not blanch excessively with pressure. This maturation usually occurs in one to one and one-half years but may take much longer in some cases. Also as previously noted, depression and/or PTSD are likely to occur at some point, and it should be monitored on a long-term basis. Many burn survivors will require surgery for functional and cosmetic restoration for many years.[9]

Burn rehabilitation is an extremely complex and difficult process, and when combined with other major trauma, is extremely challenging. The best outcome will be achieved using a multidisciplinary team that emphasizes a dynamic approach to functional restoration through aggressive wound care, scar and contracture management, pain management, mobilization, and psychological support.

## REFERENCES

1. Pruitt BA, Wolf SE. Epidemiological, demographic, and outcome characteristics of burn injury. In: Herndon DN, editor. Total burn care. 3rd edition. Philadelphia: Saunders Elsevier; 2007. p. 14–32.
2. Herndon DN, Blakeney PE. Teamwork for total burn care: achievements, direction, and hopes. In: Herndon DN, editor. Total burn care. 3rd edition. Philadelphia: Saunders Elsevier; 2007. p. 9–13.
3. American Burn Association. Burn incident fact sheet. 2016. Available at: http://www.cdc.gov/nchs/ahcd/web_tables.htm#2011. Accessed January 22, 2015.
4. Chou TD, Lee TW. The management of white phosphorus burns. Burns 2001; 27(5):492–7.
5. United States Nuclear Regulatory Commission. Lethal dose (LD). 2017. Available at: https://www.nrc.gov/reading-rm/basic-ref/glossary/lethal-dose-ld.html. Accessed April 10, 3017.
6. Singh M, Alavi A, Wong R, et al. Radiodermatitis: a review of our current understanding. Am J Clin Dermatol 2016 Jun;17(3):277–92.
7. Purdue GF, Arnoldo BD. Electrical injuries. In: Herndon DN, editor. Total burn care. 3rd edition. Philadelphia: Saunders Elsevier; 2007. p. 513–20.
8. Ahrenholz DH, Schubert W. Creatine kinase as a prognostic indicator in electrical injury. Surgery 1988;104(4):741–7.
9. Young AW. Rehabilitation of burn injuries. In: Shannon S, editor. Physical medicine and rehabilitation clinics of North America. Philadelphia: W.B. Saunders Co; 2002. p. 85–108.
10. Haberal M, Abali AES. Fluid management in major burn injuries. Indian J Plast Surg 2010;43(Suppl):S29–36.
11. Burk JF. Primary excision and prompt grafting as routine therapy for the treatment of burns in children. Surg Clin North Am 1976;56:477.
12. Sterling JP, Heimbach DM. Management of the burn wound. ACS Surgery: Principles and Practice 2010. https://doi.org/10.2310/7800.S0713.
13. PBS News Hour. Why this Brazilian city uses fish skin to treat burn victims. Available at: https://www.pbs.org/newshour/health/brazilian-city-uses-tilapia-fish-skin-treat-burn-victims. Accessed March 3, 2017.
14. Woodroof A, Phipps R, Woeller C, et al. Evolution of a biosynthetic temporary skin substitute: A preliminary study. Eplasty 2015;15:e30. Available at: https://www.ncbi.nlm.nih.gov/pmc/articles/PMC4511025/.
15. Lundy JB, Chung KK. Update on severe burn management for the intensivist. J Intensive Care Med 2016;31(8):499–510.
16. Clark DE, Lowman JD, Griffin RL, et al. Effectiveness of an early mobilization protocol in a trauma and burns intensive care unit: a retrospective cohort study. Phys Ther 2013;93:186–96.
17. Kress J. Clinical trials of early mobilization of critically ill patients. Crit Care Med 2009;37(10):S442–7.
18. Needham DM. Mobilizing patients in the intensive care unit: improving neuromuscular weakness and physical function. JAMA 2008;300:1685–90.

19. TEAM Study Investigators, Hodgson C, Bellomo R, Berney S. Early mobilization and recovery in mechanically ventilated patients in the ICU: a bi-national, multicentre, prospective cohort study. Crit Care 2015;19:81.
20. Taylor S, Manning S, Quarles J. A multidisciplinary approach to early mobilization of patients with burns. Crit Care Nurs Q 2013;36:56–62.
21. Hopkins R, Spuhler V. Strategies for promoting early activity in critically ill mechanically ventilated patients. AACN Adv Crit Care 2009;20:277–89.
22. Perme C, Chandrashekar R. Early mobility and walking program for patients in intensive care units: creating a standard of care. Am J Crit Care 2009;18:212–21.
23. Schweickert W, Pohlman M, Pohlman A, et al. Early physical and occupational therapy in mechanically ventilated, critically ill patients: a randomized controlled trial. Lancet 2009;373:1874–82.
24. Morris P. Moving our critically ill patients: mobility barriers and benefits. Crit Care Clin 2007;23:1–20.
25. Hodgson C, Bailey M, Bellomo R, et al. A binational multicenter pilot feasibility randomized controlled trial of early goal-directed mobilization in the ICU. Crit Care Med 2016;44:1145–52.
26. Deng H, Chen J, Li F, et al. Effects of mobility training on severe burn patients in BICU: a retrospective cohort study. Burns 2016;42:1404–12.
27. Abrams D, Javidfar J, Farrand E, et al. Early mobilization of patients receiving extracorporeal membrane oxygenation: a retrospective cohort study. Crit Care 2014;18(1):R38.
28. Richard R, Jones J, Parshley P. Hierarchical decomposition of burn body diagram based on cutaneuous functional units and its utility. J Burn Care Res 2015;36:33–43.
29. Nedelac B, Serghiou M, Niszczak J, et al. Practice guidelines for early ambulation of burn survivors after lower extremity grafts. J Burn Care Res 2012;33:319–29.
30. Gawaziuk J, Peters B, Logsetty S. Early ambulation after-grafting of lower extremity burns. Burns 2018;44:183–7.
31. Lorello D, Peck M, Albrecht M, et al. Results of a prospective randomized controlled trial of early ambulation for patients with lower extremity autografts. J Burn Care Res 2014;35:431–6.
32. Richard RL, Baryza MJ, Carr JA, et al. Burn rehabilitation and research: proceedings of a consensus summit. J Burn Care Res 2009;30:543–73.
33. Schneider JC, Holavanahalli R, Helm P, et al. Contractures in burn injury: defining the problem. J Burn Care Res 2006;27:508–14.
34. Leblebici B, Adam M, Bagis S, et al. Quality of life after burn injury: the impact of joint contracture. J Burn Care Res 2006;27:864–8.
35. Parry I, Walker K, Niszczack J, et al. Methods and tools used for the measurement of burn scar contracture. J Burn Care Res 2010;31:888–903.
36. Edgar D, Finlay V, Wu A, et al. Goniometry and linear assessments to monitor movement outcomes: are they reliable tools in burn survivors? Burns 2009;35:58–62.
37. Richard R, McGlinchey P, Parry I. Challenging standard goniometric measurements for patients with burn injuries: a suggested paradigm shift to move beyond practice as usual. J Burn Care Res 2013;34(2):S131.
38. Dewey WS, Richard RL, Parry IS. Positioning, splinting & contracture management. In: Esselman P, Kowalske K, editors. Physical medicine and rehabilitation clinics of North America, vol. 22. Philadelphia: WB Saunders; 2011. p. 229–47.
39. Helm PA, Kevorkian CG, Lushbaugh M, et al. Burn injury: rehabilitation management in 1982. Arch Phys Med Rehabil 1982;63:6–16.
40. Hedman TL, Quick CD, Richard RL, et al. Rehabilitation of burn casualties. In: Lenhart MK, editor. Textbooks of military medicine, care of the combat amputee.

Falls Church (VA): Office of the Surgeon General, Department of the Army; 2009. p. 277–380.

41. Richard R, Lester M, Miller S, et al. Identification of cutaneous functional units related to burn scar contracture development. J Burn Care Res 2009;30:625–31.
42. Vocke S, Ware L. Cutaneous functional units and their clinical implications on the treatment and evaluation of the burned upper extremity. ASHT Times 2016;23(1): 1–3.
43. Schneider J, Holavanahalli R, Helm P, et al. Contractures in burn injury part II: investigating joints of the hand. J Burn Care Res 2008;29:606–13.
44. Chapman T, Richard R, Hedman T, et al. Military return to duty and civilian return to work factors following burns with focus on the hand and literature review. J Burn Care Res 2008;29:756–62.
45. Richard RL, Dewey WS, Anyan WR III, et al. Increased burn rehabilitation treatment time improves patient outcome. J Burn Care Res 2014;35(3):S100.
46. Richard RL, Jones JA, Dewey WS, et al. Small and large burns alike benefit from lengthier rehabilitation time. J Burn Care Res 2015;36:S85.
47. Richard RL, Dewey WS, Anyan III, et al. Cutaneous functional unit is a better index than total body surface area related to burn patient outcomes. J Burn Care Res 2014;35(3):S77.
48. Richard R, Staley M. Biophysical aspects of normal skin and burn scar. In: Richard R, Staley M, editors. Burn care and rehabilitation: principles and practice. Philadelphia: F.A. Davis; 1994. p. 49–69.
49. Jacobson K, Fletchall S, Dodd H, et al. Current concepts burn rehabilitation, Part I: care during hospitalization. Clin Plast Surg 2017;44:703–12.
50. Arem A, Madden J. Effects of stress on healing wounds. Intermittent noncyclical tension. J Surg Res 1976;20:93–102.
51. Godleski M, Oeffling A, Bruflat A, et al. Treating burn-associated joint contracture: results of an inpatient rehabilitation stretching protocol. J Burn Care Res 2013;34: 420–6.
52. Schutlz-Johnson K. Static progressive splinting. J Hand Ther 2002;15(2):163–78.
53. Flowers K. A proposed decision hierarchy for splinting a stiff joint, with an emphasis on force application parameters. J Hand Ther 2002;15(2):158–62.
54. Richard R, Miller S, Staley M, et al. Multimodal versus progressive treatment techniques to correct burn scar contractures. J Burn Care Rehabil 2000;21:506–12.
55. Huang T, Blackwell S, Lewis S. Ten years of experience in managing patients with burn scar contractures of axilla, elbow, wrist and knee joints. Plast Reconstr Surg 1978;61(1):70–6.
56. O'Brien L, Jones DJ. Silicone gel sheeting for preventing and treating hypertrophic and keloid scars. Cochrane Database Syst Rev 2013. https://doi.org/10.1002/14651858.CD003826.
57. Sever C, Uygur F. Treatment of facial burn scars with CO2 laser resurfacing and thin skin grafting. J Craniofac Surg 2010;21(4):1024–8.
58. Young AW, Graves C, Kowalske KJ, et al. Guideline for burn care under austere conditions: pain management. J Burn Care Res 2017;38(2):e497–509.
59. Rimaz S, Alavi CE, Sedighinejad A, et al. Effect of gabapentin on morphine consumption and pain after surgical debridement of burn wounds: a double-blind randomized clinical trial study. Arch Trauma Res 2012;1(1):38–43.
60. Blankeney PE, Rosenberg L. Psychosocial recovery and reintegration of patients with burn injuries. In: Herndon DN, editor. Total burn care. 3rd edition. Philadelphia: Saunders Elsevier; 2007. p. 829–43.

61. Giannoni-Pastor A, Eiroa-Orosa FJ. Prevalence and Predictors of posttraumatic stress symptomatology among burn survivors: a systematic review and meta-analysis. J Burn Care Res 2016;37(1):e79–89.
62. Rodriguez DJ. Nutrition in patients with severe burns: state of the art. J Burn Care Rehabil 1996;17(1):62–70.
63. Wesner ML, Hickie J. Long-term sequelae of electrical injury. Can Fam Physician 2013;59(9):935–9.
64. Tamam Y, Tamam C, Tamam B, et al. Peripheral neuropathy after burn injury. Eur Rev Med Pharmacol Sci 2013;17(Suppl 1):107–11.
65. Goutos I, Eldardiri M. Comparative evaluation of antipruritic protocols in acute burns. The emerging value of gabapentin in the treatment of burns pruritis. J Burn Care Res 2010;31(1):57–63.
66. Pandit SK, Maliaaa CN. A study of bone and joint changes secondary to burns. Burns 1993;19(3):227–8.
67. Fricke NB, Omnell ML. Skeletal and dental disturbances in children after facial burns and pressure garment use: a four year follow-up. J Burn Care Rehabil 1999;20(3):239–49.
68. Goel A, Shrivastava P. Post-burn scars and scar contractures. Indian J Plast Surg 2010;43(Suppl):S63–71.
69. Lester ME, Young AW. Incidence of heterotopic ossification among military and civilian burn casualities: a preliminary analysis. Platform Presentation 2011 American Burn Association Meeting, Chicago, IL, March 29-April 1, 2011.
70. Tsionos I, Leciercq C. Heterotopic ossification of the elbow in patients with burns. Results after early excision. J Bone Joint Surg Br 2004;86(3):396–403.
71. Burns Open. Sinha S, Biernaskie JA. Nitrogen-containing bisphosphonates for burn-related heterotopic ossification. Available at: https://doi.org/10.1016/j.burnso.2017.12.004. Accessed December 23 2017.

# Neurobehavioral Management of the Polytrauma Veteran

Bryan P. Merritt, MD[a,b,]*, Tracy Kretzmer, PhD[a,c],
Tamara L. McKenzie-Hartman, PsyD[a,d], Praveen Gootam, MD[a,e]

## KEYWORDS

- Mild TBI • Concussion • Post-concussive symptoms • Veteran • Polytrauma
- Interdisciplinary

## KEY POINTS

- Holistic treatment approaches that include a coordinated care approach to address the complex needs of this population should be the gold standard of care.
- Despite underlying etiology, patients can benefit from cognitive rehabilitation approaches that focus on teaching compensatory skills and strategies that over time can become automatic via rehearsal and reinforcement.
- The potential benefits of successful treatment of sleep-wake disorders in the population with traumatic brain injury include improvement in functional outcomes, cognition, mood, perceived pain, headache, and quality of life.
- When patients and family members witness communication between providers, the effect becomes that of improved trust and confidence with the treatment team, as well as increased insight into their symptom presentation and functioning.

## INTRODUCTION

In 2005, the Department of Veterans Affairs (VA) health care system established the Polytrauma System of Care to provide specialized care to both active-duty service members (ADSMs) and veterans experiencing deployment-related injuries. This system of care was established to better address the unique injuries military service

[a] James A. Haley Veterans Hospital, 13000 Bruce B Downs Boulevard #117, Tampa, FL 33612, USA; [b] Department of Neurology, University of South Florida Medical School, 4202 E Fowler Avenue, Tampa, FL 33620, USA; [c] Department of Psychology, University of South Florida Medical School, 4202 E Fowler Avenue, Tampa, FL 33620, USA; [d] Defense and Veterans Brain Injury Center (DVBIC), Silver Spring, MD, USA; [e] Department of Psychiatry and Behavioral Neurosciences, University of South Florida Medical School, 4202 E Fowler Avenue, Tampa, FL 33620, USA
* Corresponding author. James A. Haley Veterans Hospital, 13000 Bruce B Downs Boulevard #117, Tampa, FL 33612.
E-mail address: Bryan.Merritt@va.gov

Phys Med Rehabil Clin N Am 30 (2019) 133–154
https://doi.org/10.1016/j.pmr.2018.09.003
1047-9651/19/Published by Elsevier Inc.
pmr.theclinics.com

members experienced as a result of their service in the Afghanistan and Iraq wars. There are now more than 2.7 million Iraq and Afghanistan veterans and Reserve/National Guard members eligible for care in the VA system.[1] Approximately 62% of those eligible have used the VA health care system, with the vast majority of these individuals (92%) receiving their health care through outpatient services. Many of these veterans present to polytrauma outpatient clinics seeking treatment for a variety of physical, cognitive, and behavioral complaints. For many, these symptoms negatively impact their ability to reintegrate into civilian life and may even rise to level of service-connected disability. Injuries resulting from combat exposure, such as blast-related traumatic brain injury (TBI) or traumatic stress are complex in that symptoms across conditions often overlap and exacerbate other comorbid conditions, making differential diagnosis and treatment planning challenging.

It was with the increased use of improvised explosive devices (IEDs) that blast-related injuries, particularly TBI, became known as the "hallmark" or "signature" injury of the wars. Of the 379,519 service members diagnosed with TBI between 2000 and 2017, 82% of these injuries were characterized as mild in nature.[14] Individuals suffering a mild TBI (mTBI) or concussion may or may not experience postconcussive symptoms (PCSs), such as headache, dizziness, light/noise sensitivity, fatigue, insomnia, and/or irritability. PCSs are expected to fully resolve within a few hours to weeks after the event. However, some individuals continue to experience PCSs for years after injury,[15] with symptoms often remaining refractory despite multiple treatment paradigms. Factors underlying continued symptomology remain under debate, but studies have consistently demonstrated that the presence of untreated mental health sequelae or other psychosocial stressors are often the more primary contributing factor to persistent or chronic PCS reporting.[6,16,17] For a military population, the presence of posttraumatic stress, chronic pain, insomnia, and other postdeployment adjustment difficulties are often comorbidly present with TBI. Prevalence studies estimate up to 20% of the 2.7 million Iraq and Afghanistan veterans have posttraumatic stress disorder (PTSD) and/or depression,[18] and 7% of this veteran cohort carry a diagnosis of TBI and PTSD.[18] In a seminal article by Hoge and colleagues,[16] PTSD and depression were found to be important mediators in the relationship between mTBI and somatic health complaints.

Aside from TBI and PTSD/depression diagnoses, the most commonly diagnosed condition within this cohort is "musculoskeletal ailments."[1] Therefore, when examining the polytrauma veteran with a history of mTBI, PTSD/depression, and chronic pain, it can be challenging to determine underlying etiology (Fig. 1), make appropriate triage decisions, and initiate the most efficacious treatment paradigm, particularly given these various conditions tend to be managed by different specialty providers (eg, neurologist, physiatrist, psychology). Although the VA/Department of Defense (DoD) has established clinic practice guidelines for each of these conditions, when there are multiple comorbid conditions present, there is limited empirical evidence to provide guidance to polytrauma providers.

The focus of this article was to examine some of the most common neurobehavioral symptoms presented in the polytrauma veteran with a history of mTBI and PTSD and to review the optimal treatment approach within an interdisciplinary team setting. Although recommended interventions discussed may be appropriate to all types of veteran treatment settings, the impact of a specialized inpatient mTBI and postdeployment program is reviewed. In 2006, the Post-Deployment Rehabilitation and Evaluation Program (PREP) was developed to address the unique needs of this population. It is an inpatient rehabilitation team consisting of multiple interdisciplinary providers that conducts clinically indicated evaluations and treatment for mTBI and

## Post-Deployment Triad

| Symptoms | Mild TBI | PTSD/ Depression | Pain |
|---|---|---|---|
| Memory Impairment | X | x | x |
| Concentration Problems | x | x | x |
| Irritability | x | x | x |
| Insomnia/Sleep Problems | x | x | x |
| Fatigue | x | x | x |
| Headaches | x | x | x |
| Dizziness | x | x | x |
| Affective disturbance | x | x | x |
| Personality Change | x | x | x |
| Apathy | x | x | x |

**Fig. 1.** Post deployment triad.

postdeployment-related issues, including PCS, chronic pain, sleep difficulties, multisensory symptoms, orthopedics injuries, cognitive complaints, and psychological difficulties. It is the unique aspects that are provided within an inpatient setting by interdisciplinary providers that has assisted with significant symptom reduction, even in a population that is often refractory to multiple treatment paradigms.

## NEUROBEHAVIORAL SYMPTOMS
### Cognitive Difficulties

Cognitive difficulties, including inattention, slowed processing speed, and poor memory are commonly reported by polytrauma veterans. Despite knowledge of the well-established recovery trajectory following concussion, many individuals continue to report cognitive difficulties years after injury. Comorbid medical and behavioral conditions (ie, depression, anxiety, chronic pain, sleep difficulties, psychosocial stressors, substance misuse, multisensory symptoms) can negatively impact cognition,[19,13] and have been demonstrated to be more primary etiologic factors underlying cognitive complaints than a history of remote concussion(s).[15,20,21] Additional factors also complicating the clinical picture and contributing to worsening cognitive outcomes may include litigation/compensation involvement, overestimates of premorbid functioning, iatrogenic effects/misattribution of symptoms to head injury history, and medications.[15,17] Given the myriad of other potential contributing factors, determining primary causes of poor cognition can be complicated. As such, a thorough clinical interview begins with evaluating injury history (including, eg, both training and deployment history, blast and weapons exposures, airborne operations), and details about symptom presentations (eg, onset, timeline, frequency, and triggers). The history and symptoms are then assessed within the context of other factors, such as overall physical health, developmental history, occupational/academic functioning (eg, via objective reports from supervisors, performance reviews), pain, sleep, mood/stress, family/social support, medications, and substance use, and beliefs about current functioning are crucial in helping to uncover contributing factors of persistent PCS.

Numerous studies confirm poorer neuropsychological performance (ie, attention, memory, processing speed, executive functioning), among Operation Enduring Freedom/Operation Iraqi Freedom/Operation New Dawn service members and veterans with comorbid PTSD and sleep difficulties when compared with combat controls.[22] As such, interventions aimed at reducing combat stress and improving sleep are strongly encouraged, and a large part of most treatment plans within PREP, when addressing chronic cognitive complaints among patients with mTBI.[10,23] Expectedly, ADSMs and veterans within PREP are initially reluctant to accept the relationship between other factors, especially mental health factors, and their cognitive complaints. However, numerous PREP team providers, including neuropsychology, psychiatry, psychology, and speech pathology, are well-versed and essential in explaining how, PTSD and sleep problems, for example, uniquely impact cognitive skills such as attention and processing speed that further impact higher-order abilities such as memory and executive functioning. Conversations about how cognitive deficits can have considerable impact on quality of life, return to work/school, job performance, community reintegration, and relationships are also had by numerous PREP team members at various time points throughout treatment.[11]

It is easy to see how seemingly straightforward cognitive complaints, without such information offered and consistently reinforced by various disciplines, can lead patients with complex polytrauma, and perhaps individual providers alike, to erroneously blame TBI history only and direct care toward cognitive concerns only without adequately addressing other important driving factors. Unfortunately, this misinformed perspective also can be further exacerbated by the unfortunate stigma mental health diagnosis and treatment carry for many individuals. Logically then, whether a provider within an interdisciplinary team, or an outpatient TBI clinic, first-line treatments of postconcussive cognitive complaints should be nonpharmacological and center around providing education, treating comorbid symptomatology, and using cognitive rehabilitation (**Table 1**). Specifically, interventions using psychoeducation to increase TBI knowledge and understanding of factors that impact cognition, facilitate lifestyle/environmental modifications, and set realistic expectations regarding recovery timelines are among the most effective.[5–8] Such education is oftentimes vital when significant symptoms are presented against the backdrop of "normal" neurodiagnostic tests and neuropsychological functioning, which can be frequently

**Table 1**
**Evidence-Based approach to treatment of Cognitive Symptoms in Mild Traumatic Brain Injury**

| Symptom | Medication | Rehabilitation Therapies | Behavioral Interventions | Adjunctive Approaches |
|---|---|---|---|---|
| Cognition | Not recommended | Cognitive rehabilitation:<br>• Adjunctive skills[2–4]<br>• Compensatory strategies[2–4] | Psychoeducation[5–8]<br>Mental health treatment to address:<br>• Underlying psychiatric conditions<br>• Sleep<br>• Chronic pain<br>• Marital/family functioning<br>• Occupational distress<br>• Substance abuse | Biofeedback[9]<br>Sleep[10–12] Interventions<br>Multisensory treatments[13] |

perceived as frustrating and/or inaccurate. This type of education or feedback is often best received when it is provided by a trusted provider with well-established rapport, and then periodically reinforced by other members of the interdisciplinary team who also have well-established rapport. Furthermore, the message that their neuro-diagnostic findings are "normal" despite their daily experience of cognitive difficulties, and that their difficulties are better attributed to "PTSD, chronic pain, and poor sleep," may be received as an invalidating message, such that their cognitive deficits are somehow less true or just "all in their head." Spending additional time validating the patient's experience(s) and negative functional impacts it has on his or her daily living will help to bolster the patient's willingness to engage in more efficacious therapies that often carry a stigma or represent a path that can be anxiety provoking (ie, psychotherapy).

Despite underlying etiology, patients can benefit from cognitive rehabilitation approaches that focus on teaching compensatory skills and strategies that over time can become automatic via rehearsal and reinforcement. Compensatory strategy training is thought to help organize behavior and improve efficiency by teaching "cognitive prosthetics" (ie, the use of task lists, calendars with reminders, memory notebooks, and alarms),[2] implementing environmental modifications (eg, verbal and nonverbal cues, signs within the environment), and using cognitive assistive technology (eg, wristwatches, smartphones, tablets with alarm and note-taking functions, GPS devices), to support daily functioning, work, and school activities.[3,4] Within PREP, engagement from numerous team members, including speech pathology, audiology (for assistive hearing devices), and occupational therapy, are used when incorporating various cognitive prosthetics into a treatment plan. In contrast, cognitive rehabilitation emphasizes adaptive approaches that use specific cognitive skills to accomplish functional tasks/processes.[3] For example, strategies may include learning to engage in more cognitively challenging tasks at the beginning of the day, or when the most alert/rested. Other strategies include breaking complex tasks down into smaller components, resetting expectations regarding time to complete tasks (ie, teaching pacing and the incorporation of breaks), and reducing distractions (eg, turning off phone and TV, closing the door, making the room quiet). Expectedly, most PREP providers are involved in either implementing or reinforcing such adaptive approaches across their individual treatments (eg, breaking down a complex vocational rehabilitation goal into multiple steps across appointments), as well as within conversations about how to best adjust the treatment plan for the individual patient (eg, coordinating among providers to schedule cognitive testing early in the morning when most alert; or planning to have art or recreation therapy after a stressful psychotherapy session). Early evidence supports biofeedback as a mechanism for improving cognitive functioning among those with mTBI,[9,24,25] although there is no evidence to support computer-based rehabilitation (ie, rote repetition of tasks on a computer) without the involvement of a clinician.[26]

Multisensory challenges, such as vestibular symptoms (eg, dizziness, balance difficulties, gaze stability), and ocular-motor impairments (eg, convergence/accommodation insufficiencies, saccadic dysfunction) have also been linked with cognitive fatigue and worse neuropsychological outcomes.[19] As these difficulties are largely overlooked when it comes to managing PCS, and certainly contribute to sustained cognitive complaints, evaluation and interventions aimed at addressing such problems are strongly supported. PREP providers, including optometry/vision rehabilitation, audiology, physical/vestibular therapy, speech pathology, and neuropsychology, routinely discuss multisensory complaints and treatments as they pertain to cognitive performance and functional difficulties at work, home, or school. Qualitatively within PREP, as improvements with a patient's ability to hear better or use assistive devices to help block out high-pitched tones (ie, tinnitus), or even rely less on their visual system secondary to improvements in vestibular functioning, providers are able to also see correlated improvements in mood and overall cognitive functioning.

## Headaches

Posttraumatic headaches (PTH) are one of the most common symptoms following TBI, occurring in 30% to 90% of cases, regardless of TBI severity.[27] The identification, characterization, and management of headaches have implications for management of both acute and chronic TBIs. Within the polytrauma patient population, headaches are a very common symptom and sequalae of other co-occurring etiologies (eg, insomnia, chronic pain, anxiety), which can therefore lead to some confusion and frustration of both patients and providers when headaches become refractory to treatment.

PTHs are defined as secondary headache disorders that start within 7 days after head trauma according to the International Classification of Headache Disorders.[28] A history of primary headache disorders before TBI and female gender have been found to be risk factors for the development of PTHs, although many ADSMs and veterans without such histories also present with PTH. Most patients suffering from PTH can expect resolution within 3 months postinjury; however, approximately 18% to 33% of PTHs can persist beyond 1 year.

PTH can present as several types, including migraines, tension, mixed tension/migraine, or cervicogenic headaches. This classification of the distinct types of headaches is important to identify during the clinical evaluation, as it will guide appropriate treatment and management. The process should begin with a detailed headache history and discussion of its temporal relationship with head trauma. A description of the location, severity, intensity, frequency, and associated symptoms (nausea, vomiting, photosensitivity) and a focused neurologic and musculoskeletal physical examination will help classify the type of the headache and thereby inform appropriate treatments.[4] Careful consideration should be given to identification of any potential "red flags" for headaches, including fever, weight loss, abrupt onset, awakening from sleep, or focal neurologic symptoms. Presence of red flags during the clinical history and examination should prompt more aggressive acute care management.

Comorbid symptoms and conditions also should be carefully discussed and considered before initiation of treatment. Comorbid symptoms, such as dizziness, cognitive difficulties, and visual difficulties, can complicate maintenance of treatment programs, whereas comorbid conditions such as pain, sleep, and psychological difficulties, may also significantly contribute to the headache syndrome and prevent efficacious treatment.[29] The presence of significant comorbid symptomology and conditions in patients with PTH is common among military service members and usually will necessitate careful coordination among providers so that a patient-centered approach is maintained.

Treatment and management of PTH should begin with an identification of the frequency, duration, and severity of the headaches. The use of headache logs is beneficial for both patient and provider, as they provide objective evidence to analyze headache characteristics; examine trends, patterns, and triggers; and monitor the success or failure of various treatment modalities. Treatment of PTH should include consideration of both pharmacologic and nonpharmacologic treatments. Pharmacologic treatment of PTH should be guided by the type of PTH (tension, migraines, cervicogenic, or mixed). Consideration should be given o the use of both abortive medications (eg, acetaminophen, nonsteroidal anti-inflammatory, triptans), as well as potential initiation of a preventive medication (eg, antiepileptics, tricyclic antidepressants, beta-blockers). When initiating abortive medications, caution should be made to avoid overuse of short-acting medications, particularly given the role they play in the development of rebound headaches. Consideration of other comorbidities and symptoms should be made when selecting a potential preventive medication to promote treatment of multiple symptoms with the same medication.[4] The use of a headache log is very useful when a preventive medication is initiated, as it will guide titration of the dose and provide feedback on its effectiveness.

Nonpharmacologic treatment should not be overlooked, as it will aid in reducing the reliance on medications as the primary treatment modality and will promote other more active strategies that patients can use. Such nonpharmacologic treatments include education on lifestyle modifications, physical therapy, relaxation therapy, mindfulness training, treatment for insomnia, biofeedback, and cognitive behavior therapy (CBT).

### Dizziness and Disequilibrium

One of the more complex neurobehavioral symptoms, especially in the chronic stage, is the development of dizziness and disequilibrium symptoms. The differential diagnosis of dizziness and disequilibrium is broad ranging and includes benign paroxysmal positional vertigo, central and/or peripheral vestibulopathy, peri-lymphatic fistulas, labyrinthine concussion, migraines, visual dysfunction, cervicogenic or vertebral-basilar insufficiency, temporal bone fractures, dysautonomia, psychological disorders, medication side effects, and idiopathic etiologies.[30] This broad scope of potential etiologies therefore requires a careful, deliberate approach that, as always, begins with a careful assessment to discuss the characteristics of the symptoms, a description of the onset and frequency patterns, identification of triggers, and a review of systems and comorbidities, followed by a physical examination. This careful approach will then determine necessary next steps in the assessment stage (eg, imaging, visual assessments, mental health referrals) and will also determine the need to request further vestibular assessments (via otolaryngology, audiology, or vestibular rehabilitation) if an underlying vestibular etiology is suspected. Pharmacologic treatments (ie, meclizine, scopolamine, dimenhydrinate) for dizziness are generally not recommended due to their tendency to increase the likelihood of reliance on medications, rather than allowing physiologic central compensation to develop.[31]

### Visual Difficulties

Visual difficulties are commonly overlooked symptoms after mTBI. However, visual difficulties can significantly impact frequency of headaches, reading and comprehension, and concentration, and can also contribute to dizziness/balance symptoms. Common visual difficulties in veterans with TBI include photosensitivity, convergence insufficiency, accommodative dysfunction, oculomotor dysfunction, and visual field defects.[32] Assessment should include inquiry about functional impacts on daily activities as well as review of medications and other comorbidities that may be contributing factors to visual difficulties. Consideration should be made to referral to optometry, neuro-ophthalmology, neurology, and/or visual rehabilitation if difficulties persist and continue to contribute to daily functioning. It is also important to approach visual difficulties in conjunction with other disciplines that may be treating symptoms impacted by vision. including headaches and cognitive and vestibular symptoms.

Consistent education and communication across disciplines will help to prevent patient confusion as improvements and/or setbacks occur during various treatment approaches.

### Posttraumatic Stress Disorder/Depression

Compared with the general population, individuals diagnosed with TBI are at an increased risk of developing depression, PTSD, anxiety,[33–36] changes in relationship status,[37] employment stability,[38] worse global outcomes and health-related quality of life,[39] and poorer overall satisfaction with life.[40] Specifically, polytrauma veterans and ADSMs have been found to struggle with multiple psychiatric and medical conditions, including depression, anxiety, substance misuse, chronic pain, and sleep disorders, with estimates ranging from 25% to 50% for major depression within the first year following injury,[35,41] and 12% to 20% for PTSD.[42] Inversely, those with mTBI and comorbid mood disorders are also more likely to report higher levels of PCS, such as fatigue, frustration, somatic complaints, and concentration difficulties,[23,43–45] which further contribute to poorer TBI recovery, increased disability beliefs/rates, and more complicated treatment needs (ie, increased medical visits).[23,42,46,47]

Despite the common occurrence of overlapping complex medical and psychiatric conditions, a lack of standardized practices for assessing and treating comorbid mood and TBI have yet to be established. The DoD/VA Clinical Practice Guidelines for the Management of Concussion (2016)[4] asserts that comorbid conditions, including anxiety, depression, and substance abuse, should be treated both pharmacologically and psychotherapeutically, regardless of etiology.

Oftentimes, this approach leads to silos of care in which ADSMs and polytrauma veterans are treated separately and perhaps independently by medical, rehabilitation, and mental health providers. For example, mental health providers may be reluctant to provide treatment because of unfamiliarity with the polytrauma population and/or beliefs that certain treatments are contraindicated among those with comorbid TBI. Similarly, medical and rehabilitation providers may send polytrauma veterans to clinics to separately address cognitive complaints (eg, poor attention, memory), pain/orthopedic issues, multisensory problems (eg, vestibular, oculomotor), not knowing that comorbid mood disorders also contribute to worse/prolonged PCS including cognitive problems, sleep difficulties, somatic complaints, as well as vestibular symptoms.[19,22,48,49]

To date, interventions such as prolonged exposure and cognitive processing therapy, which involve a combination of cognitive restructuring and exposure to the trauma memory have a well-established evidence base for treating PTSD and mTBI.[50,51] A recent study by Wolf and colleagues[23] revealed preliminary evidence (with large treatment effect sizes) for the use of a trauma-focused treatment among polytrauma veterans in reducing symptoms of PTSD, as well as PCS, regardless of their etiology. Results also revealed that injury severity, treatment setting (ie, inpatient vs outpatient), and active-duty versus veteran status were unrelated to reductions in PCS. This finding is also supported among PREP patients, as well as via PREP outcome data (see **Fig. 3**). Outcome data have shown statistically significant improvements in mood symptomatology as well as overall neurobehavioral symptom scores (ie, PCS) secondary to engagement in trauma-focused therapy. Qualitatively, PREP patients also typically report improvements in overall cognitive functioning, sleep difficulties, pain complaints, and so forth after engaging in rehabilitation therapy with a behavioral health/trauma–focused treatment component.

There are numerus other treatment modalities also gaining evidence-based support for the treatment of PTSD (**Table 2**). These include skills training in affective and

**Table 2**
Evidence-Based approach to treatment of co-occurring Depression & Post-traumatic Stress Disorder

| Symptom | Medications | Rehabilitation Therapies | Behavioral Interventions | Adjunctive Approaches |
|---|---|---|---|---|
| Depression | Selective serotonin reuptake inhibitors (SSRIs)[52]<br>Serotonin norepinephrine reuptake inhibitors (SNRIs)<br>Tricyclic antidepressants (TCAs)<br>Dopamine reuptake inhibitors (DRIs)<br>Mood stabilizers | PT approved daily exercise | Cognitive behavior therapy for depression (CBT-D)[53]<br>Supportive psychotherapy[54]<br>Behavioral therapy: Behavioral activation[53]<br>Interpersonal therapy (IPT)<br>Mindfulness-based treatments[55] | Acceptance and commitment therapy (ACT)[56]<br>Biofeedback or neurofeedback[57]<br>Motivational interviewing (MI)[58]<br>Mental health treatment to address:<br>• Sleep<br>• Chronic pain<br>• Marital/family functioning<br>• Occupational distress<br>• Substance abuse |
| Posttraumatic stress disorder | SSRIs[52] (sertraline and paroxetine)<br>SNRIs[52] (fluoxetine and venlafaxine)<br>TCAs<br>Mood stabilizers<br>Prazosin[52] | Physical therapy approved daily exercise<br>Art therapy[25] | Prolonged exposure (PE)[51]<br>Cognitive processing therapy (CPT)[50] | Eye movement desensitization and reprocessing (EMDR)[59]<br>MI[60]<br>Dialectical behavior therapy (DBT)[60]<br>Acceptance and commitment therapy (ACT)[61,62]<br>Mindfulness-based treatments[63]<br>Trauma-informed guilt reduction therapy (TrIGR)[64]<br>Skills training in affective and interpersonal regulation (STAIR)[65]<br>Written exposure therapy (WET)[66]<br>Biofeedback and neurofeedback[57]<br>Mental health treatment to address:<br>• Sleep<br>• Chronic pain<br>• Marital/family functioning<br>• Occupational distress<br>• Substance abuse |

interpersonal regulation (STAIR), particularly for veterans with military sexual trauma and childhood trauma,[65] and dialectical behavioral therapy, which is effective in treating veterans with PTSD who are high risk for suicide.[60] However, such treatments, among others, remain as adjunctive treatments until evidence of their effectiveness among a polytrauma population is established.

Research also supports therapies including CBT, behavioral activation, supportive therapy, interpersonal therapy, and mindfulness, to be effective in treating depression and PCS among those with mTBI.[53–55,67] Additional therapy modalities effective with the treatment of depression also remain as adjunctive (see **Table 2**) until further evidence supporting their effectiveness among a polytrauma population is gleaned.

Currently there are no treatments approved by the Food and Drug Administration (FDA) for treating PCS, and study results assessing medication use among comorbid TBI and mood are limited. That said, selective serotonin reuptake inhibitors are generally supported as first-line medications in the treatment of PTSD and depression by the FDA, although studies evaluating the effectiveness among TBI populations is mixed.[39,52,67] Additional medications, including fluoxetine, venlafaxine, and prazosin, have also shown promise in treating comorbid PTSD and TBI.[52] In general, however, consensus among prescribers is to "start low and go slow," while being vigilant to possible drug interactions, symptom exacerbations, or medication side effects (ie, increased cognitive impairment, lowered seizure threshold, multisensory issues) that may differentially impact TBI symptomatology and recovery. Inclusion of certain medications should be reviewed with other treatment providers, as some may be contraindicated in certain treatment modalities. For example, the use of benzodiazepines, which may be used for anxiety and insomnia, are often discouraged when patients are engaged in exposure-based therapies for PTSD.

Despite high rates of comorbid depression, PTSD, and anxiety, many ADSMs and veterans do not actually receive mental health treatment.[39,42,46] Barriers to receiving effective treatment for comorbid TBI and mood include challenges such as access to VA care, work/child care demands, geographic location, lack of access to clinicians trained in treating comorbid conditions, as well as mental health stigma, military cultural biases, and other personal factors (eg, time, financial stress). The stigma associated with mental health treatment should not be underestimated. Up to 50% of veterans diagnosed with PTSD do not seek mental health treatment, and for many others who do initiate PTSD therapy, 15% to 30% do not complete treatment.[18] Understanding PTSD and the role the symptom of avoidance plays in a patient's life and daily decision making, such as avoiding socializing/crowds (eg, attending treatment appointments), fear of being exposed to triggers that may elicit trauma memories (eg, trauma exposure therapy), engagement (of any kind), or the understandable preference that their symptoms are explained by a physical or neurologic injury rather than due to a mental health condition, which, unfortunately for many, may be wrongly perceived as a personal weakness. It is because of this overlapping symptom complexity that a holistic approach including medical staff, rehabilitation providers, and mental health clinicians for the treatment of polytrauma veterans and ADSMs is strongly suggested and proven to be effective within the Tampa VA's PREP.

### Sleep Disturbances

Sleep-wake disturbances are among the most prevalent and persistent sequelae of TBI.[68] Nearly 60% of people with brain injury experience long-term difficulties with sleep. More specifically, patients suffering from TBI of any severity commonly report insomnia, excessive daytime sleepiness, increased sleep need (also known as pleosomnia), and sleep fragmentation,[69–71] as well as other unique sleep-wake sequelae.

Clinical evaluation and treatment of these sleep-wake disorders needs to be an integral component of any interdisciplinary approach in the rehabilitation of patients with mTBI/polytrauma.

Sleep-wake disturbances are common in the chronic phase of brain injury. In a meta-analysis of 1706 survivors of TBI, the most common sleep disturbances were insomnia (50%), poor sleep efficiency on polysomnography (PSG) (49%), early morning awakenings (38%), and nightmares (27%).[72] Sleep-related breathing and movement disorders are also prevalent in the chronic phases of TBI, with a reported prevalence of obstructive sleep apnea (OSA) ranging from 25% to 35%.[70,73]

Clinical insomnia refers to a group of symptoms including difficulty initiating and maintaining sleep, sleep fragmentation, and early morning awakenings. Unlike most other sleep disturbances after TBI, insomnia is more prevalent in mTBI compared with moderate or severe TBI.[74] The presence of insomnia correlates with decreased satisfaction in life, anxiety, and depression.[75] A retrospective study of 202 patients with TBI (37% with moderate to severe TBI) at a mean of 2 years postinjury found 65% of patients with mTBI complained of insomnia, compared with 41% of patients with moderate to severe TBI. Approximately one-quarter of patients with mTBI continued to complain of insomnia 5 years postinjury.[74] Among military personnel, the incidence of insomnia appears to increase in a dose-dependent fashion with the number of head injuries incurred, ranging from 6% in those with no history of TBI, 20% after a single TBI, and 50% in those with multiple episodes.[76]

There is preliminary evidence that circadian rhythm disorders, including delayed sleep phase or irregular sleep-wake type, occur with increased frequency in patients with TBI. Symptoms of a circadian rhythm disorder are easy to overlook, as they are often misattributed to insomnia. In one study, 36% of individuals who complained of insomnia after mTBI instead met criteria for a circadian rhythm disorder.[77,78] The distinction is important, because treatment approaches differ.

Excessive daytime sleepiness, distinct from fatigue and pleosomnia, is a prominent symptom after TBI. The reported frequency in patients with TBI ranges from 50% to 80%, compared with an expected rate in the general population of 10% to 25%.[79] Excessive daytime sleepiness refers to the inability to maintain wakefulness and alertness during the major waking episodes of the day, with sleep occurring unintentionally or at inappropriate times.[80] Sleepiness manifests mainly during sedentary activities, in contrast to fatigue, which typically affects pursuit of more active goals.

Pleosomnia (increased sleep need in a 24-hour cycle) is common after TBI. This term is more precise than "hypersomnia," which is often used interchangeably for both excessive daytime sleepiness and increased sleep need.[81] In a prospective case control study that included 42 patients with TBI studied 6 months after injury, patients who were post-TBI slept 1.2 hours more than matched controls.[82,83] This pattern persisted at 18 months.[83] Findings also demonstrated that these patients with TBI underestimated both excessive daytime sleepiness and pleosomnia. In addition, daytime sleepiness was more pronounced in patients with TBI with shorter sleep duration, suggesting that sleepiness might constitute an epiphenomenon of insufficient sleep in subjects needing more sleep than usual.

Sleep-related breathing disorders, including OSA and central sleep apnea (CSA), occur with increased frequency after TBI. Studies have found an OSA prevalence ranging from 25% to 35% in TBI survivors, which is higher than rates in most general population-based studies.[70,84,85] Many symptoms of OSA overlap with those of TBI as well as other sleep-wake disorders. The most common symptoms of OSA in the general population are daytime sleepiness and loud snoring. Additional symptoms include waking up gasping or choking, morning headaches, nocturia, moodiness or irritability, lack of concentration, and memory impairment. On physical examination, patients are often obese and may have evidence of a crowded oropharynx and increased neck circumference. Clinical features of CSA are similar, except that obesity is less likely to be present.

Sleep-wake disorders are common after TBI and should be suspected in patients presenting with a broad range of sleep complaints. The goals of the evaluation are to define the sleep complaint, diagnose specific treatable sleep disorders, and identify any additional medical and psychiatric comorbidities that may be contributing to the sleep disturbances. Most sleep-wake disorders are diagnosed using a combination of both subjective and objective screening tools in the clinic.[86] Subjective tools include a sleep history and questionnaires completed by patients and/or their bed partners, whereas objective tools include actigraphy, PSG, multiple sleep latency test, and the maintenance of wakefulness test. Generally, patients with TBI may overestimate insomnia complaints, and underestimate pleosomnia and/or excessive daytime sleepiness.[79,82,87,88] These observations stress the importance of objective sleep testing in patients with TBI. There are several structured and validated screening tools, including the Pittsburgh Sleep Quality Index and the Epworth Sleepiness Scale. Questions should target multiple sleep domains, including perceived sleep quality, sleep latency, sleep duration, sleep disturbances (including abnormal movements or behaviors during sleep), sleep medication use, daytime dysfunction, and daytime sleepiness. A sleep diary or log, to be completed by the patient in advance or following the initial evaluation, can be particularly helpful to supplement the history.[89] Finally, given the frequent comorbidity of psychiatric disorders in patients with TBI and their implications for treatment, the history should also probe for symptoms of depression, anxiety, and PTSD.

Pharmacologic and behavioral approaches for insomnia in patients with a history of TBI are generally similar to those in the general population, with the caveat that there may well be greater sensitivity to side effects in the latter. For example, special attention should be paid to cognitive impairment, vestibular or visual disturbances, headache exacerbation, and the like from medications.

With all pharmacologic therapies for insomnia, patients should be treated with the lowest effective dose and for the shortest time possible.[90] Limited data in patients with TBI suggest that benzodiazepine and nonbenzodiazepine receptor agonists are similarly effective but generally only for brief periods if necessary.[91] Any drug that can cross the blood-brain barrier has the potential to impact a person's sleep. Therefore, the full prescribed and over-the-counter medication list should be carefully reviewed in all patients with TBI. A wide variety of medications used in the management of TBI may contribute to daytime sleepiness or aggravate insomnia, including antiepileptics, opioids, benzodiazepines, antipsychotics, antidepressants, neurostimulants, and glucocorticoids. Also, substances of abuse, including alcohol, nicotine, caffeine, and illicit recreational drugs also are relevant.

Behavioral approaches that have been studied in the TBI population include CBT for insomnia and acupuncture.[92,93] In one small randomized study, acupuncture did not affect objective measures of sleep by actigraphy but did improve subjective sleep quality, cognitive function, and the ability to taper sleep medication use. Further, if sleep disturbances are driven by PTSD-related nightmares, then appropriate PTSD intervention should be one of the primary interventions used.

All parasomnias are exacerbated by sleep deprivation or sleep fragmentation, and therefore the first-line approach to treatment is to identify and treat causes of poor sleep quality (ie, improve sleep hygiene, avoid alcohol, and treat sleep apnea and restless legs syndrome). PTSD-related nightmares can be effectively treated with prazosin and/or image-rehearsal therapy with or without CBT for insomnia.[94]

In patients with rapid eye movement (REM) sleep behavior disorder, which can result in violent dream enactment, establishing a safe sleeping environment is the primary goal of treatment. This can be achieved through modification of the sleep environment and pharmacotherapy, if necessary. Medications known to cause or exacerbate REM sleep behavior disorder, such as serotonin reuptake inhibitors, serotonin norepinephrine reuptake inhibitors, and tricyclic antidepressants, should be discontinued or avoided if possible. Low-dose clonazepam and high-dose melatonin are effective therapies in patients with frequent, disruptive, or injurious behaviors.[94–96]

Individuals with OSA in the post-TBI setting should be treated similar to those without brain injury, including weight loss, positive airway pressure therapy, and behavioral modifications. The potential consequences of untreated OSA in patients with TBI were illustrated by a small case control study that included 19 patients with TBI with OSA and 16 patients with TBI without OSA on nocturnal PSG.[97] Patients with OSA performed significantly worse than those without OSA on tasks of sustained attention and memory.

Treatment for the various sleep-wake disorders discussed are numerous and vary according to the dominant symptom or specific sleep disorder as well as relevant comorbidities. Beyond symptomatic improvement, the potential benefits of successful treatment of sleep-wake disorders in the TBI population include improvement in functional outcomes, cognition, mood, perceived pain, headache, and quality of life.[98,99]

## Interdisciplinary Versus Silo of Care

Throughout this discussion of some of the major neurobehavioral symptoms, it is obvious that the assessment and development of a treatment plan for each symptom can quickly become complex with many variables to consider. Common comorbidities that exist in the polytrauma veteran population (ie, PTSD, depression, chronic pain, sleep difficulties) also have very similar symptom profiles (see **Fig. 1**), and therefore assessment of those comorbidities becomes imperative.[100,101] Typically, veterans first present to their primary care physicians with complaints of headaches and/or cognitive problems within the context of a recent or remote history of mTBI. From that point, a thorough assessment of the injury, symptoms, and comorbidities occurs, followed by the development of a treatment plan, which is likely to include a combination of medication initiation, diagnostic testing, and consultations. From there, the potential exists to begin a cascade of events that can lead to disjointed treatment plans (ie, independent lanes of care) and unexpected negative consequences. This cascade of events can include the following:

- Medication failure and/or the development of side effects
- Confusion or increased frustration regarding any normal diagnostic studies
- Overemphasis on incidental findings from diagnostic evaluations
- Delays in completion of consultation appointments
- Conflicting education/interpretation from consultants
- Additional medication initiation and diagnostic testing requested by consultants
- Further medication side effects, drug interactions, and potential therapeutic failures
- Unclear findings on further diagnostic evaluations
- Enlarged network of providers involved in care
- Possible confusion and increased frustration regarding lack of improvement and/ or identification of etiologies
- Increased symptomatology secondary to frustration

- Disengagement with providers
- Increased risk of self-medication and unguided trials of experimental treatments

When "Silos of Care" develop in outpatient clinical care settings, providers often treat veterans independently and without discussion/consultation from other disciplines that are involved in the care. Subsequently, veterans oftentimes become the messenger between providers, which increases the risk of conflict, confusion, and misunderstandings. Although this string of events can occur even when providers have the best intentions during evaluations/treatments, such events occur secondary to the complex overlap of symptom comorbidities, and the traditional outpatient medical care models that are not designed to allow enough flexibility (ie, due to time constraints, separate provider locations, complexity of appointment scheduling, insurance coverage) to prevent these pitfalls.

To combat the previously described series of events that is common with the neurobehavioral management of mTBI/polytrauma, an interdisciplinary approach is highly recommended.[102] The diversity of symptoms will necessitate a diverse specialized group of disciplines that can guide assessment and treatment planning for PCS, psychological difficulties, chronic pain, and sleep difficulties. Interdisciplinary teams, when designed and implemented correctly, will begin a coordinated assessment period that will lead to consistent nonconflicting education, even when diagnostic testing is unrevealing. Well-designed teams can communicate across disciplines to improve each individual provider evaluation. This might include an observation that increased anxiety triggers a dizziness episode or migraine headaches affect a patient's concentration during a session. These may be patterns the patient was not aware of and therefore never reported. When those types of observations occur, and are communicated to the other disciplines, each provider then has more information to consider for diagnostic and treatment planning. In addition, when patients and family members witness this communication between providers, the effect becomes that of improved trust and confidence with the treatment team, as well as increased insight into their symptom presentation and functioning. This can then lead the patient to begin to accept more difficult treatment protocols (ie, psychological treatments, intensive vestibular rehabilitation programs, cognitive therapies) that the same patient may have been resistant to in the past. Standard recommendations are to focus on the treatment of symptoms, regardless of the potential etiology.[102] A focus on reduction of the symptom burden and improving overall functioning are generally well-received goals for polytrauma veterans. Published literature is still limited in demonstrating effectiveness of interdisciplinary treatments in this population. However, recent studies demonstrate a reduction in self-reported neurobehavioral symptoms when an interdisciplinary approach is applied in specialty care clinics.[103]

The PREP program was specifically developed and designed to combat the effects of silos of care, and provide the ideal setting for an interdisciplinary team to guide the assessments and treatment of the patients with polytrauma/mTBI. Commonly, evaluations, education, and a few isolated treatment/therapy recommendations, is all that is required for this population. However, when evaluations lead to multiple physical, cognitive, and psychological therapy recommendations, then follow through with these extensive and intensive treatment recommendations can become burdensome and lead to treatment failures. For these situations, the PREP program would provide extension within the program to facilitate and coordinate rehabilitation and mental health treatment protocols. These would include vestibular and vision rehabilitation, cognitive therapy, pain treatments (medical

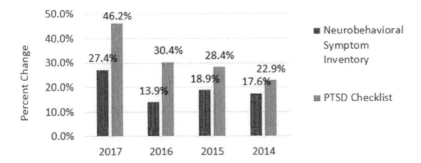

Neurobehavioral Symptom Inventory (NSI) is self-report inventory of 22 postconcussive symptoms rated on a 5-item scale (range 0 to 88) was used. Participants indicate the extent to which each symptom has disturbed them in the previous two weeks. The NSI has been shown to have high internal consistency and test-retest reliability.
PTSD Checklist (PCL)

**Fig. 2.** Advances made with neurobehavioral and PTSD symptoms.

and behavioral), sleep management, and PTSD treatment with exposure-based psychotherapies. When treated together, significant gains have been made with neurobehavioral symptoms, as well as in PTSD symptoms **(Fig. 2)**.[104] This example further emphasizes the importance of interdisciplinary approaches to managing neurobehavioral symptoms in veterans with mTBI/polytrauma. The role that the interdisciplinary team served during assessments and evaluations, also is important to maintain during treatment of these patients. As treatment and therapies proceed throughout the various disciplines, it becomes important to manage patients' expectations as well as maintain support and motivation to patients if they encounter setbacks or side effects to treatments.

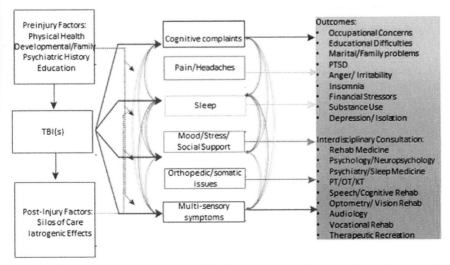

**Fig. 3.** Holistic treatment approaches. KT, kinesiotherapy; OT, occupational therapy; PT, physical therapy;

## SUMMARY

Over the past decade there has been increased recognition that more structured and empirically supported diagnostics and interventions aimed at the mTBI/polytrauma population are needed. Although effective clinical practice guidelines exist for each of these various conditions, the potential unintended negative consequence of treating comorbid conditions separately rather than holistically, raises understandable concerns. For example, if a patient's cognitive complaints or increased irritability are attributed to their history of concussion(s), providers might initiate a treatment protocol that addresses neurologic changes, such as medication or cognitive rehabilitation. However, if those same complaints were demonstrated to be the result of undiagnosed or untreated PTSD, a very different treatment protocol would be initiated. The use of interdisciplinary teams for this complex population not only improves diagnostic accuracy, but by initiating appropriate treatment protocols, patients are more likely to experience positive symptom change. By fully understanding what comorbid conditions are present, a provider is then able to identify what conditions are driving the patient's current neurobehavioral symptom complaints. The interdisciplinary team can then work toward reducing patient burden (excessive appointments and therapies), reducing overutilization of health care services for refractory symptoms, and, most importantly, assist these veterans with improved reintegration into civilian life. Holistic treatment approaches that include a coordinated care approach to address the complex needs of this population should be the gold standard of care (**Fig. 3**).

## REFERENCES

1. Department of Veterans Affairs. Cumulative from 1st qtr FY 2002 through 3rd qtr FY 2015 (October 1, 2001 – June 30, 2015). In: Department of Veterans Affairs, editor. Epidemiology program postdeployment health program. Washington, DC: Analysis of VA health care utilization among Operation Enduring Freedom (OEF), Operation Iraqi Freedom (OIF), and Operation New Dawn (OND) veterans; 2017. p. 1–11.
2. Wortzel HS, Arciniegas DB. Treatment of post-traumatic cognitive impairments. Curr Treat Options Neurol 2012;14(5):493–508.
3. Chen AJ. Optimizing cognitive functioning after TBI. New York: Syllabus for course at The American Academy of Neurology Institute; 2017.
4. Department of Defense. DoD policy guidance for management of mild traumatic brain injury/concussion in the deployed setting. 2012; DoDi 6490.11(September).
5. Bell KR, Hoffman JM, Temkin NR, et al. The effect of telephone counselling on reducing post-traumatic symptoms after mild traumatic brain injury: a randomised trial. J Neurol Neurosurg Psychiatry 2008;79(11):1275–81.
6. Mittenberg W, Tremont G, Zielinski RE, et al. Cognitive-behavioral prevention of postconcussion syndrome. Arch Clin Neuropsychol 1996;11(2):139–45.
7. Mittenberg W, Zielinski RE, Fichera S. Recovery from mild head injury: a treatment manual for patients. Psychotherapy in Private Practice 1993;12:37–52.
8. Paniak C, Toller-Lobe G, Durand A, et al. A randomized trial of two treatments for mild traumatic brain injury. Brain Inj 1998;12(12):1011–123.
9. Thornton K. Improvement/rehabilitation of memory functioning with neurotherapy/QEEG biofeedback. J Head Trauma Rehabil 2000;15(6):1285–96.
10. Fernandez-Mendoza J, Calhoun S, Bixler EO, et al. Insomnia with objective short sleep duration is associated with deficits in neuropsychological performance: a general population study. Sleep 2010;33(4):459–65.

11. Martindale SL, Morissette SB, Rowland JA, et al. Sleep quality affects cognitive functioning in returning combat veterans beyond combat exposure, PTSD, and mild TBI history. Neuropsychology 2017;31(1):93–104.
12. Verfaellie M, Lee LO, Lafleche G, et al. Self-reported sleep disturbance mediates the relationship between PTSD and cognitive outcome in blast-exposed OEF/OIF veterans. J Head Trauma Rehabil 2016;31(5):309–19.
13. Sufrinko AM, Marchetti GF, Cohen PE, et al. Using acute performance on a comprehensive neurocognitive, vestibular, and ocular motor assessment battery to predict recovery duration after sport-related concussions. Am J Sports Med 2017;45(5):1187–94.
14. Defense and Veterans Brain Injury Center (DVBIC). DoD worldwide TBI numbers, 2000-2017. 2018.
15. McCrea MA. Mild traumatic brain injury and postconcussion syndrome. New Yorks: Oxford University Press; 2008.
16. Belanger HG, Curtiss G, Demery JA, et al. Factors moderating neuropsychological outcomes following mild traumatic brain injury: a meta analysis. J Int Neuropsychol Soc 2005;11:215–27.
17. Hoge C, McGurk D, Thomas J, et al. Mild traumatic brain injury in U.S. soldiers returning from Iraq. N Engl J Med 2008;358:453–63.
18. Fischer H. In congressional research service report: a guide to U.S. military casualty statistics: operation Freedom's sentinel, operation inherent resolve, operation New Dawn, Operation Iraqi Freedom, and Operation Enduring Freedom. 2015.
19. Vanderploeg RD, Belanger HG, Curtiss G. Mild traumatic brain injury and posttraumatic stress disorder and their associations with health symptoms. Arch Phys Med Rehabil 2009;90(7):1084–93.
20. Lew HL, Otis JD, Tun C, et al. Prevalence of chronic pain, posttraumatic stress disorder, and persistent postconcussive symptoms in OIF/OEF veterans: polytrauma clinical triad. J Rehabil Res Dev 2009;46(6):697–702.
21. Mittenberg W, DiGiulio DV, Perrin S, et al. Symptoms following mild head injury: expectation as aetiology. J Neurol Neurosurg Psychiatry 1992;55:200–4.
22. Shandera-Ochsner AL, Berry DT, Harp JP, et al. Neuropsychological effects of self-reported deployment-related mild TBI and current PTSD in OIF/OEF veterans. Clin Neurospsychol 2013;27(6):881–907.
23. Wolf GK, Mauntel GJ, Kretzmer T, et al. Comorbid posttraumatic stress disorder and traumatic brain injury: generalization of prolonged-exposure PTSD treatment outcomes to postconcussive symptoms, cognition, and self-efficacy in veterans and active duty service members. J Head Trauma Rehabil 2018;33(2):E53.
24. Tinius TP, Tinius KA. Changes after EEG biofeedback and cognitive retraining in adults with mild traumatic brain injury and attention deficit hyperactivity disorder. J Neurother 2000;4(2):27–44.
25. Walker MS, Kaimal G, Gonzaga AM, et al. Active-duty military service members' visual representations of PTSD and TBI in masks. Int J Qual Stud Health Well-being 2017;12(1):1267317.
26. Cicerone KD, Langenbahn DM, Braden C, et al. Evidence-based cognitive rehabilitation: updated review of the literature from 2003 through 2008. Arch Phys Med Rehabil 2011;92(4):519–30.
27. Uomoto JM, Esselman PC. Traumatic brain injury and chronic pain: differential types and rates by head injury severity. Arch Phys Med Rehabil 1993;74(1):61–4.

28. Silberstein SD, Olesen J, Bousser MG, et al. The international classification of headache disorders, 2nd edition (ICHD-II)—revision of criteria for 8.2 medication-overuse headache. Cephalalgia 2005;25(6):460–5.
29. Theeler B, Lucas S, Riechers RG 2nd, et al. Post-traumatic headaches in civilian and military personnel: a comparative, clinical review. Headache 2013;53(6): 881–900.
30. Staab JP, Puckenstein MJ. Expanding the differential diagnosis of chronic dizziness. Arch Otolaryngol Head Neck Surg 2007;133(2):170–6.
31. Hain TC, Yacovino D. Pharmacologic treatment of persons with dizziness. Neurol Clin 2005;23(3):831–53.
32. Brahm KD, Wilgengurg HM, Kirby J, et al. Visual impairment and dysfunction in combat-injured service members with traumatic brain injury. Optom Vis Sci 2009;86(7):817–25.
33. Iverson KM, Hendricks AM, Kimerling R, et al. Psychiatric diagnoses and neurobehavioral symptom severity among OEF/OIF VA patients with deployment-related traumatic brain injury: a gender comparison. Womens Health Issues 2011;21(4 Suppl):S210–7.
34. Osborn AJ, Mathias JL, Fairweather-Schmidt AK, et al. Anxiety and comorbid depression following traumatic brain injury in a community-based sample of young, middle-aged and older adults. J Affect Disord 2016;213:214–21.
35. Scholten AC, Haagsma JA, Cnossen MC, et al. Prevalence of and risk factors for anxiety and depressive disorders after traumatic brain injury: a systematic review. J Neurotrauma 2016;33(22):1969–94.
36. Zaninotto AL, Vicentini JE, Fregni F, et al. Updates and current perspectives of psychiatric assessments after traumatic brain injury: a systematic review. Front Psychiatry 2016;7:95.
37. Stevens LF, Lapis Y, Tang X, et al. Relationship stability after traumatic brain injury among veterans and service members: a VA TBI model systems study. J Head Trauma Rehabil 2017;32(4):234–44.
38. Dillahunt-Aspillaga C, Nakase-Richardson R, Hart T, et al. Predictors of employment outcomes in veterans with traumatic brain injury: a VA traumatic brain injury model systems study. J Head Trauma Rehabil 2017;32(4):271–82.
39. Fann JR, Hart T, Schomer KG. Treatment for depression after traumatic brain injury: a systematic review. J Neurotrauma 2009;26:2383–402.
40. Gause LR, Finn JA, Lamberty GJ, et al. Predictors of satisfaction with life in veterans after traumatic brain injury: a VA TBI model systems study. J Head Trauma Rehabil 2017;32(4):255–63.
41. Bombardier CH, Fann JR, Temkin NR, et al. Rates of major depressive disorder and clinical outcomes following traumatic brain injury. JAMA 2010;303(19): 1938–45.
42. Harvey MM, Rauch SA, Zalta AK, et al. Intensive treatment models to address posttraumatic stress among post-9/11 warriors: the warrior care network. Focus 2017;15:378–83.
43. Kreutzer J, Seel RT, Gourley E. The prevalence and symptom rates of depression after traumatic brain injury: a comprehensive examination. J Head Trauma Rehabil 2002;17(1):74–5.
44. Singh R, Mason S, Lecky F, et al. Prevalence of depression after TBI in a prospective cohort: the SHEFBIT study. Brain Inj 2017;32(1):84–90.
45. Vasterling JJ, Dikmen S. Mild traumatic brain injury and posttraumatic stress disorder: clinical and conceptual complexities. J Int Neuropsychol Soc 2012; 18(3):390–3.

46. Lavoie S, Sechrist S, Quach N, et al. Depression in men and women one year following traumatic brain injury (TBI): a TBI model systems study. Front Psychol 2017;8:634.

47. Miles SR, Harik JM, Hundt NE, et al. Delivery of mental health treatment to combat veterans with psychiatric diagnoses and TBI histories. PLoS One 2017; 12(9):e0184265.

48. Scott JC, Matt GE, Wrocklage KM, et al. A quantitative meta-analysis of neurocognitive functioning in posttraumatic stress disorder. Psychol Bull 2015;141(1): 105–40.

49. Vasterling JJ, Grande L, Graefe AC, et al. Neuropsychological assessment of posttraumatic stress disorder (PTSD). In: Armstrong C, Morrow L, editors. Handbook of medical neuropsychology: applications of cognitive neuroscience. New York: Springer; 2010. p. 447–65.

50. Chard KM, Schumm JA, McIlvain SM, et al. Exploring the efficacy of a residential treatment program incorporating cognitive processing therapy-cognitive for veterans with PTSD and traumatic brain injury. J Traumatic Stress 2011;24(3): 347–51.

51. Wolf GQ, Strom TK, Kehle SM, et al. A preliminary examination of prolonged exposure therapy with Iraq and Afghanistan veterans with a diagnosis of posttraumatic stress disorder and mild to moderate traumatic brain injury. J Head Trauma Rehabil 2012;27(1):26–32.

52. Yue JK, Burke JF, Upadhyayula PS, et al. Selective serotonin reuptake inhibitors for treating neurocognitive and neuropsychiatric disorders following traumatic brain injury: an evaluation of current evidence. Brain Sci 2017;7(8) [pii:E93].

53. Waldron B, Casserly LM, O'Sullivan C. Cognitive behavioural therapy for depression and anxiety in adults with acquired brain injury. What works for whom? Neuropsychol Rehabil 2012;23(1):64–101.

54. Ashman T, Cantor J, Gordon WA, et al. A randomized controlled trial of sertraline for the treatment of depression in persons with traumatic brain injury. Arch Phys Med Rehabil 2009;90(5):733–40.

55. Hollon SD, Ponniah K. A review of empirically supported psychological therapies for mood disorders in adults. Depress Anxiety 2010;27:891–932.

56. Forman EM, Herbert JD, Moirta E, et al. A randomized controlled effectiveness trial of acceptance and commitment therapy and cognitive therapy for anxiety and depression. Behav Modif 2007;31(6):772–99.

57. Yucha CB, Montgomery D. Evidence-based practice in biofeedback and neurofeedback. Washington, DC: Faculty Publications; 2008. Paper 1.

58. Arkowitz H, Burke BL. Motivational interviewing as an integrative framework for the treatment of depression. In: Arkowitz H, Westra HA, Miller WR, et al, editors. Applications of motivational interviewing. Motivational interviewing in the treatment of psychological problems. New York: Guilford Press; 2008. p. 145–272.

59. Sharpless BA, Barber JP. A clinician's guide to PTSD treatments for returning veterans. Prof Psychol Res Pr 2011;42(1):8–15.

60. Jakupcak M, Varra EM. Treating Iraq and Afghanistan war veterans with PTSD who are at high risk for suicide. Cogn Behav Pract 2011;18:85–97.

61. Orsillo SM, Batten SV. Acceptance and commitment therapy in the treatment of posttraumatic stress disorder. Behav Modif 2005;29(1):95–129.

62. Walder RD, Hayes SC. Acceptance and commitment therapy in the treatment of posttraumatic stress disorder: theoretical and applied issues. In: Follette VM, Ruzek JI, editors. Cognitive-behavioral therapies for trauma. 2nd edition. New

York: Guilford Press; 2006. Available at: https://actmindfully.com.au/upimages/ACT_in_the_Treatment_of_PTSD.pdf.
63. King AP, Erickson TM, Giardino ND, et al. A pilot study of group mindfulness-based cognitive therapy (MBCT) for combat veterans with posttraumatic stress disorder (PTSD). Depress Anxiety 2013;30(7):638–45.
64. Norman SB, Wilkins KC, Myers US, et al. Trauma informed guilt reduction therapy with combat veterans. Cogn Behav Pract 2014;1(21):78–88.
65. Cloitre M, Jackson C, Schmidt JA. Case reports: STAIR for strengthening social support and relationships among veterans with military sexual trauma and PTSD. Mil Med 2016;181(2):e183–7.
66. Sloan DM, Marx BP, Lee DJ, et al. A brief exposure-based treatment vs cognitive processing therapy for posttraumatic stress disorder: a randomized noninferiority clinical trial. JAMA Psychiatry 2018;75(3):233–9.
67. Vasterling JJ, Jacob SN, Rasmusson A. Traumatic brain injury and posttraumatic stress disorder: conceptual, diagnostic, and therapeutic considerations in the context of co-occurrence. J Neuropsychiatry Clin Neurosci 2018;30(2):91–100.
68. Ouellet MC, Beaulieu-Bonneau S, Morin CM. Sleep-wake disturbances after traumatic brain injury. Lancet Neurol 2015;14(7):746–57.
69. Baumann CR. Traumatic brain injury and disturbed sleep and wakefulness. Neuromolecular Med 2012;14:205.
70. Castriotta RJ, Wilde MC, Lai JM, et al. Prevalence and consequences of sleep disorders in traumatic brain injury. J Clin Sleep Med 2007;3:349.
71. Ouellet MC, Beaulieu-Bonneau S, Morin CM. Insomnia in patients with traumatic brain injury: frequency, characteristics, and risk factors. J Head Trauma Rehabil 2006;21:199.
72. Mathias JL, Alvaro PK. Prevalence of sleep disturbances, disorders, and problems following traumatic brain injury: a meta-analysis. Sleep Med 2012;13:898.
73. Collen J, Orr N, Lettieri CJ, et al. Sleep disturbances among soldiers with combat-related traumatic brain injury. Chest 2012;142:622.
74. Beetar JT, Guilmette TJ, Sparadeo FR. Sleep and pain complaints in symptomatic traumatic brain injury and neurologic populations. Arch Phys Med Rehabil 1996;77:1298.
75. Cantor JB, Bushnik T, Cicerone K, et al. Insomnia, fatigue, and sleepiness in the first 2 years after traumatic brain injury: an NIDRR TBI model system module study. J Head Trauma Rehabil 2012;27:E1.
76. Bryan CJ. Repetitive traumatic brain injury (or concussion) increases severity of sleep disturbance among deployed military personnel. Sleep 2013;36:941.
77. Weitzman ED, Czeisler CA, Zimmerman JC, et al. Biological rhythms in man: relationship of sleep-wake, cortisol, growth hormone, and temperature during temporal isolation. Adv Biochem Psychopharmacol 1981;28:475.
78. Williams BR, Lazic SE, Ogilvie RD. Polysomnographic and quantitative EEG analysis of subjects with long-term insomnia complaints associated with mild traumatic brain injury. Clin Neurophysiol 2008;119:429.
79. Masel BE, Scheibel RS, Kimbark T, et al. Excessive daytime sleepiness in adults with brain injuries. Arch Phys Med Rehabil 2001;82:1526.
80. American Academy of Sleep Medicine. International classification of sleep disorders. 3rd edition. Darien (IL): American Academy of Sleep Medicine; 2014.
81. Sommerauer M, Valko PO, Werth E, et al. Excessive sleep need following traumatic brain injury: a case-control study of 36 patients. J Sleep Res 2013;22:634.

82. Imbach LL, Valko PO, Li T, et al. Increased sleep need and daytime sleepiness 6 months after traumatic brain injury: a prospective controlled clinical trial. Brain 2015;138:726.

83. Imbach LL, Büchele F, Valko PO, et al. Sleep-wake disorders persist 18 months after traumatic brain injury but remain underrecognized. Neurology 2016;86: 1945.

84. Guilleminault C, Yuen KM, Gulevich MG, et al. Hypersomnia after head-neck trauma: a medicolegal dilemma. Neurology 2000;54:653.

85. Webster JB, Bell KR, Hussey JD, et al. Sleep apnea in adults with traumatic brain injury: a preliminary investigation. Arch Phys Med Rehabil 2001;82:316.

86. Mollayeva T, Colantonio A, Mollayeva S, et al. Screening for sleep dysfunction after traumatic brain injury. Sleep Med 2013;14:1235.

87. Parcell DL, Ponsford JL, Redman JR, et al. Poor sleep quality and changes in objectively recorded sleep after traumatic brain injury: a preliminary study. Arch Phys Med Rehabil 2008;89:843.

88. Watson NF, Dikmen S, Machamer J, et al. Hypersomnia following traumatic brain injury. J Clin Sleep Med 2007;3:363.

89. Mollayeva T, Kendzerska T, Colantonio A. Self-report instruments for assessing sleep dysfunction in an adult traumatic brain injury population: a systematic review. Sleep Med Rev 2013;17:411.

90. Flanagan SR, Greenwald B, Wieber S. Pharmacological treatment of insomnia for individuals with brain injury. J Head Trauma Rehabil 2007;22:67.

91. Li Pi Shan RS, Ashworth NL. Comparison of lorazepam and zopiclone for insomnia in patients with stroke and brain injury: a randomized, crossover, double-blinded trial. Am J Phys Med Rehabil 2004;83:421.

92. Ouellet MC, Morin CM. Efficacy of cognitive-behavioral therapy for insomnia associated with traumatic brain injury: a single-case experimental design. Arch Phys Med Rehabil 2007;88:1581.

93. Zollman FS, Larson EB, Wasek-Throm LK, et al. Acupuncture for treatment of insomnia in patients with traumatic brain injury: a pilot intervention study. J Head Trauma Rehabil 2012;27:135.

94. Seda G, Sanchez-Ortuno MM, Welsh CH, et al. Comparative meta-analysis of prazosin and imagery rehearsal therapy for nightmare frequency, sleep quality, and posttraumatic stress. J Clin Sleep Med 2015;11:11.

95. Kemp S, Biswas R, Neumann V, et al. The value of melatonin for sleep disorders occurring post-head injury: a pilot RCT. Brain Inj 2004;18:911.

96. Nagtegaal JE, Kerkhof GA, Smits MG, et al. Traumatic brain injury-associated delayed sleep phase syndrome. Funct Neurol 1997;12:345.

97. Wilde MC, Castriotta RJ, Lai JM, et al. Cognitive impairment in patients with traumatic brain injury and obstructive sleep apnea. Arch Phys Med Rehabil 2007; 88:1284.

98. Makley MJ, English JB, Drubach DA, et al. Prevalence of sleep disturbance in closed head injury patients in a rehabilitation unit. Neurorehabil Neural Repair 2008;22:341.

99. Wiseman-Hakes C, Murray B, Moineddin R, et al. Evaluating the impact of treatment for sleep/wake disorders on recovery of cognition and communication in adults with chronic TBI. Brain Inj 2013;27:1364.

100. Vanderploeg RD, Belanger HG, Horner RD, et al. Health outcomes associated with military deployment: mild traumatic brain injury, blast, trauma, and combat associations in the Florida National Guard. Arch Phys Med Rehabil 2012;93(11): 1887–95.

101. Belanger H, Kretzmer T, Vanderploeg RD, et al. Symptom complaints following combat-related traumatic brain injury: relationship to traumatic brain injury severity and post-traumatic stress disorder. J Int Neuropsychol Soc 2010;16: 194–9.
102. Wicklund A, Gaviria M. Multidisciplinary approach to psychiatric symptoms in mild traumatic brain injury: complex sequelae necessitate a cadre of treatment providers. Surg Neurol Int 2013;4(1):50.
103. Janak JC, Cooper DB, Bowles AO, et al. Completion of multidisciplinary treatment for persistent postconcussive symptoms is associated with reduced symptom burden. J Head Trauma Rehabil 2017;32(1):1–15.
104. Cicerone KD, Kalmar K. Persistent postconcussion syndrome: the structure of subjective complaints after mild traumatic brain injury. J Head Trauma Rehab 1995;10:1–17.

# Rehabilitation Assessment and Management of Neurosensory Deficits After Traumatic Brain Injury in the Polytrauma Veteran

Saurabha Bhatnagar, MD[a],*, Meredith Anderson, DO[b],
Michael Chu, DO[b], Daniel Kuo, DO[b], Ogo Azuh, MD[b]

## KEYWORDS

• Traumatic brain injury • Headache • Sleep • Fatigue • Vestibular • Auditory • Vision

## KEY POINTS

• Disability after traumatic brain injury can in part be related to neurosensory deficits.
• Common neurosensory deficits include headache, sleep-related issues, fatigue and vestibular, auditory, or visual dysfunctions.
• Posttraumatic headaches often self resolve within the first year of injury and can be managed with pharmacology, interventions and therapy. Imagining not recommended for evaluation of PTH.

## INTRODUCTION

Each year, approximately 1.7 million Americans have a traumatic brain injury (TBI); more than 5 million of those hospitalized for a TBI are currently living with a disability.[1] Some have postulated this figure to be underestimated, as some patients with mild TBIs (mTBIs) do not seek medical care.[1] TBIs can be caused by a variety mechanisms, including motor vehicle accidents, falls, assaults, strikes or blows to the head, biking or sporting accidents, and blast injuries from military conflicts.[2] More than 650,000 annual cases of TBI are attributed to falls and motor vehicle accidents[3]; more than 250,000 service members have been diagnosed with a TBI from the Afghanistan and Iraq conflicts.[4]

Disclosure Statement: The authors have nothing to disclose.
a Department of Physical Medicine and Rehabilitation, Harvard Medical School, Massachusetts General Hospital, Spaulding Rehabilitation Hospital, 300 First Avenue, Charlestown, MA 02025, USA; b Department of Physical Medicine and Rehabilitation, Tufts Medical Center, 800 Washington Street, Boston, MA 02111, USA
* Corresponding author.
E-mail address: SBhatnagar1@partners.org

Phys Med Rehabil Clin N Am 30 (2019) 155–170
https://doi.org/10.1016/j.pmr.2018.08.014
1047-9651/19/Published by Elsevier Inc.

TBI is a serious problem that can lead to long-term disabilities. The prevalence of unemployment among the TBI population is 60% 2 years after injury.[5] Direct and indirect costs of TBIs have been estimated to be as high as $60 billion annually.[2] As patients can experience a wide range of symptoms (eg, headaches, sleep-cycle changes, seizure, and coma), an important factor for treating TBI is accurate diagnosis and assessment of disabilities. Current TBI management is based on sports and acceleration/deceleration injury research, and civilians as well as military veterans are managed similarly regardless of the cause of injury. However, blast-related TBI injury management is has been increasingly studied, as research has shown that service members with TBIs have a higher rate of comorbid mental health conditions compared with civilians.[6] This article reviews the diagnosis, classification, and proposed mechanisms of TBI with a focus on assessment and management of common neurosensory deficits regardless of the TBI severity.

## General Traumatic Brain Injury Pathophysiology

TBI is *a traumatically induced structural injury and/or physiologic disruption of brain function as a result of an external force.*[7] The primary insult occurs because of direct mechanical damage caused by the inciting trauma, whereas secondary injury is caused by the biomolecular or biochemical cascades that are set in motion following the initial mechanical insult.[8,9] Both injury mechanisms can disrupt the neurosensory and cognitive pathways thereby causing significant impairment and disability.

## HEADACHE
### Considerations

- Posttraumatic headache (PTH) is defined as the occurrence of a new headache, or worse headache if it is a preexisting condition, within 7 days of injury. (Delayed-onset acute and persistent headaches that develop greater than 7 days after injury are less likely but possible.)[10]
- It is more frequent after mild versus moderate to severe TBIs.[11]
- Most common patterns resemble migraines without aura and tension headaches.[10]
- Neck injuries in conjunction with TBIs may lead to cervicogenic headaches that may resemble occipital neuralgia.[10]
- Studies show that up to 80% of PTH after mTBIs resolve or show significant improvement within the first year.[12]
- Among US soldiers with PTH mainly associated with blast trauma, most are the migraine type.[11]

### Patient Evaluation Overview

PTH is diagnosed by the patients' history and is then treated based on the headache phenotype (**Table 1**).

Routine imaging studies at present do not reveal pathologic conditions and do not impact treatment and, therefore, are not recommended in the acute development of PTH.[11] There are ongoing trials of neuroimaging modalities, such as functional MRI, that may be helpful in the diagnosis of PTH.[13]

### Treatment Options

PTH is treated based on headache type. Triptans are used for abortive migraine treatment. Tricyclic antidepressants can be used prophylactically for migraine-type headaches. Amitriptyline has been effective for posttraumatic tension-type headaches.[11] Recently, it has been shown that patients with TBIs have an increased risk of stroke;

| Table 1 | |
|---|---|
| Headache types | |
| **Headache Phenotype** | **Associated Symptoms** |
| Migraine | Lateralized |
| | Pounding or throbbing |
| | May be associated with photophobia, nausea, or aura |
| Tension type | Generalized |
| | Nuchal-occipital, bifrontal, bitemporal, headband distribution |
| | Pressure, tightness, or dull aching |
| Cervicogenic | Lateralized |
| | Worsening of headache with certain neck movements |
| | Possible radiated pain from neck/back of head up |
| | and to front of the head or behind the eye |
| | Often have reduced neck range of motion |

therefore, nonvasocontracting agents like calcitonin gene-related peptide antagonists and 5HT1F (5-hydroxytryptamine [serotonin] receptor 1F) receptor agonists may be safer.[11]

Because preventative pharmacologic treatment can take weeks to become effective, it may be beneficial to create a transitional approach. This approach combines physical and cognitive activity with interventions, such as nerve blocks or physical medicine. There are few studies that have investigated whether physical therapy, massage, spinal manipulation, and mobilization are effective in treating PTH; however, there is anecdotal evidence that has shown that those who undergo adjunctive neuromuscular/PT have a significant improvement in PTH as compared with those who do not.[14] Patients with daily headaches secondary to mTBIs who meet the International Headache Society's 3 criteria for chronic migraine show a good response to botulinum toxin. For those who do not respond to botulinum toxin, peripheral neurostimulation is a promising interventional therapy that still needs further study.[13]

## SLEEP-RELATED ISSUES
### Considerations

- Approximately 75% of patients who are hospitalized for TBIs develop sleep-wake disturbances by 6 months after the injury.[15]
- Hypersomnia, or excessive daytime sleepiness, refers to the inability to maintain wakefulness and alertness during the day with sleep occurring at inappropriate times or unintentionally.[16]
- Insomnia involves trouble initiating and maintaining sleep and is associated with daytime sleepiness and depressed mood.
- Insomnia is more prevalent in mild compared with moderate or severe TBIs, unlike most other sleep disturbances after TBIs.[17]
- The incidence of insomnia among military personnel increases with the number of head injuries incurred.[18]
- Sleep-wake dysfunction may be caused by pain, injury to regulatory nuclei and brain pathways (ventrolateral preoptic nucleus or its projections), posttraumatic stress disorder (PTSD), or maladaptive behaviors.
- Patients with TBIs with comorbidities, such as PTSD, have greater sleep disturbances.

- Low to intermediate hypocretin-1 levels (also seen in narcolepsy and cataplexy) have been found in moderate to severe TBI cases but normalize 6 months after the injury. This finding may partially explain why sleep disturbances, such as hypersomnia, resolve in many patients over time.[13]

### Patient Evaluation Overview

A significant amount of information can be obtained from a good history. A sleep diary is useful to differentiate a circadian-rhythm disorder from other sleep-wake disorders, which have different treatment approaches.[19]

Other causes of sleep dysfunction include obstructive sleep apnea (OSA) and side effects of medications.

Circadian rhythm disorders are when people are unable to go to sleep and awaken at times required for work/school and social life. However, people with circadian rhythm disorders are able to get enough sleep and have normal quality of sleep. Sleep-wake disorders include insomnia and hypersomnia, which are described earlier. Questionnaires may also be useful in identifying a sleep disorder and its severity. The following 3 questionnaires have been validated in the TBI population[20]:

- Epworth sleepiness scale
- Pittsburgh sleep quality index
- Insomnia severity index

Despite subjective testing, differentiating between fatigue and a sleep disorder can be challenging. Fatigue and sleep are interrelated; subjective improvement in sleep correlates with subjective improvement in fatigue.[17] Therefore, objective tests can help to determine the presence of sleep disorders:

- Polysomnography
- Actigraphy
- Multiple sleep latency testing (MSLT)
- Maintenance of wakefulness test (MWT)

In patients with TBI, polysomnography has shown less efficient sleep, longer sleep-onset latencies, and shorter rapid eye movement–onset latency.[21] Actigraphy has not been as useful; because of mobility impairments in patients with TBI, the test may miss arousals after sleep onset and, therefore, overestimate sleep.[19]

The MSLT and MWT monitor patients' sleep with electroencephalography (EEG), electrooculography, mental or submental electromyography, and electrocardiography. The MSLT, which measures an individual's tendency to fall to sleep, is helpful in evaluating patients suspected of having hypersomnia and is not indicated for those suspected of having insomnia or circadian rhythm disorders.[22] The MWT, which measures the ability of an individual to remain awake for a period of time, is used to assess a person's response to treatment. A mean sleep latency less than 8 minutes on the MSLT supports the diagnosis of hypersomnia.[14]

### Treatment Options

Initial management should include education and lifestyle modifications, such as discussion about sleep hygiene. It is also recommended that patients trial cognitive behavioral therapy (CBT) as a first-line treatment.[17] Behavioral approaches, such as relaxation techniques, mental imagery, and/or anticipatory awakenings, may be useful for management of parasomnias.

Pharmacologic management will depend on the primary sleep complaint (**Table 2**).[13]

| Table 2 | |
|---|---|
| **Pharmacologic management of sleep disorders** | |
| Insomnia | Sleep aids: zolpidem, zaleplon, eszopiclone, ramelteon, suvorexant<br>Antihistamines: hydroxyzine, doxepin<br>Antipsychotics/antidepressants: quetiapine, doxepin, mirtazapine |
| Hypersomnia | Wakefulness promoting: modafinil, methylphenidate, amphetamines class |

It is also important to consider other comorbidities. Patients with TBI with insomnia who also have depression may benefit from trazodone or mirtazapine. Similarly, patients with hypersomnia and anxiety may have a positive effect from taking a selective serotonin reuptake inhibitor.

## FATIGUE
### Considerations

- It is defined as persistent mental or physical exhaustion and an inability to perform voluntary activities.
- It can be accompanied by cognitive dysfunction, sensory overstimulation, pain, and sleepiness.
- It is frequently associated with negative outcomes, such as decreased level of functioning and reduced quality of life and increased institutionalization and mortality.[23]
- Patients experience minimal improvement in fatigue if symptoms persist past the first year after a TBI.[24]
- Mental fatigue in patients with TBIs is most pronounced during sensory stimulation or with prolonged cognitive tasks; most have a long recovery time after performing such tasks.
- Two-thirds of patients report a clear diurnal variation in mental fatigue.

### Patient Evaluation Overview

Diagnosis is based on history and subjective scales. It is important to investigate whether fatigue limits common activities, such as taking part in conversations, reading a book, shopping, or using a computer. It is helpful to further characterize fatigue as physical or mental and consider other possible contributors, such as endocrine abnormalities or OSA.

The Multidimensional Fatigue Inventory evaluates different aspects of fatigue, including general, physical, mental, reduced activity, and reduced motivation. The Mental Fatigue Scale is the most widely used; however, daytime variation in fatigue is not included in the total score.[22] The fatigue subscale of the Profile of Mood States (POMS) and the Fatigue Severity Scale have also been used to assess general fatigue.

### Treatment Options

Nonpharmacologic treatment options include physical interventions, such as aquatic therapy, CBT, and biofeedback. Aquatic therapy has both cognitive and functional benefits as observed via the fatigue subscale of the POMS.[25] CBT has also improved cognitive function, particularly in processing speed and attention.

Pharmacologic treatment options include the following[22]:

- Methylphenidate: It is used for deficits in attention and processing speed.
- Modafinil: Studies have shown a positive effect on daytime sleepiness but no improvement on the Fatigue Severity Scale.

## VESTIBULAR DYSFUNCTION
### Considerations

- Vestibular dysfunction following TBIs can be some of the most problematic sequelae contributing to a prolonged recovery.[26]
- The incidence of dizziness that results from mTBIs can range from 24% to 83%.[27]
- Active-duty service members and veterans exposed to blast injuries have reported high rates of vestibular symptoms, including dizziness, clumsiness (15%–40%), imbalance (7%), and vertigo (24%).[28]
- Individuals with TBIs who experience vestibular symptoms have been found to have impaired performance in activities of daily living, diminished quality of life, increased mood disorders, and diminished tolerance for rehabilitation in polytrauma centers.[29]
- One method of differentiating the numerous causes of dizziness is to categorize the underlying cause of TBI-associated vestibular disorders into their origin (**Table 3**).[24,30]

### Patient Evaluation Overview

In the TBI population, vestibular symptoms commonly manifest as complaints of dizziness and imbalance. To provide the most suitable treatment options, one must accurately identify the source of these symptoms with a systematic evaluation[28,31]:

- History
- Physical examination and office-based vestibular testing
- Laboratory vestibular and balance studies
- Targeted neuroradiographic testing
- Formal audiometric testing

The history can be extremely useful for differentiating between the various peripheral disorders. For example, patients complaining of feeling dizzy for a few seconds when rolling or turning in bed is a characteristic feature of benign paroxysmal positional vertigo. A report of sudden onset vertigo triggered by sound is the hallmark complaint of superior semicircular canal dehiscence.[32] Questions important in TBI-related dizziness include the following[29]:

- Details of the head injury causing the TBI
- Description of dizziness
- Association of headache
- Past medical and surgical history, family history, medications (prescription, over the counter, herbal, illicit)

**Table 3**
**Peripheral and central causes of vestibular symptoms after traumatic brain injury**

| Peripheral | Central |
|---|---|
| • Benign paroxysmal positional vertigo | • Direct trauma to brainstem and/or cerebellum |
| • Labyrinthine concussion | • Concussion of vestibular nuclei and/or central vestibular pathways |
| • Perilymph fistula/superior semicircular canal dehiscence | • Posttraumatic seizure |
| • Delayed endolymphatic hydrops/Meniere disease | • Posttraumatic stress syndrome |
| • Temporal bone fracture | • Posttraumatic migraine headache |

- Dietary history
- History of consumption of ototoxic agents (eg, aminoglycosides, salicylates, loop diuretics, quinine)

Physical examination should include the evaluation of the head, eyes, ears, nose, and throat. In addition, specialized office-based clinical tests for dizziness (**Box 1**) help identify the extent and location of the lesion.[28–30,33,34]

Otovestibular laboratory studies (**Box 2**) provide clinicians with tools to quantify suspected vestibular deficits and/or to establish a baseline measure before undertaking any interventions.[29,30]

Typically, in patients who have had a TBI, a computed tomography (CT) scan has already been performed at the time of the injury with or without an MRI.[29,35] CT of the head is normal in 90% of cases of mTBIs despite the alarming neuropsychological signs and symptoms present in this population.[36] However, there are instances when specific imaging is indicated (**Table 4**).[29]

## Treatment Options

With the exception of migraines and psychological disorders, medications are typically used for acute symptom control.[28,29] Chronic use of medications for suppression of vestibular symptoms should be avoided, as they can also suppress the central nervous system response and impair central vestibular system recovery.[37] The most commonly used medications for managing symptoms of dizziness, vertigo, migraines, and nystagmus include the following[38–40]:

---

**Box 1**
**Targeted clinical tests for dizzy patients**

- Spontaneous nystagmus
- Gaze nystagmus
- Saccades
- Vergence test
- Head thrust test
- Headshake test
- Dynamic visual acuity test
- Fixation suppression test
- Dix-Hallpike test
- Aural pressure/sound tests
- Cerebellar limb coordination tests
  - Finger-to-nose
  - Heel-shin
  - Rapid alternating motion
- Somato-sensation tests
- Posture tests
- Romberg test
- Sharpened/tandem Romberg test
- Gait observation

---

**Box 2**
**Otovestibular laboratory tests**

- Electronystagmography
- Rotary chair
- Postural control assessment
- Computerized dynamic posturography
  ○ Sensory organization test
  ○ Motor control test
  ○ Adaptation test
- Postural evoked responses

---

- Antihistamines
- Anticholinergics
- Phenothiazine
- Benzodiazepines
- L-channel calcium channel blockers
- Tricyclic antidepressants
- Selective serotonin reuptake inhibitors
- Antiepileptics

The mainstay of the treatment of dizziness and balance dysfunction is vestibular physical therapy (VPT). This exercise-based program is designed specifically to reduce vestibular symptoms and improve function and general activity in patients with TBIs and dizziness.[41,42] The major components of VPT include gaze stabilization, balance-retraining, adaptation, substitution, and habituation techniques that target the vestibuloocular reflex (VOR), cervico-ocular reflex (COR), depth perception, somatosensory retraining, dynamic gait, and aerobic function.[28,39,40] A comprehensive VPT program should include a multidisciplinary team and typically incorporates the following principles of recovery for vestibular lesions:

- *Adaptation*: When there is hypofunction of the VOR, the vestibular system is unable to generate sufficient eye movements in response to head movement, resulting in reduced gain and gaze instability.[28,43] Exercises to maintain visual fixation on a single target are used to increase VOR gain and promote vestibular adaptation.[39,44,45]
- *Habituation*: The goal of habituation exercises is to reduce position-induced dizziness over time through repeated exposure to symptom-provoking stimuli.[31,39]

---

**Table 4**
**Indications for targeted radiographic studies**

| Indication | Radiography |
|---|---|
| Vestibular/cochlear concussion | • MRI of brainstem with and without gadolinium– diethylenetriamine pentaacetic acid enhancement<br>• Contrast-enhanced CT of brainstem |
| Superior semicircular canal dehiscence<br>Skull fractures | CT of temporal bones |
| Pulsatile tinnitus with dizziness | • Magnetic resonance angiography<br>• CT angiography |

- *Substitution*: Substitution exercises are used to enhance postural control and decrease the incidence of falls by using other sensory stimuli, such as visual or somatosensory signals, to substitute for vestibular hypofunction.[39,42]

## AUDIOLOGICAL DYSFUNCTION
### Considerations

- Peripheral otologic trauma is frequently observed in patients with temporal bone fracture.[46]
- In individuals who have had a TBI from a blast exposure, rupture of the tympanic membrane was the most frequent cause of audiological dysfunction.[47]
- Auditory system damage can also be noise induced due to damaged cochlear hair cells.[45]
- Common otologic complaints include hearing loss, otalgia, tinnitus, aural fullness, and dizziness.
- The most common symptoms driving patients to seek audiologic evaluation include increased difficulty understanding speech in the presence of background noise and difficulty following rapidly spoken or long-running speech.[48]

### Patient Evaluation Overview

Patients presenting with otologic symptoms after TBIs should receive a comprehensive audiometric evaluation that can include the following:

- Otoscopy
- Tympanometry
- Audiometry
- Acoustic reflex thresholds
- Acoustic reflex decay
- Speech reception thresholds
- Speech intelligibility

No standard test battery or procedures exist for evaluating otologic and central auditory processing (CAP) disorders in patients with TBIs because these individuals frequently have multiple injuries, altered levels of consciousness, and contraindications that can impede an auditory assessment. Symptoms can be mistaken for PTSD, mental health issues, and neurocognitive deficits, which can lead to inappropriate therapies and increase frustration and emotional distress in patients with TBIs.[45,46]

Tests are often omitted or modified to accommodate for patients' injuries.[45] Routine clinical audiometric testing is normally adequate to evaluate peripheral otologic disorders. However, CAP disorders resulting from TBIs require additional nonstandard evaluation techniques, including standardized questionnaires.[45,46] The Hearing Handicap Inventory for Adults can be used to assess the emotional and social consequences of hearing loss.[49] The Tinnitus Impact Screening Interview is a questionnaire that can be used to rapidly assess the severity of patients' tinnitus.[50]

### Treatment Options

Hearing loss resulting from peripheral audiologic injuries, such as tympanic membrane rupture or ossicular disruption, typically resolve within a few months of injury.[45] Hearing aids and other assistive listening devices are used in individuals with permanent sensorineural hearing loss.

Tinnitus treatment uses the Progressive Tinnitus Management method, which is an educational approach to promote self-management and involves 5 levels of clinical services[45]:

1. Triage
2. Audiologic assessment
3. Group educational counseling
4. Interdisciplinary evaluation
5. Individualized support

Other forms of tinnitus therapy include CBT, neuromonics tinnitus treatment, tinnitus masking, and tinnitus retraining therapy.[51]

Current clinical guidelines for the treatment of CAP involve a 2-step approach that includes auditory training and general management options.[45,52] Auditory training programs are designed to capitalize on the plasticity of the auditory system by altering the neural encoding of sound and subsequent timing of brainstem responses to improve detection, discrimination, and recall of auditory information.[45,46] General management strategies use compensatory techniques and environmental modifications, such as frequency modulation, television captioning, teletext, volume-control telephones, and alerting devices, that use visual or tactile signals to alert the person of acoustical events in his or her surrounding environment.[45]

## VISUAL DYSFUNCTION
### Considerations

More than 50% of the brain is involved in the visual processes[2]; thus, it is of little surprise that 50% to 90% of patients who have a TBI have visual symptoms and are diagnosed with at least one oculomotor dysfunction.[2,6] Injury to any part of the visual pathways, such as optic nerve, optic tract, chasm, optic radiation, occipital cortex, cranial nerves, oculomotor obstructions, and retina, can lead to various visual deficits[1,2,5,6]:

- Visual acuity deficits can be a summation of several visual deficits.[3]
- Approximately 55% report issues with light sensitivity (photophobia).[4,53]
- A retrospective study reported that approximately 38.75% of patients with TBIs experienced visual field defects with the most common defect in a scattered pattern (58.06%), followed by homonymous hemianopia (22.58%).[54]
- Approximately 13% of patients have double vision after a TBI.[4]
- Vergence dysfunction is the inability for the eyes to converge or diverge to align the fovea on objects and maintain binocular vision.[51]
  - A total of 56.3% of patients with TBIs have vergence dysfunction with convergence insufficiency as the most common type (42.5%).[5,7,51]
  - Symptoms include eye strain, blurry vision, double vision, headaches, loss of concentration, difficulty reading, difficulty remembering what was read, and visual fatigue.[1,2,51]
- Versional deficiency is defined as conjugate eye movements that encompass saccades, pursuits, and fixation.[5,8]
  - Roughly 51.7% of patients with TBIs have versional deficiency, with approximately 38.9% experiencing saccadic dysfunction and 32.5% with pursuit dysfunction.[3,5]
  - Symptoms include reading difficulties, such as reduced speed and patients frequently losing their place causing them to reread text.[51]
- Accommodative insufficiency is the inability to focus or maintain focus on an object at near or far distances.

| Table 5 | |
|---|---|
| Ocular dysfunction clinical examination and tests | |
| **Visual Deficit** | **Testing** |
| Visual acuity deficit | Snellen chart: initial screen<br>Standard ophthalmoscopic examination<br>CT if concern for retrobulbar hemorrhage<br>CSV-1000 or Pelli-Robson charts: test for<br>subtle changes (ie, contrast sensitivity) |
| Photophobia | Ophthalmoscopic examination: rule<br>out inflammatory processes |
| Vergence dysfunction | Prism adaptation (best)<br>Phoropter<br>Cranial nerve testing (eg, H-pattern test) |
| Versional dysfunction | Smooth pursuit: H-pattern and VOR cancellation tests |
| Accommodative insufficiency | Measure amplitude: minus lens (best),<br>push up, modified push up, push down methods |
| Visual field deficits | Confrontation testing: initial screen<br>Perimetry tests |
| Diplopia | Monocular vs binocular: cover 1 eye<br>and if resolves, it is binocular<br>Vertical: Parks 3-step test<br>Horizontal: Hess Lancaster or red lens test |

- Roughly 40% of patients have accommodative insufficiency after TBIs.[3,5]
- It is controlled by the autonomic nervous system and vulnerable to diffuse axonal injury and focal lesions.[5,7]
- Symptoms include blurry vision, visual fatigue, asthenopia (eye strain), and headaches and are usually worse when doing activities at near distances, such reading and typing.[51]

These deficits can affect activities of daily living, such as reading, which can impact educational or occupational pursuits.[3,6,51,55]

### Patient Evaluation Overview

All patients with a TBI should have a general vision screening because of the high frequency of visual deficits and resulting diminished functional ability. In one study, a team of optometrists and occupational therapists created a screening guideline to address most visual deficits associated with TBIs. The screening guidelines include a questionnaire for self-reported symptoms and performance and 8 vision tests, which investigate for acuity, reading, accommodation, convergence, eye alignment/binocular vision, saccades, pursuits, and visual fields.[56] A detailed history should be taken, as symptoms can provide important information into the specific deficit. A more focused clinical examination can then be performed (**Table 5**).[1,3,51,57–60]

### Treatment Options

The mainstay of treatment of photophobia after TBIs includes filters, visors, wraparound framed polarized lenses, tints, and awareness of different types of ambient lighting.[4,51] Specifically, one study showed that the optical tint FL-41 is most beneficial, reducing patients' frequency of blinks and sensitivity to light.[61] It should be noted that patients should not wear sunglasses indoors, as this will foster their retinas to adapt to darker environments further exacerbating photophobia.[59] The goal is to optimize the patients' comfort.

The management of vergence dysfunction with oculomotor rehabilitation in non-TBI and mTBI populations has been established.[62,63] The goal is to attain a clear binocular field of view by improving the speed and accuracy of all integrated oculomotor functions.[61] Ciuffreda and colleagues[64] observed a 50% improvement in final binocular eye position with conversion and diversion using a computer oculomotor rehabilitation program for mTBI.

Versional dysfunction can be treated with pursuit and saccadic therapies. Pursuit rehab consists of having patients track an object in horizontal and vertical planes. As patients' tracking ability improves, the target distance and velocity can be adjusted to increase the difficulty. In the same way, saccadic rehabilitation involves presenting targets in all 4 visual quadrants and then having patients focus on the targets when the target switches from quadrant to quadrant.[57]

Accommodative insufficiency is generally treated with reading glasses or bifocal/progressive lenses and accommodative exercises. Ramp accommodative exercises consist of placing a target at arms' length and slowly moving an object closer to patients until blur occurs. The object is then placed back at arm's length and the exercise is repeated. Step exercises involve asking patients to focus on an object at a distance for 3 seconds and then focus on an object at near distance for 3 seconds. The patients continue to switch between far and near to strengthen their accommodative ability.[57]

Visual field rehabilitation consists of optical assistance and visual compensatory strategies. Optical assistance uses prisms to relocate the blind visual field toward the functional visual field.[56,57,65] Visual compensatory strategies include the following:

- Use rehabilitation that stresses peripheral awareness and teaches patients to continuously scan their environment.[51,54]
- Scroll or tilt reading material away from the field of loss.[51]
- Typoscope or line guides assist with tracking.[51]
- Visual anchors, such as using tape or colored markers, can help patients perceive boundaries of field cut and cue patients to complete the scan toward the blind side.[56]
- Technology, such as Dynavision (Dynavision International LLC, West Chester Ohio), enhances patients' scanning ability by using contrast, timed response, and auditory feedback.[57]

Binocular diplopia is treated with ocular occlusion via an eye patch or tinted lens as well as monovision optical correction. Monovision optical correction uses glasses or contacts that focus one eye for near objects and one eye for distance objects and requires patients to have good vision in both eyes and the ability to switch ocular fixation from near to distant objects.[58] The most successful treatment involves using prisms to redirect the light pathway to focus on the fovea.[58] More invasive options include botulinum toxin injections to extraocular muscles or surgical realignment via lengthening/shortening of the muscles.[58] Any of these treatment modalities can be combined with ocular rehabilitation to strengthen oculomotor function.

## SUMMARY

Neurosensory deficits after TBIs can frequently lead to disability and, therefore, are important to properly diagnose and treat. Current TBI management is similar between civilian and military populations regardless of the cause of injury. However, new research is on the horizon, as military veterans have higher rates of comorbid mental health conditions compared with civilians and show poor long-term clinical out-comes.[6] PTH most commonly resembles migraines and is managed similarly. A transitional approach that involves adjuvant physical therapy may also be beneficial. Sleep-related issues, including hypersomnia and insomnia, are treated pharmacologically based on the specific sleep-related complaint. Fatigue after TBIs is difficult to treat; but medications, such as methylphenidate and modafinil, have been used. CBT and aquatic therapy have been shown to be beneficial. There are many different clinical tests used to diagnose peripheral versus central causes of vestibular dysfunction. The mainstay of treatment of dizziness and balance dysfunction is vestibular physical therapy, but there are also many different classes of medications used to treat specific vestibular symptoms. Visual dysfunction incorporates numerous different diagnoses, which are frequently treated with specific rehabilitation programs.

## REFERENCES

1. Mandese M. Oculo-visual evaluation of the patient with traumatic brain Injury Maria Mande. Optom Vis Dev 2009;40(1):37–44.
2. Alvarez T, Kim E, Vicci V, et al. Concurrent vision dysfunctions in convergence insufficiency with traumatic brain injury. Optom Vis Sci 2012;89(12):1740–51.
3. Brahm K, Wilgenburg H, Kirby J, et al. Visual impairment and dysfunction in combat-injured servicemembers with traumatic brain injury. Optom Vis Sci 2009;86(7):817–25.
4. Magone T, Kwon E, Shin S. Chronic visual dysfunction after blast-induced mild traumatic brain injury. J Rehabil Res Dev 2014;51(1):71–80.
5. Cuthbert JP, Harrison-Felix C, Corrigan JD, et al. Unemployment in the United States after traumatic brain injury for working-age individuals: prevalence and associated factors 2 years postinjury. J Head Trauma Rehabil 2015;30(3):160–74.
6. MacDonald C, Barber J, Jordan M, et al. Early clinical predictors of 5-year outcome after concussive blast traumatic brain injury. JAMA Neurol 2017;74(7): 821–9.
7. Department of Veterans Affairs, Department of Defense, USA. VA/DoD Clinical practice guideline for the management of concussion-mild traumatic brain injury. Version 2.0. 2016.
8. Thiagarajan P, Ciuffreda KJ, Ludlam DP. Vergence dysfunction in mild traumatic brain injury (mTBI): a review. Ophthalmic Physiol Opt 2011;31:456–68.
9. Cockerham G, Goodrich G, Weichel E, Orcutt James, Rizzo Joseph, Bower Kraig, Schuchard Ronald. Eye and visual function in traumatic brain injury.(JRRD at a Glance)(Brief article). J Rehabil Res Dev 2009;46(6):811–8.
10. Stacey A, Lucas S, Dikmen S, et al. Natural history of headache five years after traumatic brain injury. J Neurotrauma 2017;34:1558–64.
11. Ruff RL, Blake K. Pathophysiological links between traumatic brain injury and post-traumatic headaches. 2016.
12. Holtkamp MD, Grimes J, Ling G. Concussion in the military: an evidence-base review of mTBI in US military personnel focused on posttraumatic headache. Curr Pain Headache Rep 2016;20(6):37.
13. Dean PJ, Sato JR, Vieira G, et al. Multimodal imaging of mild traumatic brain injury and persistent postconcussion syndrome. Brain Behav 2015;5(1):45–61.
14. Conidi, Francis X. Interventional treatment for post-traumatic headache. Curr Pain Headache Rep 2016;20(40):1–8.
15. Viola-Saltzman M, Watson NF. Traumatic brain injury and sleep disorders. Neurol Clin 2012;30(4):1299–312.

16. American Academy of Sleep Medicine. International classification of sleep disorders. 3rd edition. Darien, IL: American Academy of Sleep Medicine; 2014.
17. Beetar JT, Guilmette TJ, Sparadeo FR. Sleep and pain complaints in symptomatic traumatic brain injury and neurologic populations. Arch Phys Med Rehabil 1996; 77:1298.
18. Bryan CJ. Repetitive traumatic brain injury (or concussion) increases severity of sleep disturbance among deployed military personnel. Sleep 2013;36:941.
19. Vermaelen J, Greiffenstein P, deBoisbland B. Sleep in traumatic brain injury. Crit Care Clin 2015;31:551–61.
20. Werner J, Baumann C. TBI and sleep-wake disorders: pathophysiology, clinical management, and moving towards the future. Semin Neurol 2017;37:419–32.
21. Viola-Saltzman M, Musleh C. Traumatic brain injury-induced sleep disorders. Neuropsychiatr Dis Treat 2016;12:339–48.
22. Littner MR, Kushida C, Wise M, et al. Practice parameters for clinical use of the multiple sleep latency test and the maintenance of wakefulness test. Sleep 2005;28:113.
23. Ulrichsen KM, Kaufmann T, Dørum ES, et al. Clinical utility of mindfulness training in the treatment of fatigue after stroke, traumatic brain injury and multiple sclerosis: a systematic literature review and meta-analysis. Front Psychol 2016;7:912.
24. Johansson B, Ronnback L. Assessment and treatment of mental fatigue after a traumatic brain injury. Neuropsychol Rehabil 2017;27(7):1047–55.
25. Xu G-Z, Li Y-F, Wang M-D, et al. Complementary and alternative interventions for fatigue management after traumatic brain injury: a systematic review. Ther Adv Neurol Disord 2017;10(5):229–39.
26. Wallace B, Lifshitz J. Traumatic brain injury and vestibulo-ocular function: current challenges and future prospects [review]. Eye Brain 2016;8:153–64.
27. Akin FW, Murnane OD. Head injury and blast exposure: vestibular consequences [review]. Otolaryngol Clin North Am 2011;44(2):323–34, viii.
28. Franke LM, Walker WC, Cifu DX, et al. Sensorintegrative dysfunction underlying vestibular disorders after traumatic brain injury: a review [review]. J Rehabil Res Dev 2012;49(7):985–94.
29. Scherer MR, Burrows H, Pinto R, et al. Evidence of central and peripheral vestibular pathology in blast-related traumatic brain injury. Otol Neurotol 2011;32(4): 571–80.
30. Zasler ND, Katz DI, Zafonte RD. Brain injury medicine: principles and practice. New York: Demos; 2007.
31. Chandrasekhar SS. The assessment of balance and dizziness in the TBI patient [review]. NeuroRehabilitation 2013;32(3):445–54.
32. Ward BK, Carey JP, Minor LB. Superior canal dehiscence syndrome: lessons from the first 20 years [review]. Front Neurol 2017;8:177.
33. Scherer MR, Schubert MC. Traumatic brain injury and vestibular pathology as a comorbidity after blast exposure [review]. Phys Ther 2009;89(9):980–92.
34. Goebel JA. The ten-minute examination of the dizzy patient. Semin Neurol 2001; 21(4):391–8.
35. Gizzi M, Riley E, Molinari S. The diagnostic value of imaging the patient with dizziness. A Bayesian approach. Arch Neurol 1996;53(12):1299–304.
36. Toth A. Magnetic resonance imaging application in the area of mild and acute traumatic brain injury: implications for diagnostic markers? [Chapter 24]. In: Kobeissy FH, editor. Brain neurotrauma: molecular, neuropsychological, and rehabilitation aspects. Boca Raton (FL): CRC Press/Taylor & Francis; 2015. p. 329–40.

37. Bronstein AM, Lempert T. Management of the patient with chronic dizziness [review]. Restor Neurol Neurosci 2010;28(1):83–90.

38. Huppert D, Strupp M, Mückter H, et al. Which medication do I need to manage dizzy patients? [review]. Acta Otolaryngol 2011;131(3):228–41.

39. Hain TC, Uddin M. Pharmacological treatment of vertigo [review]. CNS Drugs 2003;17(2):85–100.

40. Han MH, Craig SB, Rutner D, et al. Medications prescribed to brain injury patients: a retrospective analysis [review]. Optometry 2008;79(5):252–8.

41. Whitney SL, Alghwiri AA, Alghadir A. An overview of vestibular rehabilitation [review]. Handb Clin Neurol 2016;137:187–205.

42. Gottshall K. Vestibular rehabilitation after mild traumatic brain injury with vestibular pathology [review]. NeuroRehabilitation 2011;29(2):167–71.

43. Herdman SJ. Role of vestibular adaptation in vestibular rehabilitation [review]. Otolaryngol Head Neck Surg 1998;119(1):49–54.

44. Schubert MC, Migliaccio AA, Clendaniel RA, et al. Mechanism of dynamic visual acuity recovery with vestibular rehabilitation [review]. Arch Phys Med Rehabil 2008;89(3):500–7.

45. Han BI, Song HS, Kim JS. Vestibular rehabilitation therapy: review of indications, mechanisms, and key exercises. J Clin Neurol 2011;7(4):184–96.

46. Patel A, Groppo E. Management of temporal bone trauma. Craniomaxillofac Trauma Reconstr 2010;3(2):105–13.

47. Fausti SA, Wilmington DJ, Gallun FJ, et al. Auditory and vestibular dysfunction associated with blast-related traumatic brain injury. J Rehabil Res Dev 2009; 46(6):797–810.

48. Gallun FJ, Papesh MA, Lewis MS. Hearing complaints among veterans following traumatic brain injury. Brain Inj 2017;31(9):1183–7.

49. Newman CW, Weinstein BE, Jacobson GP, et al. The hearing handicap inventory for adults: psychometric adequacy and audiometric correlates. Ear Hear 1990; 11(6):430–3.

50. Henry JA, Schechter MA, Zaugg TL, et al. Outcomes of clinical trial: tinnitus masking versus tinnitus retraining therapy. J Am Acad Audiol 2006;17(2):104–32.

51. Lew HL, Jerger JF, Guillory SB, et al. Auditory dysfunction in traumatic brain injury. J Rehabil Res Dev 2007;44(7):921–8.

52. American Speech-Language-Hearing Association. Guidelines for the audiologic management of individuals receiving cochleotoxic drug therapy. Am Speech Lang Hear Assoc 1994.

53. Suhr C, Shust M, Prasad R, et al. Recognizing TBI-related vision disorders: these visual signs and symptoms can help uncover concussions and will guide your approach to intervention. Review of Optometry 2015;152(12):56.

54. Suchoff K, Kapoor N, Ciuffreda KJ, et al. The frequency of occurrence, types, and characteristics of visual field defects in acquired brain injury: a retrospective analysis. Optometry 2008;79(5):259–65.

55. Capó-Aponte JE, Urosevich TG, Temme LA, et al. Visual dysfunctions and symptoms during the subacute stage of blast-induced mild traumatic brain injury. Mil Med 2012;177(7):804–13.

56. Radomski MV, Finkelstein M, Llanos I, et al. Composition of a vision screen for service members with traumatic brain injury: consensus using a modified nominal group technique. Am J Occup Ther 2014;68(4):422–9.

57. Wallace B, Lifshitz J. Traumatic brain injury and vestibulo-ocular function: current challenges and future prospects. Eye Brain 2016;8:153–64.

58. Berryman A, Rasavage K, Politzer T. Practical clinical treatment strategies for evaluation and treatment of visual field loss and visual inattention. NeuroRehabilitation 2010;27(3):261–8.

59. Barnett B, Singman P. Vision concerns after mild traumatic brain injury. Curr Treat Options Neurol 2015;17(2):1–14.

60. Phillips PH. Treatment of diplopia. Semin Neurol 2007;27(03):288–98.

61. Katz BJ, Digre KB. Diagnosis, pathophysiology, and treatment of photophobia. Surv Ophthalmol 2016;61(4):466–77.

62. North RV, Henson DB. The effect of orthoptic treatment upon the vergence adaptation mechanism. Optom Vis Sci 1992;69:294–9.

63. Ciuffreda KJ. The scientific basis for and efficacy of opto- metric vision therapy in non-strabismic accommodative and vergence disorders. Optometry 2002;73: 735–62.

64. Ciuffreda KJ, Yadav NK, Thiagarajan P, et al. A novel computer oculomotor rehabilitation (cor) program for mild traumatic brain injury (MTBI). MDPI, Multidisciplinary Digital Publishing Institute; 2017. Available at: www.mdpi.com/2076-3425/7/8/99.

65. Pouget MC, Lévy-Bencheton D, Prost M, et al. Acquired visual field defects rehabilitation: critical review and perspectives. Ann Phys Rehabil Med 2012;55(1): 53–74.

# Vision Rehabilitation After Traumatic Brain Injury

Check for updates

Sandra M. Fox, OD[a],*, Paul Koons, MS, OMS, CLVT, CBIS[b], Sally H. Dang, OD[c]

## KEYWORDS

- Traumatic brain injury • Visual dysfunction • Vision rehabilitation • Vision therapy
- Concussion

## KEY POINTS

- Visual dysfunctions and symptoms are commonly experienced after even mild traumatic brain injury (TBI) despite excellent visual acuity.
- All individuals who have experienced a TBI/concussion should be screened for vision symptoms and visual dysfunction.
- A TBI-specific eye examination is necessary to identify the visual sequelae of TBI as well as address any vision/ocular issues that may be contributing to other post-TBI complaints, such as headache, photosensitivity, and vertigo.
- Recognizing and establishing your local vision rehabilitation network of professionals will offer a comprehensive approach for the patient experiencing visual dysfunction and visual deficits due to TBI.
- Combining office-based and home-based vision therapy training will maximize visual potential and functional results.

## INTRODUCTION

Visual dysfunction and vision-related symptoms are common but often overlooked sequelae of traumatic brain injury (TBI). Approximately 70% of the brain is either directly involved with visual processing or is a component for other sensory processing.[1,2] Six of the 12 cranial nerves pertain to vision and visual/ocular functions. In addition, the areas of the brain that are most likely to be injured during a TBI (frontal,

Disclosure Statement: The views, opinions and/or findings expressed herein are those of the authors and do not necessarily reflect the views or the official policy of the Department of Veterans Affairs or the US government.
[a] Surgical Service, Ophthalmology, Polytrauma Rehabilitation Center, South Texas Veterans Healthcare System, 7400 Merton Minter, San Antonio, TX 78229, USA; [b] Blind Rehabilitation Service, Major Charles Robert Soltes, Jr. O.D. Blind Rehabilitation Center (BRC), Tibor Rubin VA Medical Center, 5901 East 7th Street, Long Beach, CA 90822, USA; [c] Optometry Service, VA Long Beach Healthcare System, 5901 East 7th Street, Long Beach, CA 90822, USA
* Corresponding author.
E-mail address: Sandra.fox2@va.gov

occipital, temporal, and parietal lobes, as well as the long axonal fibers connecting the midbrain to the cortex) are vision related.[1] Thus, it is not surprising that even a mild TBI/concussion can lead to significant visual sequelae that will adversely affect rehabilitation and quality of life.

Much of what we now know about how brain injury affects the visual system was gleaned from research performed within the Department of Defense (DoD) and the Department of Veterans Affairs (VA) systems. Although earlier research postulated a different mechanism of action for blast-related TBI than non–blast-related TBI, more recent research has found minimal difference in the visual sequelae between blast-related and non–blast-related TBI.[1,3,4] This suggests that VA and DoD research concerning the assessment and management of the visual sequelae of mild TBI can be applicable to those sustaining a mild TBI/concussion in the civilian setting.

## VISUAL IMPAIRMENT VERSUS VISUAL DYSFUNCTION

*Visual impairment* or blindness occurs when visual acuity is decreased and or the visual field is constricted. The incidence of diagnosed visual impairment and blindness resulting from TBI ranges from approximately 9% to 38% depending on the definition used, the mechanism of injury (blast vs non-blast) and the severity of the TBI, with most cases occurring in blast-related moderate to severe TBI.[3,5-7]

*Visual dysfunction* refers to a disorder of any visual function, such as oculomotor and accommodation, visual spatial deficits, and photosensitivity. Visual dysfunctions and symptoms are commonly experienced after TBI despite excellent visual acuity.[1,2,4,5,7,8] They can contribute to headache and dizziness; cause diplopia, eye fatigue, and an inability to focus; adversely affect reading and all near tasks; and contribute to photophobia.[4,6,8-10] Undiagnosed, the visual sequela can affect school, work, and other activities of daily living.

### Visual Symptoms and Dysfunction in Traumatic Brain Injury

Self-reported vision complaints, including blurry vision distance and near, eye strain, eye pain, double vision, bumping into objects, difficulty reading, and light sensitivity, range from 65% to 79% depending on the study design and patient population.[1,3,4,6,8-10] Difficulty reading was a common complaint (32%–66%),[1] as was light sensitivity (33%–69%).[1,4,8-10]

The visual dysfunctions most often identified were convergence insufficiency, accommodative dysfunction, and photosensitivity.[3,4,6,7,9-11]

Other visual anomalies, such as visual field loss, cranial nerve disorder, strabismus, pursuit/saccade disorder, diplopia, and ocular injuries, are less frequently diagnosed and are more often found in moderate to severe TBI. The wide range in the frequency of visual dysfunction in people with TBI is most likely due to differences in settings and patient populations. Studies reporting data on unscreened individuals with TBI report much lower rates of visual dysfunction than studies that use self-report measures to screen for visual symptoms, highlighting the value of screening for visual dysfunction in patients with TBI.

## MILD TRAUMATIC BRAIN INJURY
### Screening for Visual Dysfunction in Mild Traumatic Brain Injury

Not all rehabilitation settings will have optometrists/ophthalmologists on staff to provide an eye examination for persons who have experienced a mild TBI. In such cases, a method to screen patients with TBI for possible visual symptoms should be implemented.

***Brain injury vision symptom survey questionnaire***

The Brain Injury Vision Symptom Survey (BIVSS) Questionnaire is a 28-item self-administered survey for vision symptoms related to TBI.[12] It probes multiple dimensions of vision-related behaviors, including eyesight clarity, visual comfort, diplopia, depth perception, dry eye, peripheral vision, light sensitivity, and reading and is the screening tool of choice for visual symptoms related to mild TBI.

***Screening protocol for therapists***

Although symptom surveys are quite useful in identifying individuals who have visual symptoms, a more in-depth screening protocol is necessary to determine if the visual symptoms are such that an additional evaluation by an optometrist or ophthalmologist is required. Occupational therapists, vision rehabilitation therapists, and blind rehabilitation outpatient specialists within the VA system can perform additional screening tests to facilitate the appropriate referrals. A consensus panel of occupational therapists and optometrists suggested a screening protocol designed to identify TBI-related vision disorders in adults.[13] **Table 1** uses their recommendations with a few updated modifications.

In addition, although the consensus of this group did not include computerized vision screening programs, such as the Home Therapy System (HTS) Binocular Vision Assessment (HTS Inc, Gold Canyon, AZ) and VERA vision screening software (Visual Technology Applications, Philadelphia, PA), the computerized vision screening programs do show promise, and in one small study showed excellent validity and repeatability for assessing near-related binocular vision problems and pursuit and saccadic eye movements.[14,15] HTS Vision Therapy is a computer program that can be used as an in-office screening tool for accommodation, vergence, and eye movements (pursuits and saccades). It also contains the Computerized Perceptual Therapy System, which evaluates visual perceptual areas including visual concentration, visual closure, visual processing, and visual sequential memory.

## The Traumatic Brain Injury–Specific Vision Evaluation

A TBI-specific vision evaluation is indicated when a patient has experienced a TBI. Before the TBI vision evaluation, a comprehensive baseline refractive and ocular health examination is important to address non–TBI-related vision issues. It is

**Table 1**
**Screening tests for visual sequelae in mild traumatic brain injury**

| Test with corrective lenses if appropriate: older than 40, may need reading glasses | |
| --- | --- |
| Symptom self-report | Brain Injury Vision Symptom Survey |
| Distance visual acuity | Distance Snellen chart |
| Near visual acuity chart | Any near single letter/number chart |
| Accommodation | Accommodative amplitude test |
| Convergence | Near point of convergence |
| Eye alignment and binocular vision | Stereo test |
| Saccades | Developmental eye movement test |
| Pursuits | Northeastern State University College optometry oculomotor test |
| Visual Fields | Confrontation visual fields finger Counting |

*Courtesy of* Sandra Fox, OD, San Antonio TX, USA.

common to have refractive error, such as latent hyperopia that is often symptomatic after the TBI. A thorough damp refraction with dilation is helpful to detect latent hyperopia, which will cause near or accommodative vision challenges. Ruling out any pre-existing ocular disease is important. Patients with TBI often have dry eye syndrome that adds to fluctuations in vision. It is recommended that patients with TBI have a baseline screening visual field test.

In addition to visual sequelae such as oculomotor dysfunction and photosensitivity, common complaints after mild TBI include headaches, vertigo, and difficulty reading and concentrating while reading. The role of the optometrist/ophthalmologist is to address any vision/ocular issues that may be contributing to these complaints.

**Box 1** from the Walter Reed National Military Medical Center Vision Center of Excellence includes the eye/vision tests that are included as the basic components of an eye examination.

## Patient History

Considering what we now know about mild TBI/concussion, a question pertaining to military service and a history of high-impact sports should be a part of every medical/social history. Any positive responses should prompt additional TBI-related questions designed to determine if there is a possible oculomotor dysfunction. See **Box 2** for additional TBI-related questions.

## Additional Testing

### Oculomotor dysfunction

If a patient is symptomatic for oculomotor dysfunction, additional clinical testing must be performed to evaluate visual efficiency to determine the specific types and

---

**Box 1**
**Basic eye care/vision examination by an eye care provider**

History[a]

Visual acuity

Refractive error measurement

External examination

Pupillary testing

Extraocular muscle testing/pursuits

Cover test (distance and near)

Confrontation visual field testing

Tonometry

Slit lamp biomicroscopy: anterior segment, cornea, macula, lens, and optic nerve

Binocular indirect ophthalmoscopy with scleral depression[b]

Gonioscopy[b]

[a] It is recommended that assessment of medical history also include the question, "Have you been exposed to blast or sustained a head injury, concussion, or traumatic brain injury (TBI)?" A positive response to this question would be a sufficient rationale to ask TBI-related ocular history questions and conduct supplemental testing.
[b] If patient history indicates exposure to blast, head injury, concussion, and/or TBI.
Previously published materials from Walter Reed National Military Medical Center/Vision Center of Excellence. 2016; with permission.

---

**Box 2**
**TBI-related ocular history questions**

Did you have any neurologic problems or symptoms before your TBI (multiple sclerosis, stroke, brain tumor, severe headaches, other)?

When did your TBI occur (on what date)?

Did you lose consciousness during or after your TBI incident?

Were you disoriented or confused during or after your TBI incident?

Do you bump into objects and walls more now than before your injury?

Were your eyes, eyelids, or area around your eyes injured when your TBI event occurred?

Do you cover or close one eye at times since your injury?

Have you noticed a change in your vision since your injury?

Are you more sensitive to light, either indoors or outdoors, since your injury?

Have you had any double vision since your injury?

Have you noticed any changes in your peripheral vision since your injury?

Is your vision blurry at distance or near since your injury?

Have you noticed a change in your ability to read since your injury?

Do you lose your place while reading more now than before your injury?

How long can you read continuously before you need to stop?

Do you get headaches during/after reading more now than before your injury?

Do you have more difficulty remembering what you have read now than before your injury?

*Data from* Goodrich G, Martinsen G. Development of a mild traumatic brain injury-specific vision screening protocol: a Delphi study. J Rehabil Res Dev 2013;50(6):757–68; and Previously published materials from Walter Reed National Military Medical Center/Vision Center of Excellence. 2016; with permission.

---

severities of oculomotor dysfunction. **Table 2** lists the oculomotor dysfunction parameters that need to be tested and methods that can be used.

### Visual information processing

Visual information processing, which includes visual spatial information, visual analysis, and visual motor integration, also needs to be evaluated. **Table 3** pertains to visual information processing function, description, and testing methods.

Simple observation of the patient's gait and balance can diagnose spatial localization problems. This may or may not be present with motion sensitivity, which is common in crowded places. Patients may report feeling dizziness, nausea, and unsteadiness.

### Treatment Strategies

Once the visual dysfunction has been identified, a treatment plan will need to be developed to improve the visual efficiency. **Box 3** describes the treatment strategies used for oculomotor dysfunction.

### Rehabilitation Team

As with any rehabilitation plan, it is often necessary to have coordination of subsequent referrals to other services. The goal is to understand how various vision

| Table 2 Recommended tests to evaluate for oculomotor dysfunctions | |
|---|---|
| **Oculomotor Parameter** | **Testing** |
| Eye alignment | *Distance and near cover test in multiple positions of gaze and head tilt* *Phorias (vertical and horizontal)* Maddox rod Modified Thorington |
| Vergence | *Vergence ranges (vertical and horizontal)* *Vergence facility* |
| Convergence amplitude | *Near point of convergence* Repeated measures |
| Accommodation | *Push-up method* Repeated measures *Minus lens* Repeated measures *Accommodative facility (monocular and binocular)* *Negative relative accommodation/Positive relative accommodation (NRA/PRA)* *Near retinoscopy* Accommodative convergence/accommodation (AC/A) ratio |
| Eye movements | *Ductions* *Versions* *Pursuit* *Saccades* Developmental eye movement (DEM) King-Devick |
| Suppression check | *Worth 4 Dot (distance and near)* Random dot stereopsis |
| Vestibulo-ocular reflex | (If positive, refer to audiology, otolaryngology, or vestibular physical therapist) Dynamic visual acuity Head thrust Low-frequency head shake |

Note: not all tests are required; italicized tests provide more comprehensive results as recognized by our expert panel, but selection of tests is left to the clinical judgment of the eye care provider.

Previously published materials from Walter Reed National Military Medical Center/Vision Center of Excellence. 2016; with permission.

problems affect function. See **Table 4** for additional specialties that may need to be consulted.

### Plan of Care of Oculomotor Dysfunctions Associated with Traumatic Brain Injury

**Fig. 1** is an algorithm outlining the process for the care of the patient with oculomotor dysfunctions associated with TBI.

### Vision Rehabilitation for Mild Traumatic Brain Injury

Vision rehabilitation after mild TBI can be further complicated by comorbidities and must be considered when developing the rehabilitative plan.

### Comorbidities

In the military/veteran TBI population, there is a high prevalence of comorbid drug/ substance abuse and mental illness, further complicating the diagnosis and treatment of visual symptoms. Among veterans with TBI, 89% had a comorbid psychiatric

| Table 3<br>Recommended tests to evaluate visual information processing | | |
|---|---|---|
| Function | Description | Tests |
| Visual spatial | Ability to tell where objects are in space and in relation to yourself | Draw a clock from memory<br>Line bisection (2 levels)<br>Copy picture (2 levels)<br>Letter cancellation |
| Visual analysis | Ability to determine awareness of size and color | Test of Visual Perceptual Skills: form constancy, visual closure, visual memory |
| Visual motor integration | Hand-eye coordination<br>Ability to control hand movement guided by vision | Writing skills<br>Pen and paper tests<br>Tangrams<br>Parquetry block designs |
| Spatial localization | The reference of a visual sensation to a definite locality in space | Dynavision<br>Walking obstacle course<br>Walking gait testing<br>Balance testing (TUG, POMA) |

*Abbreviations:* POMA, tinetti performance oriented mobility assessment; TUG, timed up and go.

diagnosis, most commonly with posttraumatic stress disorder (PTSD),[16] in which the prevalence has been found to be as high as 89%.[17]

### Posttraumatic stress disorder
PTSD is associated more often with mild TBI than in more severe TBI[18,19] and can complicate the clinical presentation. A study comparing the *visual function* of veterans with TBI only with that of veterans with TBI and PTSD found high rates of oculomotor dysfunction in both groups with no difference between patients with or without PTSD, indicating that the oculomotor dysfunction is a sequela of the TBI.[18] Those with co-morbid PTSD did have more self-reported visual symptoms and higher complaints of photosensitivity and there is some thought that hypersensitivity could play a role in the increased reporting of visual symptoms.[20]

### Posttraumatic headaches
Headache is one of the most common and persistent symptoms after TBI and is more likely to persist after mild TBI than moderate or severe TBI. The chronic symptom-atology of service members and veterans following TBI is an overlap of chronic post-traumatic headaches, PTSD, and other psychiatric disorders.[21]

### Vertigo
A TBI can disrupt the coordination of sensory input from the visual, vestibular, and so-matosensory pathways necessary for balance and stabilization in the visual environ-ment. Dizziness and vertigo are common complaints after a TBI.

### Photosensitivity
Photosensitivity is more common in mild blast-related TBI. Approximately 50% will experience a decrease in photosensitivity over time and those who do not wear darkly tinted lenses are more likely to notice a decrease in sensitivity over time. The factors that were associated with hindering or inhibiting photosensitivity reductions included dry eye, migraines, hyperacusis, and loss of consciousness,[22] all common conditions in the military/veteran population. In addition, veterans with PTSD and mild TBI endorse photosensitivity much more frequently than those without PTSD.

---

**Box 3**
**Treatment strategies for oculomotor dysfunction**

Correction of refractive error to improve vision, binocular alignment, and accommodative function

Added lenses to improve binocular alignment and accommodative function

When necessary, prism therapy to eliminate double vision and restore visual comfort

Office-based oculomotor rehabilitation (with home-reinforcement) using a variety of procedures to improve oculomotor function

When necessary, surgery for associated strabismus or other relevant oculomotor problems

Previously published materials from Walter Reed National Military Medical Center/Vision Center of Excellence. 2016; with permission.

---

*Before vision rehabilitation, it is important to rule out any visual or ocular conditions that may be contributing to headaches, vertigo, and photosensitivity, as well as whether PTSD may be contributing to the symptomatology.*

### Vision Rehabilitation Team

The ideal setting for providing the patient with TBI with appropriate vision care and vision therapy is a team of providers working together in a vision clinic.[23] Because most rehabilitation services for the population with mild TBI occur in an outpatient setting, it is vital to establish a professional support network that evaluates and treats vision-related issues.

Vision rehabilitation specialists may include occupational therapists, certified low-vision therapists, optometrists, and typically other trained blind rehabilitation specialists with knowledge in vision therapy training. It is imperative that the vision therapists work closely with the eye care practitioner's plan of care and provide regular updates as to the patient's therapy progression, regression, and/or plateau of skills, as this may require reevaluation of the vision therapy treatment plan.

### Types of Vision Rehabilitation Programs

Vision rehabilitation settings in mild TBI may include an optometrist/ophthalmologist office or facilities with inpatient and/or outpatient rehabilitation clinics. Within Veterans Affairs Medical Centers, inpatient and outpatient clinics exist that offer specialty rehabilitation programs aimed at evaluating and training those with visual dysfunctions resulting from TBI.

---

**Table 4**
**Referral to appropriate facility-specific provider**

| | |
|---|---|
| Audiology/Otolaryngology/Vestibular Physical Therapy | Speech/Language Therapy |
| Blind/Low-Vision Rehabilitation | Neurology/Neuro-Ophthalmic Care |
| Occupational Therapy | Psychology/Psychiatry/Neuro-Psychiatry |
| Physical Therapy | |

Previously published materials from Walter Reed National Military Medical Center/Vision Center of Excellence. 2016; with permission.

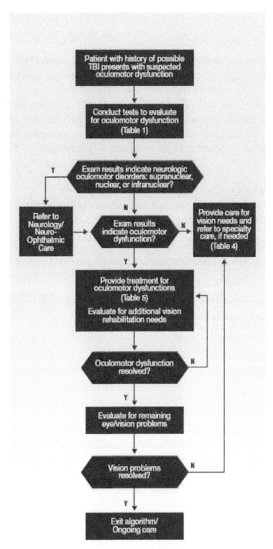

**Fig. 1.** Algorithm for the care of oculomotor dysfunctions associated with TBI. (*From* Walter Reed National Military Medical Center/Vision Center of Excellence. 2016; with permission.)

## Vision Therapy

The American Optometric Association defines vision therapy as a sequence of neuro-sensory and neuromuscular activities individually prescribed and monitored by the doctor to develop, rehabilitate, and enhance visual skills and processing.[24] The goal of vision therapy is to improve the speed, accuracy, and integration of oculomotor functions.

Eye movements include motions that shift the direction of eye gaze, such as saccades, pursuits, and vergences.[25] Oculomotor dysfunctions associated with TBI may affect many areas of daily living, including reading, visual learning, and ability to concentrate. Vision therapy is an accepted treatment of choice for the most common TBI-related visual dysfunctions. See **Table 5** for management and treatment options for common oculomotor dysfunctions associated with TBI.

### Office-based and home-based vision therapy treatment strategies

Once a vision therapy plan of care is developed, the patient (and family) should be educated about the relationship between the visual deficit and dysfunction and the ability to complete a visual task. A schedule should be created for regular inpatient training (office visit) with a home exercise program (HEP) for therapy reinforcement. The HTS program can be provided to the patient as an excellent home therapy tool for those individuals with access to computers. Complying with the HEP is crucial for success.

### Duration of vision therapy and frequency

A patient's motivation and commitment are key to success for any vision therapy training program. The average duration for most vision therapy programs range

**Table 5**
**Management and treatment options for common oculomotor dysfunctions associated with traumatic brain injury**

| Condition | Primary Treatment | Secondary Treatment |
| --- | --- | --- |
| Accommodative insufficiency Ill-sustained accommodation | Plus-powered lenses | Oculomotor rehabilitation |
| Accommodative excess | Oculomotor rehabilitation | |
| Convergence Insufficiency | Oculomotor rehabilitation | Prism lenses Extraocular muscle surgery |
| Convergence excess | Plus-powered lenses | Oculomotor rehabilitation |
| Fusional vergence dysfunction | Oculomotor rehabilitation | |
| Divergence insufficiency | Prism lenses | Oculomotor rehabilitation |
| Divergence excess/basic exophoria | Oculomotor rehabilitation | Extraocular muscle surgery |
| Basic esophoria | Prism lenses | Oculomotor rehabilitation |
| Vertical phoria | Oculomotor rehabilitation and prism lenses | Extraocular muscle surgery |
| Saccadic dysfunction | Oculomotor rehabilitation | |
| Cranial nerve (CN) III palsy | Fresnel prism, ptosis crutch, near lenses | Extraocular muscle surgery |
| CN IV palsy | Fresnel prism, distance and near glasses, base down near yoked prism, reading stands, sector occlusion, and/or full field occlusion Prisms likely ineffective if significant torsion | Oculomotor rehabilitation Extraocular muscle surgery |
| CN VI palsy | Fresnel prism | Oculomotor rehabilitation Medications Extraocular muscle surgery |

*Adapted from* Scheiman M. Understanding and managing vision disorders after traumatic brain injury. A guide for military optometrists. Washington, DC; Office of the Surgeon General: 2011; and Previously published materials from Walter Reed National Military Medical Center/Vision Center of Excellence. 2016; with permission.

between 4 and 6 weeks, depending on the patient's goals. It is recommended that patients attend weekly in-office therapy in addition to home vision therapy to make certain they are accurately performing the therapy.

Office-based vision therapy training should resemble a "fitness center" for the eyes, using a multitude of devices or techniques aimed at isolating and improving the specific visual function.

### Tint Evaluation

Based on the patient's self-report or symptom checklist, the vision therapist should evaluate each type of glare experienced by the patient, including outdoor, indoor, computer screen/iPhone, and night glare. Distant acuity charts may prove beneficial to evaluate visual clarity during indoor and outdoor tint evaluations. For those patients using darker tints, the goal is to decrease the tint level over time (increase light transmission levels) and improve their tolerance of brighter environments. Exceptions would be patients who experience migraines and patients who have abnormally large pupil size (often secondary to medication). *PTSD as a comorbidity can complicate the tint assessment and the goal of decreasing tint over time.*

## MODERATE TO SEVERE TRAUMATIC BRAIN INJURY

Individuals who experience a moderate or severe TBI will have visual sequelae like those with mild TBI; however, in addition to oculomotor/accommodative dysfunction and photosensitivity, they are more likely to experience ocular trauma whereby visual impairment is more common. Also, the more severely the brain has been damaged, the more likely a visual field deficit will be present. The frequency of ocular injuries in moderate to severe TBI ranges from 30% to 38% and includes orbital fractures, lid lacerations, traumatic cataracts, traumatic maculopathy, retinal hemorrhages, optic neuropathy, globe ruptures, angle recession, hyphema, and corneal injuries.[4,6] Blindness or legal blindness in moderate to severe TBI was found in 13% to 14%[3,6] and 18% to 32% were found to have visual field deficits.[3,4]

### The Traumatic Brain Injury–Specific Eye Examination in Moderate to Severe Traumatic Brain Injury

The level of cognition may make a subjective evaluation challenging so the eye care provider may need to rely on objective findings only. The initial evaluation is likely to take place at bedside and the goal of this evaluation is to evaluate ocular health because the patient with moderate/severe TBI is more likely to have ocular trauma. More severe patients may be nonverbal or in a low level of consciousness. Assessing visual potential is crucial because visual tracking is a part of the Coma Recovery Scale and visual impairment/blindness is more likely in the patient with more severe TBI. One study found that 65% of patients with disorder of consciousness misdiagnosed as being in a vegetative state were blind or vision impaired.[26]

The visual potential is assessed by examining the ocular health, determining the refractive error, and using objective methods of assessing visual acuity, such as the optokinetic drum and preferential looking (Teller Cards).

### Vision Rehabilitation in Moderate to Severe Traumatic Brain Injury

Addressing the ocular health concerns and ensuring that any refractive error is corrected is primary in the acute setting. Frequent follow-up is indicated as the patient progresses and more subjective testing can be performed. Diplopia, visual impairment/blindness, and visual field deficits may become more apparent as the patient's cognition improves.

Cotreatment among therapists often may prove beneficial due to incorporation of multiple rehabilitation techniques that maximize training efforts and keep goals relevant to daily activities.

Examples:

- Occupational therapist reviews patient's daily task calendar, and vision therapist reinforces eye movement pursuit and fixation
- Vision therapist practices patient's visual scanning techniques on white board to locate letter, whereas speech and language pathologist practices pronunciation of letter/word
- Physical therapy provides training to patient for improved walking posture/gait and walking endurance, whereas vision therapist incorporates bilateral scanning to locate wall targets

### Diplopia

Cranial nerve palsies are common after moderate to severe TBI and the resultant diplopia will adversely affect rehabilitation. Patching is not ideal, especially for mobility. Using a Fresnel press-on prism to eliminate the diplopia is preferable because the press-on prism eliminates the diplopia without significantly compromising vision. The prism power can be changed as the palsy improves over time.

### Visual impairment/blindness

Determining if the patient has suffered vision loss is critical to the rehabilitation process. Once it has been determined that a patient is visually impaired, low-vision eye care providers and therapists with experience in low-vision rehabilitation will need to be consulted to partner with the patient's TBI rehabilitation team. The rehabilitation team should provide modifications and compensatory strategies that will be used for rehabilitation purposes.

The VA provides blind and vision rehabilitation programs to eligible veterans and active duty service members who are visually impaired. These training programs offer veterans the opportunity to acquire the skills necessary to regain independence and successfully integrate into their family and community life. For more information on blind rehabilitation services within the VA see http://www.prosthetics.va.gov/blindrehab/BRS_Coordinated_Care.asp.

### Visual field loss

Visual field deficits have been found in 35% of patients with TBI in a sample clinic population having a range of visual symptoms.[27] Deficits of all types may be present, ranging from hemianopia to small, scattered regions of reduced sensitivity (**Table 6**).[27]

**Fig. 2** is an algorithm that outlines the steps and clinical decision points in the eye care and rehabilitation process for patients with visual field loss associated with TBI/acquired brain injury.

### Testing for visual field loss

**Box 4** outlines the screening tests recommended to evaluate the type of vision problem the patient may be experiencing. These tests will indicate whether the visual disturbance is related to possible visual field loss.

| Table 6 |
|---|
| **Types of visual field loss** |

The following types of visual field loss and their extent can be measured using visual field testing (perimetry):

| | |
|---|---|
| Hemianopia/ Quadrantanopia | Characterized by the complete loss of the left or right half of the field of vision, or a smaller segment due to injury within the visual projections of one hemisphere and that may impact patient mobility |
| Central scotoma | Characterized by a centrally located area or areas of vision loss that reduce visual acuity |
| Peripheral scotoma | Characterized by focal loss of portions of the peripheral field of vision, including hemianopia, quadrantanopia, ring scotoma, and arcuate field defects that may impact patient mobility |
| Monocular vision | Characterized by the total loss of vision in one eye |

Previously published materials from Walter Reed National Military Medical Center/Vision Center of Excellence. 2016; with permission.

If initial screening testing indicates that there may be visual field loss, more extensive visual field testing should be performed. **Box 5** lists the accepted methods for visual field testing (perimetry).

*Additional tests*
In addition to visual field deficits, patients with TBI may experience visual neglect and other visual processing deficits that will affect activities of daily living. To evaluate for the presence of neglect as well as assess the impact of the visual field deficit on function, additional testing procedures can be used. See **Table 7**.

*Rehabilitation for Visual Field Loss*

Vision rehabilitation for the patient with visual field loss requires a team approach. The specific provider(s) recommended for the patient will depend on the clinical management and rehabilitation required. **Box 6** also lists providers to whom the patient may be referred if the clinical condition(s) require additional specialized management.

Visual field loss may cause one to miss words along one side of a sentence (static), or to bump into objects on the side of the visual deficit while ambulating in a hallway (dynamic). Rehabilitation techniques for visual field loss can be categorized as either "optical management" (eg, prisms, magnifiers, telescopes, reverse telescopes) or "compensatory strategies" (eg, scanning, head movement, eye movement, awareness, mobility training). Compensatory strategies are often effective because these procedures help the individual to learn to better use their remaining vision to overcome their visual field loss. Training the patient to conduct systematic visual scanning techniques and fuller head movements can improve object detection in the missing visual field and enable the individual to learn to better use their remaining vision in static and dynamic environments. **Table 8** outlines the specific rehabilitation techniques and strategies recommended for each type of visual field loss.

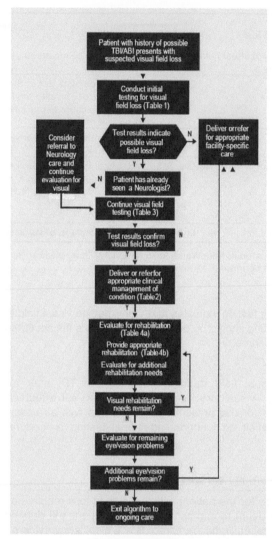

**Fig. 2.** Algorithm for rehabilitation process for visual field loss. ABI, acquired brain injury. (*From* Walter Reed National Military Medical Center/Vision Center of Excellence. 2016; with permission.)

---

**Box 4**
**Initial screening tests for visual field loss**

Confrontation field testing (nonseeing to seeing)[a]

Central visual acuity measurement

Amsler grid/facial recognition testing

Tangent screen

[a] If not already completed as part of basic eye/vision examination.
  Previously published materials from Walter Reed National Military Medical Center/Vision Center of Excellence. 2016; with permission.

---

**Box 5**
**Visual field testing (perimetry)**

Humphrey/Humphrey Esterman

Octopus

Goldmann

Previously published materials from Walter Reed National Military Medical Center/Vision Center of Excellence. 2016; with permission.

---

## REHABILITATION OVERVIEW

Visual dysfunction is commonly associated with TBI and often identified through visual symptom questionnaires, such as the BIVSS. Recognizing the visual symptomology requiring a TBI-specific eye examination is a crucial starting point toward successful patient rehabilitation. Assessments must address a patient's strengths, limitations, needs, preferences, and desired outcomes. Identifying and developing your rehabilitative referral network is vital when dealing with a TBI patient population experiencing deficits in visual function. Therapists or other rehabilitation clinicians may be the first to

---

**Table 7**
**Functional visual impact tests/procedures**

| Functional Task | Visual Impact Test |
|---|---|
| Scanning | • biVABA (portion)<br>• DEM (adult)<br>• King-Devick |
| Visual attention | • biVABA<br>• Rivermead (will rule out presence or absence of neglect)<br>• Dynavision<br>• Wayne fixation<br>• Useful field of view |
| *Reading/Near vision* | • biVABA<br>• Smith-Kettlewell reading test (SK Read)<br>• Pepper test<br>• Minnesota low-vision reading test (MN Read)<br>• Visagraph |
| *Visual perception* | • Motor-free visual perception test (vertical is recommended but not always available)<br>• Test of Visual Perceptual Skills (TVPS)<br>• DVPT-Adult<br>• Home Therapy System CPT Program |
| Functional independence | • Functional Independence Measure (FIM) |
| Quality of life (QOL) | • National Eye Institute Visual Functioning Questionnaire (NEI-VFQ-25) with 10-item euro-ophthalmic supplement<br>• College of Optometrists in Vision Development (COVD) Quality of Life Assessment |

*Abbreviations:* biVABA, brain injury visual assessment battery for adults; CPT, computer perceptual therapy; DEM, developmental eye movement; DVPT, developmental visual perception test.
Previously published materials from Walter Reed National Military Medical Center/Vision Center of Excellence. 2016; with permission.

> **Box 6**
> **Providers for clinical management and rehabilitation of visual field loss and related conditions**
>
> Optometrist/Ophthalmologist
>
> Neurologist/Neuro-Ophthalmologist
>
> Occupational/Physical therapist
>
> Audiologist[a]
>
> Low-Vision or Blind Rehabilitation Specialist (Veterans Affairs facilities)
>
> Certified Driver Evaluation Specialist
>
> [a] Hearing loss may compound spatial awareness difficulties caused by visual field loss.
> Previously published materials from Walter Reed National Military Medical Center/Vision
> Center of Excellence. 2016; with permission.

notice a problem, therefore, 2-way communication (between medical and rehabilitation teams) is vital.

Once an eye care provider identifies the visual deficits and/or dysfunction, a vision rehabilitation plan of care should be offered to improve visual functioning and quality of life. Successful vision rehabilitation training begins with education of the visual dysfunction to both the patient and family members. A combination of office and home therapy will offer a comprehensive approach to improving function. Vision therapy training may appear repetitive to the patient; therefore, it is important to provide multiple therapeutic activities to keep the patient engaged in therapy and minimize missed appointments.

It is equally important for the rehabilitative team to continually update the eye care practitioner regarding the patient's progress, as the plan of care may need to be altered (ie, therapist informs that patient does not wear the prism

**Table 8**
**Rehabilitation of visual field loss**

| Rehabilitation | Hemianopia/ Quadrantanopia | Central Scotoma | Peripheral Scotoma | Monocular Vision |
|---|---|---|---|---|
| Awareness/Sensory integration | x | x | x | x |
| Environment training | x | x | x | x |
| Scanning | x | x | x | x |
| Reading strategies | x | x | — | — |
| Compensatory aids | x | x | x | — |
| Prisms | x | — | — | — |
| Near optical aids (magnifiers) | — | x | — | — |
| Telescopes | — | x | — | — |
| Reverse telescopes | — | — | x | — |
| Eccentric viewing | x | x | — | — |
| Mobility training | x | x | x | x |
| Fitness to drive | x | x | x | x |

x, appropriate rehabilitation strategy; —, not appropriate.
Previously published materials from Walter Reed National Military Medical Center/Vision Center of Excellence. 2016; with permission.

enses). Finally, goals should be realistic and aligned with the patient's everyday tasks.

## SUMMARY

The goal of *all* rehabilitation is to improve function and retain independence, thereby improving quality of life. Vision is a major component in every aspect of rehabilitation. Speech language pathologists and neuropsychologists administer cognitive tests that require reading. Physical therapists are working to improve mobility and balance, which are affected by vision. Occupational therapists are evaluating the ability to perform activities of daily living, and recreation therapists use games and crafts as part of therapy, all highly dependent on vision.

Knowledge of the patient's visual acuity, visual fields, and oculomotor function is crucial information for the rehabilitation team to accurately assess mobility and balance or the higher-level visual skills, such as visual tracking and scanning, visual memory, and visual cognition. Unfortunately, this information is often not available, and the patient's rehabilitation success can be significantly hampered.

The optometrist's role is to provide the rehabilitation team with this valuable information. Knowing your eye care provider and rehabilitation network will provide a team approach to identifying and improving potential visual dysfunctions caused by TBI.

## REFERENCES

1. Capo-Aponte J, Jorgensen-Wagers K, Sosa J, et al. Visual dysfunctions at different stages after blast and non-blast mild traumatic brain injury. Optom Vis Sci 2017;94(1):7–15.
2. Sutter P. Rehabilitation and management of visual dysfunction following traumatic brain injury. In: Ashley MJ, Krych DK, editors. Traumatic brain injury rehabilitation. New York: CRC Press; 1995. p. 187–219.
3. Brahm KD, Wilgenburg HM, Kirby J, et al. Visual impairment and dysfunction in combat-injured service members with traumatic brain injury. Optom Vis Sci 2009;86(7):817–25.
4. Goodrich GL, Flyg HM, Kirby JE, et al. Mechanisms of TBI and visual consequences in military and veteran populations. Optom Vis Sci 2013;90(2):106–12.
5. Bulson R, Jun W, Hayes J. Visual symptomology and referral patterns for Operation Iraqi Freedom and Operation Enduring Freedom veterans with traumatic brain injury. J Rehabil Res Dev 2012;49(7):1075–82.
6. Goodrich GL, Kirby J, Cockerham G, et al. Visual function in patients of a polytrauma rehabilitation center: a descriptive study. J Rehabil Res Dev 2007;44(7): 929–36.
7. Alvarez TL, Kim EH, Vicci VR, et al. Concurrent vision dysfunctions in convergence insufficiency with traumatic brain injury. Optom Vis Sci 2012;89(12): 1740–51.
8. Stelmack JA, Frith T, Van Koevering D, et al. Visual function in patients followed at a Veterans Affairs polytrauma network site: an electronic medical record review. Optometry 2009;80:419–24.
9. Magone MT, Kwon E, Shin SY. Chronic visual dysfunction after blast-induced mild traumatic brain injury. J Rehabil Res Dev 2014;51(1):71–80.
10. Lew HL, Poole JH, Vanderploeg RD, et al. Program development and defining characteristics of returning military in a VA Polytrauma Network Site. J Rehabil Res Dev 2007;44(7):1027–34.

11. Ciuffreda KJ, Kapoor N, Rutner D, et al. Occurrence of oculomotor dysfunctions in acquired brain injury: a retrospective analysis. Optometry 2007;78(4):155–61.
12. Laukkanen H, Scheimann M, Hayes JT. Brain Injury Vision Symptom Survey (BIVSS) questionnaire. Optom Vis Sci 2017;94:43–50.
13. Radomski M, Finkelstein M, Llanos I, et al. Composition of a vision screen for service members with traumatic brain injury: consensus using a modified nominal group technique. Am J Occup Ther 2014;68(4):422–9.
14. Gallaway M, Mitchell GL. Validity of the VERA visual skills screening. Optometry 2010;81:571–9.
15. Capo-Aponte JE, Tarbett AK, Urosevich TG, et al. Effectiveness of computerized oculomotor vision screening in a military population: pilot study. J Rehabil Res Dev 2012;49:1377–98.
16. Barker F, Cockerham G, Goodrich G, et al. Brain injury impact on the eye and vision. Optom Vis Sci 2017;94(1):4–6.
17. Bahraini N, Breshears R, Hernandez T, et al. Traumatic brain injury and post traumatic stress disorder. Psychiatr Clin North Am 2014;37:55–75.
18. Goodrich GL, Martinsen GL, Flyg HM, et al. Visual function, traumatic brain injury and posttraumatic stress disorder. J Rehabil Res Dev 2014;51(4):547–58.
19. Zatzick DF, Rivara FP, Jurkovich GJ, et al. Multisite investigation of traumatic brain injuries, posttraumatic stress disorder and self-reported health and cognitive impairments. Arch Gen Psychiatry 2010;67(12):1291–300.
20. Ragsdale KA, Neer SM, Beidel DC, et al. Posttraumatic stress disorder in OEF/OIF veterans with and without traumatic brain injury. J Anxiety Disord 2013;27:420–6.
21. Theeler B, Erickson J. Posttraumatic headache in military personnel and veterans of the Iraq and Afghanistan conflicts. Curr Treat Options Neurol 2012;(14):36–49.
22. Truong J, Cuiffreda K, Han E, et al. Photosensitivity in mild traumatic brain injury (mTBI): a retrospective analysis. Brain Inj 2014;28(10):1283–7.
23. Ripley D, Politzer T, Berryman A, et al. The vision clinic: an interdisciplinary method for assessment and treatment of visual problems after traumatic brain injury. NeuroRehabilitation 2010;27:231–5.
24. American Optometric Association Board of Trustees, 2009. Available at: www.aoa.org/Documents/optometrists/QI/definition-of-optometric-vision-therapy.pdf. Accessed October 12, 2018.
25. Sutter P. Rehabilitation and management of visual dysfunction following traumatic brain injury. In: Sutter P, editor. Vision rehabilitation: multidisciplinary care of the patient following brain injury. Boca Raton (FL): CRC Press; 2011. p. 309–46.
26. Andrews K, Murphy L, Munday R, et al. Misdiagnosis of the vegetative state: retrospective study in a rehabilitative unit. BMJ 1996;313:13–6.
27. Suchoff IB, Kapoor N, Ciuffreda KJ, et al. The frequency of occurrence, types and characteristics of visual field defects in acquired brain injury: a retrospective analysis. Optometry 2008;79:259–65.

# Rehabilitation of Cognitive Dysfunction Following Traumatic Brain Injury

Inbal Eshel, MA, CCC-SLP[a],*, Amy O. Bowles, MD[b,c],
Melissa R. Ray, MS, CCC-SLP[d]

## KEYWORDS

- Cognitive • Rehabilitation • Service members • Veterans • Concussion • Moderate
- Severe • Traumatic brain injury

## KEY POINTS

- Clinicians treating service members and veterans with cognitive challenges following mild, moderate, and severe traumatic brain injuries should consider comorbidities, communication with command, military culture and context, and linking treatment directly to duty activities.
- The authors provide specific evidence-based strategies and interventions across several cognitive domains, including attention, memory and new learning, executive functions, and cognitive-communication challenges including social communication, reading, and writing.
- Patients' willingness to engage in treatment is a primary factor influencing their overall response to cognitive rehabilitation. Treatment resistance may be secondary to a patient's difficulty recognizing deficits, difficulty with motivation, acceptance or adjustment, and/or outside social and environmental factors.
- Motivational interviewing and goal attainment scaling can be used to enhance motivation and minimize resistance.

## INTRODUCTION

Cognition is critical to who we are and how we function in the world, and it is commonly affected by trauma or other neurologic insults. Traumatic brain injuries of

Disclosure Statement: The view(s) expressed herein are those of the author(s) and do not reflect the official policy or position of Brooke Army Medical Center, the U.S. Army Medical Department, the U.S. Army Office of the Surgeon General, the Department of the Army, Department of Defense, Department of Veterans Affairs or the U.S. Government.

[a] General Dynamics Health Solutions (GDHS), Contractor Employee Supporting the Defense & Veterans Brain Injury Center, Clinical Affairs Division, 1335 East West Highway, 4th Floor, Silver Spring, MD 20910, USA; [b] Brain Injury Rehabilitation Service, Department of Rehabilitation Medicine, Brooke Army Medical Center, JBSA Fort Sam Houston, Texas, USA; [c] Uniformed Services University of the Health Sciences, Bethesda, MD 20814, USA; [d] Brain Injury Rehabilitation Service, Brooke Army Medical Center, JBSA, MCHE-ZPM-B, Fort Sam Houston, TX 78234, USA
* Corresponding author. 1335 East West Highway, 4th Floor, Silver Spring, MD 20910.
E-mail address: Inbal.eshel.ctr@mail.mil

Phys Med Rehabil Clin N Am 30 (2019) 189–206
https://doi.org/10.1016/j.pmr.2018.08.005
1047-9651/19/© 2018 Elsevier Inc. All rights reserved.

all severities are often accompanied by subjective and/or objective difficulties in various aspects of cognition including attention, memory and new learning, executive functions, and social communication. Most of the traumatic brain injuries in the military population fall into the "mild" category, so that has been a particular focus of the United States Department of Defense (DoD) and Department of Veterans Affairs (VA) for research as well as the development of clinical resources. Although many people describe post–brain injury cognitive dysfunction as a "spectrum," implying a continuous distribution of increasingly severe deficits, there are some general differences between findings in those who sustained a concussion and those with more severe injuries (**Table 1**). Mild traumatic brain injury, for example, is commonly characterized by subjective complaints in the absence of objective findings beyond the first few days to weeks,[1] whereas patients with more severe injuries may be unaware of their very significant objective abnormalities. Regardless of the severity of the initial injury, however, it is the functional impact that brings these patients to our attention, and cognitive rehabilitation is an important tool used to help them.

Although a variety of definitions are available, the most commonly used definition of cognitive rehabilitation was created by the American Congress of Rehabilitation Medicine's Brain Injury Special Interest Group:

> *Cognitive rehabilitation is a systematic, functionally oriented service of therapeutic cognitive activities, based on an assessment and understanding of the person's brain-behavior deficits. Services are directed to achieve functional changes by (1) reinforcing, strengthening, or reestablishing previously learned patterns of behavior, or (2) establishing new patterns of cognitive activity or compensatory mechanisms for impaired neurological systems*
>
> —*Harley and colleagues, 1992.*[2]

Today, the authors wish to consider a semantic change from the traditional "cognitive rehabilitation" to the "rehabilitation of cognitive dysfunction." This terminology more accurately represents the scope and purpose of rehabilitation by pivoting from the rehabilitation of cognition to the rehabilitation of the individual with cognitive challenges. Similarly, new frameworks have emerged to attempt to operationalize the complexities and nuances of rehabilitation. For example, the taxonomy for rehabilitation interventions developed by Dijkers and colleagues[3] divides rehabilitation treatments into ingredients (what the provider does), targets (the aspects of functioning those ingredients are known or hypothesized to change), and mechanism of action (how the ingredients work). The 3 types of targets include (1) tissues and organs (ingredient example: stretching to relieve neck tension), (2) skills and habits (ingredient example: teaching a mnemonic device to remember names), and (3) representations (ingredient example: coaching). This framework may prove particularly useful in the rehabilitation of cognitive dysfunction when clinicians clearly and deliberately identify and differentiate the targets, thus facilitating the application of more appropriate and helpful ingredients.

Cognitive rehabilitation uses a wide variety of approaches and can be delivered by several professionals including occupational therapists, speech-language pathologists, neuropsychologists, and others. There are a variety of excellent resources and clinical tools available, some specifically developed for military and/or veteran populations (Appendix 1). The Defense and Veterans Brain Injury Center has been tasked with developing many of these tools, and Clinical Recommendations, including one on cognitive rehabilitation, can be found on their Website (www.dvbic.dcoe.mil).

**Table 1**
General differences between symptoms following mild traumatic brain injuries and moderate/severe/penetrating traumatic brain injuries

| Symptoms/Findings | Mild TBI | Moderate/Severe/ Penetrating TBI |
|---|---|---|
| Subjective cognitive complaints | Often prominent. Most often include symptoms of impaired attention, concentration, and memory. | Varies; some survivors may have limited insight and thus few complaints. Symptoms often involve many cognitive domains, with executive functions being particularly vulnerable. |
| Objective cognitive findings | Normal objective neuropsychological testing after the first wk or 2 in most studies.[1] | Most survivors have objective abnormalities in one or more domains. Varies by location and type of injury. |
| Duration of symptoms | Generally transient, lasting days to months; symptoms may persist in a small subset. | Most people will have some sort of deficits for their lifetime, ranging from mild to profound. Recovery/ improvement can be expected to slow significantly by 12–18 mo postinjury. |

Although there is no reason to expect the principles of cognitive rehabilitation to differ significantly among populations, there are some unique characteristics in military and veteran populations that merit consideration. These include comorbidities (eg, post-traumatic stress), setting of care (eg, within the military workplace), family and social supports/stressors (eg, moving entire families to the site of care), and a unique disability context. A recent study looking at civilian and VA inpatient rehabilitation cohorts also identified important differences in level of education, employment, preinjury utilization of mental health services, and traumatic brain injury (TBI) severity.[4]

## PATIENT EVALUATION OVERVIEW

Assessment of the functional impact of cognitive dysfunction is a precursor to treatment. This is a complex topic because assessment begins when the instant emergency medical personnel are engaged, that is, with the use of the Glasgow Coma Scale. There are specific assessments appropriate for patients with emerging consciousness as well as those in the posttraumatic confusional state (posttraumatic amnesia). Specific discussions of those topics are well beyond the scope of this document, which is focused on the postacute (7–12 weeks after injury) and chronic (>12 weeks after injury) stages of injury[5] and should not differ in military/veteran patients.

The 2016 VA/DoD Clinical Practice Guideline on Concussion—Mild Traumatic Brain Injury laid out principles of assessment (**Tables 2** and **3**).

## OUTPATIENT TREATMENT

Treatment of cognitive dysfunction should be functionally oriented and directly related to real-life context as much as possible. Treatment for cognitive dysfunction is typically characterized as compensatory or restorative (**Table 4**).

**Table 2**
**Postacute and chronic mild traumatic brain injuries**

| Assessment: Postacute and Chronic Mild TBI | | | |
|---|---|---|---|
| When to Assess | Focus | Tools | Next Steps |
| If cognitive complaints (eg, losing track of personal items, forgetting appointments) persist 30–90 days past the injury | Motivational interview and case history, followed by functional cognitive assessment | Reliable and valid tools, self-report, and ecologically-relevant measures that require higher levels of sustained effort or are similar to everyday environments of the patient | Use assessment to determine clinical indications for treatment, need for referral to other rehabilitation specialists, and/or a treatment plan based on functional needs |

*Data from* Department of Veterans Affairs (VA) & Department of Defense (DoD). VA/DoD clinical practice guideline for the management of concussion-mild traumatic brain injury. Version 2. 2016. Available at: https://www.healthquality.va.gov/guidelines/Rehab/mtbi/mTBICPGFullCPG50821816.pdf. Accessed December 21, 2017; with permission.

## OVERARCHING PRINCIPLES: INTERVENTION IN INDIVIDUALS WITH MODERATE-SEVERE INJURIES

When treating individuals with moderate-severe TBI, engaging in complex therapeutic activities (eg, more advanced than the patient's current level of functioning) may be more beneficial to the patient's recovery and long-term outcomes than focusing on basic activities (eg, Ref.[6]). Although more complex activities may need to be broken down into chunks or tackled in stages, patients may be better served by incorporating

**Table 3**
**Postacute and chronic moderate-severe traumatic brain injuries**

| Assessment: Postacute and Chronic Moderate-Severe TBI | | | |
|---|---|---|---|
| When to Assess | Focus | Tools | Next Steps |
| Assessment should be completed as soon as the patient has sufficient arousal and alertness to participate and should be appropriate to their level of care (eg, inpatient/outpatient). | Case history, interview with patient and family/caregivers, and formal and informal assessment of linguistic and cognitive processing, including the use of language in social contexts that affect the potential to return to premorbid functioning in activities of daily living. | Reliable and valid norm-referenced standardized and nonstandardized assessments, considering ecological validity, modality, and context. As possible, the assessments should be relevant to the everyday environment of the patient. | Use assessment to determine clinical indications for treatment frequency and intensity, need for referral to other rehabilitation specialists, and/or a treatment plan based on functional needs. |

*Adapted from* American Speech-Language Hearing Association Practice Portal: traumatic brain injury in adults. Available at: https://www.asha.org/PRPSpecificTopic.aspx?folderid=8589935337&section=Assessment. Accessed February 21, 2018; with permission.

| Table 4 | |
|---|---|
| **Comparison of compensatory and restorative treatment** | |
| **Compensatory Treatment** | **Restorative Treatment** |
| Compensatory approaches seek to provide internal mental strategies (eg, mnemonics) or external devices or aides (eg, memory notebooks) to support activity performance despite the presence of a cognitive impairment. | Restorative approaches seek to enhance the overall operation of a cognitive system with the goal of improving performance of a wide range of activities that depend on that system. |

*From* Institute of Medicine (IOM). Cognitive rehabilitation therapy for traumatic brain injury: evaluating the evidence. Washington, DC: The National Academies Press; 2011; with permission.

more functional, multicomponent, complex tasks as compared with simple, unidimensional tasks. Although not fully understood, a possible explanation for this counterintuitive principle is that engaging in complex tasks more closely mirrors those found in daily living and thus may be more inherently meaningful, acting as a motivator to engage in treatment.[6] Using the therapeutic milieu as a stepping stone toward community reentry also supports the generalization of strategies; therapeutic engagement should be as functional as possible to support integration into daily life. Other strategies that support generalization of strategies include practicing the skill and strategy in a variety of environments, and emphasizing self-management (with family/caregiver and environmental support as needed) as much as possible from the onset of treatment.

## OVERARCHING PRINCIPLES: INTERVENTION IN INDIVIDUALS WITH MILD INJURIES

Although the treatment domains will mirror those for moderate-severe deficits, patients with a history of mild TBI usually have greater insight and can develop an improved understanding of the injury and treatment strategies. For individuals with mild TBI, treatment often focuses on self-reported cognitive symptoms in the absence of identified deficits on standardized assessment. Several military-centric resources have been developed to support the treatment of this population (see Appendix 1). As with intervention for moderate-severe injuries, therapy should draw explicit connections to functional tasks to support generalization and maximize outcome. Self-management should be a major focus from the onset of treatment (**Table 5**).

## SPECIAL CONSIDERATIONS FOR SERVICE MEMBERS AND VETERANS

- Comorbidities
- Communication with command
- Understanding of military culture and context
- When possible, treatment should directly link to duty activities

Good rehabilitation programming recognizes and integrates the unique situation of the individual patient, and this strategy is particularly important when providing rehabilitation for military and veteran populations. Much has been said about the impact of posttraumatic stress disorder (PTSD) on cognitive symptomatology, particularly in the postconcussion population, because of symptom overlap. It is important to recognize that military and veteran populations may also live with depression or anxiety or any of the myriad behavioral health challenges that affect the broader population, not just PTSD. These other disorders may also be associated with cognitive dysfunction. Clinicians must balance addressing cognitive complaints with reinforcing the importance of appropriate behavioral health interventions. Some military and veteran patients

**Table 5**
Select specific interventions and strategies by domain

| Domain | Interventions and Strategies | Examples | Considerations for Mild TBI/ Concussion |
|---|---|---|---|
| Awareness/insight | Awareness training | Awareness Intervention Protocol—Predict-Perform (eg, Ref.[a]). This technique asks patients to predict their performance before undertaking a task (associated with a measurable outcome—eg, speed, accuracy) and then compares the prediction to the actual outcome. Other strategies include clear and consistent feedback from providers, peers, and family and clear and structured opportunities for the patient to evaluate their performance.[22] | Awareness intact; often hyperaware of deficits Strategies: Validate the persons' experience; Provide education on expectations of recovery and impacts of other symptoms on cognition; Increase metacognitive awareness. |

| Attention | A combination of restorative (eg, Attention Process Training) and compensatory strategy training (metacognitive strategies, environmental management). Restorative training should not occur in isolation; treatment for attention should include focus on generalization via metacognitive strategy use and environmental management | Attention Process Training (eg, Ref.[9]): structured drills and exercises (paper or computer based) stimulating specific domains of attention. The exercises provide opportunities for patients to apply strategies and focus on improving performance (ie, listening for a target sound for a sustained period of time with background distractions present). Training on generalization of strategies used in functional settings is essential. Environmental modifications and compensatory strategies should be used to support self-management of symptoms (eg, decreasing background noise and distractions, using alerts and alarms, implementing self-talk and active listening) | See moderate-severe population Consider Attention Process Training if assessment reveals attention deficits and patient is able to participate in the recommended treatment frequency |
|---|---|---|---|

(continued on next page)

**Table 5**
*(continued)*

| Domain | Interventions and Strategies | Examples | Considerations for Mild TBI/Concussion |
|---|---|---|---|
| Memory and new learning | Errorless learning, external memory strategies/aids, spaced retrieval (eg, Ref.[10]) | Errorless learning: teaching in a way that keeps the learner from making mistakes as they learn. Errorless learning is in contrast to "trial and error" or errorful learning, in which the learner attempts a task and benefits from feedback. For example, modeling how to enter appointments appropriately into a device and guiding the patient step-by-step as they practice, keeping them from making any mistakes (errorless learning) vs allowing them to attempt independently and then self-correct errors ("trial and error" learning) <br><br> Spaced retrieval: practicing learning information (eg, a medication name) over progressively longer intervals of time starting with immediate recall; questions may be dispersed throughout the session <br><br> External memory strategies: developing routine and adapting environments; application of high or low-technology aids such as smartphones, calendars, and notebooks | Internal and external strategies/aids. External aids include but are not limited to smartphones, notebooks, calendars, and alarms. Internal aids include but are not limited to repetition, association, and visual imagery |

| Executive functions | Metacognitive strategies, problem-solving, goal management training | Goal, Plan, Do, Review[11]: | See moderate-severe population |
|---|---|---|---|
| | | Goal: For example, "What are you trying to accomplish?" | |
| | | Plan: For example, "What are the steps? What do you need? How long will this take?" | |
| | | Do: Execute the plan. | |
| | | Review: For example, "How'd it work out?" | |
| | | Problem-solving strategy, for example, DBESTE[12]: | |
| | | 1. Define the problem. | |
| | | 2. Brainstorm solutions to the problem. | |
| | | 3. Evaluate each solution in terms of ease of implementation, costs and benefits, and likely consequences. | |
| | | 4. Select a solution to try. | |
| | | 5. Try the solution. | |
| | | 6. Evaluate the solution: Did it work? Do you need to try another one? If so, go back to step 4. | |
| | | Goal Management Training—5 step method (eg, Ref.[13] | |
| | | 1. "Stop—what am I doing?," | |
| | | 2. "Define the goal," | |
| | | 3. "List the steps," | |
| | | 4. "Learn the steps," then | |
| | | 5. "Check—am I doing what I planned?" | |

*(continued on next page)*

**Table 5**
*(continued)*

| Domain | Interventions and Strategies | Examples | Considerations for Mild TBI/Concussion |
|---|---|---|---|
| Cognitive-communication: pragmatics/social communication | Two primary types of treatment: social communication skills treatment and treatment of emotion perception deficits<br><br>Group-based treatment provides ample opportunities for learning, practicing, and rehearsing social behaviors | Treatment of social communication skills may include but is not limited to: using and interpreting nonverbal messages; working with peers to solve problems; conforming to social boundaries and rules; and communication of thoughts, wants, and needs[14]<br><br>Treatment of emotional perceptual challenges may include but is not limited to: recognition of nonverbal emotional expression including facial expression, eye contact, tone of voice, and body posture[11] | See moderate-severe population |
| Cognitive-communication: reading | NOTE: strategies do not apply if significant language/visual disturbance present<br><br>Strategies can be conceptualized as pre-, during, and post-reading | Pre-reading: anticipate content; activate prior knowledge<br><br>While reading: organize information; select, highlight, and summarize key ideas; take notes; use internal strategies to improve attention; ask yourself the 5 "Wh-questions" (Who? What? Where? When? Why?) or use the PQRST strategy (Preview; Question; Read; State; Test)<br><br>Post-reading: integrate knowledge and test for recall | See moderate-severe population |
| Cognitive-communication: writing | NOTE: strategies do not apply if significant language/visual disturbance present<br><br>Note-taking; diagrams | Mindmapping, concept mapping, or spider diagrams can arrange information on paper before writing to help with organization | See moderate-severe population |

think that rehabilitation providers "blame" the cognitive symptoms on behavioral health conditions, whereas behavioral health providers "blame" the symptoms on brain injury, each clinician requiring that the other issue be addressed first. This leaves patients feeling confused and not cared for. Clinicians should be sensitive to this type of situation and optimize provider-to-provider communication to mitigate its impact. Clinicians may also recognize that some cognitive compensatory strategies can be helpful to patients with functional complaints regardless of cause. That being said, cognitive rehabilitation is not an appropriate substitute for evidence-based behavioral health interventions for behavioral health diagnoses.

Military culture and context are unique and extend well beyond just the donning of a uniform. Military populations receive care within their workplace and may be in the uncomfortable position of having their supervisors and peers aware of their medical conditions. In some situations, this can be an asset where the work-group is actively involved and supportive of return to duty activities. It can be especially helpful to use duty-related activities as a context for therapies, which can be useful for relevance, engagement, and self-efficacy. Multiple protocols have been developed specifically for this population, including SCORE and CogSMART.[8,12] In other situations, it can be very challenging for Service Members to recover within the context of their workplace. Military Service Members regularly move to another post and another job about every 2 years. A Service Member may find him or herself recovering from injury and trying to learn a new job/new place and/or learning to work with a new supervisor or peer group. Sometimes, Service Members need to be relocated to a military installation or VA for more comprehensive or specialized services. In these situations, the entire household is often uprooted and moved along with the Service Member. Although this provides a certain amount of social support, it is also associated with stress and sometimes increases social isolation.

## INTERDISCIPLINARY TREATMENT MODALITIES

Because of the importance of cognition in almost all aspects of human functioning, it is often best to address cognition from a variety of different perspectives. Team members may include neuropsychologists, psychologists, occupational therapists, speech language pathologists, recreational therapists, and all other members of the rehabilitation team. These professionals often work together for collaborative goal setting and generalization.

For example, memory can be assessed and addressed in paper-and-pencil or office-based activities, which are then transferred to a more functional approach within the clinic (eg, kitchen-based activity) and finally to a community-based experience (eg, outing). Communication among team members is critical for consistent carry-over and reinforcement of strategy use. This nesting approach often helps patients and families understand how basic skills and exercises relate to their real-world goals (**Fig. 1**).

## TREATMENT RESISTANCE/COMPLICATIONS

There are many factors that can influence treatment outcomes. Patients' willingness to engage in treatment is a primary factor influencing their overall response to cognitive rehabilitation. Treatment resistance may be secondary to a patient's:

1. Difficulty recognizing deficits
2. Difficulty with motivation, acceptance, or adjustment
3. Outside social and environmental factors

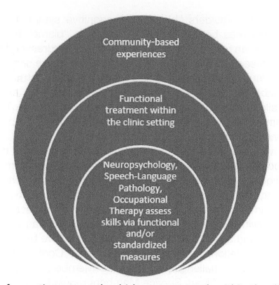

**Fig. 1.** Example of a nesting approach which connects work within the clinic to real-world goals.

The provider and rehabilitation teams' ability to identify these deficiencies in awareness early on during the rehabilitation process can ensure the team applies the appropriate therapeutic interventions that facilitate in the recovery process.[15] Each of these factors is described in more detail:

### Patient's Difficulty Recognizing Deficits (Awareness and Insight)

Crosson and colleagues[16] defined 3 primary levels of awareness: intellectual, emergent, and anticipatory. Without intellectual awareness, the patient may be aware of a problem but unable to identify it. With emergent awareness, patients recognize when impairment affects their ability to perform a task as they are attempting to perform that task. With anticipatory awareness, patients anticipate when impairment will affect performance and implement strategies to maximize success. Anticipatory awareness training teaches patients to identify when they need to use a specific strategy, increasing self-monitoring and self-management of symptoms. Challenges at any of these levels should be directly addressed as part of an intervention plan.

Formal neuropsychological assessment along with other standardized assessment from specialties such as speech-language pathology or occupational therapy will help identify strengths and weaknesses and further define rehabilitation goals. Although these initial sessions may provide information on performance, frequent and consistent monitoring of progress in treatment may occur through many modalities and be beneficial in providing direct feedback to a patient on his or her current functioning.

Specific strategies to increase awareness and self-monitoring include the following:

a. Identify functional tasks that are important to the patient, in their functional environment, which will provide opportunities for building awareness
b. Provide clear and consistent feedback as a provider (rating forms, video feedback)
c. Allow for feedback in the environment (peers in group therapy, providers in interdisciplinary team, family)
d. Provide clear and structured opportunities for the patient to self-evaluate their performance (eg, self-monitoring forms)

Patients with brain injury are often more accurate at assessing their strengths and weaknesses in concrete, observable areas such as physical limitations, but experience difficulty assessing more abstract, higher-level cognitive skills (eg, executive functioning, social communication).[17] As such, detailed and objective records, including graphs and charts that clearly define performance, may support awareness. The example in **Table 6** tracks a patient's performance by date, with a score to bolster awareness and allow the therapist to track changes to further identify the patient's response to treatment and strategies.

During treatment, patients may engage in errorless learning and modeling to build strategies. However, patients may also benefit from addressing errors when provided structured opportunities for failure. These opportunities may occur when the therapist tapers cues during structured settings or increases participation in less structured settings (group, outings) where the environment cannot be controlled.

### Difficulty with Motivation, Acceptance, or Adjustment

Cultivating a therapeutic alliance and identifying functional and meaningful goals for the patient early in the rehabilitation process can affect outcomes. Motivation plays a key role in a patient's success and has been known to affect a patient's adjustment to injury and desire and ability to return to work or identify future vocational or avocational plans, and it can improve general psychosocial functioning. Identifying the patient's values, plans, and desire or willingness to change can be enhanced through a process called motivational interviewing.[18] One technique to facilitate motivational interviewing is represented by the acronym OARS (Open-ended questions and statements, Affirmations, Reflective listening, Summaries) (**Table 7**).

### Outside Social and Environmental Factors

Outside environmental factors that may affect treatment include family dynamics, changes in roles and responsibilities, financial concerns that arise following the injury, and the impact of caregiver burden on the caregiver and patient. As a patient transitions from acute care to rehabilitation, the patient and family play a more active role in the overall rehabilitation process, including making future decisions and setting goals. It is the treatment team's responsibility to build an understanding of family dynamics and roles, including their cultural background. The rehabilitation team can benefit from developing an alliance with the patient and family and including all necessary members of the patient's team in assessment, treatment and goal-setting. Consistent communication can ensure all members of the team are focused on functional and relevant goals.

Recommendations:

- Meet regularly with patient, family, and team
- Provide ongoing education and documentation for the patient and family
- Discuss prognosis and realistic expectations for recovery to initiate future planning
- Provide information on additional patient and family resources (ie, family therapy)
- Provide information on community resources and support groups

### EVALUATION OF OUTCOME AND LONG-TERM RECOMMENDATIONS
#### Outcomes

Treatment is typically concluded when the patient has met their goals and returned to their highest level of functioning following an injury. Formal assessment and self-report measures are frequently incorporated to identify initial strengths and weaknesses,

**Table 6**
**Sample tracking chart for monitoring rehabilitation goals**

**Patient Instructions:**
Please utilize the tracking charts below to monitor progress on your selected rehabilitation goals. In the far left column list each goal individually, and in the columns to the right, make of note of how much time (in minutes) you have spent each day working on that goal either with a therapist or on your own time. Please make time every day to track your progress.

| Rehabilitation Goals | | #1 | #2 | #3 | #4 | #5 |
|---|---|---|---|---|---|---|
| **1. Visual Scanning (predriving skill building)** | Date | 9 Aug | 14 Aug | 21 Aug | — | — |
| Complete user-paced reaction time with central fixation for 1 min with reaction time of 1 s or less, 95% or higher general accuracy, and central accuracy of 75% or higher | Reaction time | 1.13 | 1.21 | 1.08 | — | — |
| | General accuracy % | 98.15 | 97.86 | 95.54 | — | — |
| | Central accuracy % | 82.76 | 90.03 | 89.26 | — | — |
| | Parameters: 1 min, size 6 circles, cent fix, cent flash | — | — | — | — | — |
| **2. Conversational skills** | Date | 9 Aug | 14 Aug | 21 Aug | | |
| Participate in a 10-min conversation with 2 others, losing conversational thread <3 times, inappropriately changing topic <1 time, and using inappropriate language <2 times | Number of interruptions of conversation partner | 5 | 6 | 4 | — | — |
| | Number of times topic or thread was lost/forgotten | 2 | 3 | 1 | — | — |
| | Number of times topic was changed inappropriately (abruptly, without transition, or obvious relevance) | 3 | 4 | 4 | — | — |
| | Inappropriate language (curse words, name-calling, etc) | 3 | 3 | 3 | — | — |
| | Parameters: 10 min, 2 conversational partners, in-clinic environment | — | — | — | — | — |
| **3. Strategy use–smart phone calendar** | Date | 9 Aug | 14 Aug | 21 Aug | | |
| Use smartphone calendar for appointments, entering 100% of appointments with 1 cue (only to initiate task) with 90% initial accuracy, double-checking appointments and correcting with 99% accuracy | Number of cues required to initiate schedule entry | 2 | 3 (initiate task × 2, cue for app) | 2 | — | — |
| | Number (%) of appointments entered correctly | 10 | 10 | 12 | — | — |
| | Number (%) of errors self-identified | 3 | 4 | 3 | — | — |
| | Number (%) of errors missed but found by therapist/helper | 4 | 4 | 2 | — | — |
| | Number (%) of appointments entered correctly after 2nd attempt | 15 | 12 | 15 | — | — |
| | Parameters: number of appointments for the wk | 17 | 18 | 16 | — | — |

**Table 7**
**Examples of OARS**

| | | |
|---|---|---|
| Open-ended questions and statements | • Invite clients to share their stories and express their concerns and needs without constraining their responses<br>• Questions may be broad or slightly more specific | "What are your most important concerns at this time?"<br>"How do you feel about this difficulty you are experiencing?"<br>"Tell me a little more about your work day, what is happening?" |
| Affirmations | • Recognize and validate the client's strengths<br>• Acknowledge positive behaviors, change and contribute to self-efficacy | "You really demonstrated great creativity and problem-solving skills identifying and applying those strategies."<br>"I appreciate all of the hard work you have done practicing the skills you have learned." |
| Reflective listening | • Demonstrates the clinicians listening and understanding of what the client stated<br>• Allows the patient to hear the reflection and correct or clarify if needed<br>• May be a brief paraphrase of what the client stated<br>• May be more complex to allow for shaping goals or introducing reflections of deeper meanings | "So I hear you say that you are..."<br>"You are expressing to me that you are..." |
| Summaries | • A series of reflections used to associate information received during the session<br>• Allows the patient to modify information as needed<br>• Can be used to highlight goals or identify plans to take steps toward change | "So I heard you say you want to start using a calendar more to help with remembering tasks and work and at home. You also stated that..." |

assist in goal-setting, and measure change and outcomes throughout the rehabilitation process.

Patients with complex injuries may be engaged in rehabilitation for a longer period of time and require measures of change that are not standardized. These may include self-report measures, questionnaires, and measurement of individual goal attainment. One method often used in rehabilitation settings to track progress toward functional outcomes is Goal Attainment Scaling (GAS).[19] Through GAS, the patient and therapist identify individualized goals, scaling them using 5 numerical values (−2 to +2). The patient identifies their expected level of outcome (−1) and where they are performing at the current time (0). GAS has been shown to help facilitate the process of planned intervention and has also been used to measure patient and clinical outcomes (**Table 8**).

| Table 8 Goal attainment scaling example | |
|---|---|
| Level of Attainment | Scale Assistive Technology |
| +2 Much more than expected | I remember to check my smartphone calendar 7 of 7 days a week. |
| +1 Somewhat more than expected | I remember to check my smartphone calendar 6 of 7 days a week. |
| 0 Expected level of outcome | I remember to check my smartphone calendar 5 of 7 days a week. |
| −1 Somewhat less than expected | I remember to check my smartphone calendar 4 of 7 days a week. |
| −2 Much less than expected | I remember to check my smartphone calendar <4 days a week. |

Formal assessment following discharge may only be necessary when there is a significant change in function or to meet a need, such as returning to work or school or to provide information to support accommodations for work, school, or returning to driving.

### Long-Term Recommendations

There are no specific evidence-based recommendations regarding long-term cognitive rehabilitation. In general, survivors of TBI should not expect to require continuous formal life-long rehabilitation of cognitive functions. After all, the purpose of rehabilitation is to get on with life and not to prepare for more rehabilitation. Nonetheless, there are some situations in which additional formal rehabilitation might be required. For example, if there is a change in function or a change in the environment or the identification of a new and unanticipated goal, reassessments may be helpful. That being said, many military and veteran traumatic brain injury survivors have long-term difficulties with employment, social relationships, psychological functioning, and general health, even more so than their civilian counterparts.[20,21] The Departments of Defense and Veterans' Affairs have several programs designed to assist with transitions, vocational rehabilitation needs, and other community reintegration challenges, and some of these programs are designed specifically for TBI survivors.

### SUMMARY

The rehabilitation of military personnel and veterans with cognitive dysfunction secondary to or attributed to traumatic brain injury has much in common with rehabilitation provided to their civilian counterparts. However, there are some important considerations for these populations including the military milieu and the frequent comorbidities that make this population unique.[4] Several specific tools and resources have been designed and empirically evaluated with these populations, and several of these are listed in Appendix 1. These materials and strategies may be particularly helpful in these populations in part because of their ecological validity and incorporation of military priorities, terms, and culture. Many military and veteran TBI survivors have additional, non-TBI-related issues, so optimizing cognition may be particularly important for their successful community reintegration and to help them resume a normal, meaningful, and full life.

## REFERENCES

1. Karr JE, Areschenkoff CN, Garcia-Barrera MA. The neuropsychological outcomes of concussion: a systematic review of meta-analyses on the cognitive sequelae of mild traumatic brain injury. Neuropsychology 2014;28(3):321–36.
2. Harley JP, Allen C, Braciszewski TL, et al. Guidelines for cognitive rehabilitation. NeuroRehabilitation 1992;2(3):62–7.
3. Dijkers MP, Ferraro MK, Hart T, et al. Toward a rehabilitation treatment taxonomy: summary of work in progress. Phys Ther 2014;94(3):319–21.
4. Nakase-Richardson R, Stevens LF, Tang X, et al. Comparison of the VA and NI-DILRR TBI model system cohorts. J Head Trauma Rehabil 2017;32(4):221–33.
5. Department of Veterans Affairs (VA) & Department of Defense (DoD). VA/DoD clinical practice guideline for the management of concussion-mild traumatic brain injury. Version 2. 2016. Available at: https://www.healthquality.va.gov/guidelines/Rehab/mtbi/mTBICPGFullCPG50821816.pdf. Accessed December 4, 2017.
6. Horn SD, Corrigan JD, Beaulieu CL, et al. Traumatic brain injury patient, injury, therapy, and ancillary treatments associated with outcomes at discharge and 9 months postdischarge. Arch Phys Med Rehabil 2015;96(8 Suppl 3):S304–29.
7. Cheng SK, Man DW. Management of impaired self-awareness in persons with traumatic brain injury. Brain Inj 2006;20(6):621–8.
8. Cooper DB, Bowles AO, Kennedy JE, et al. Cognitive rehabilitation for military service members with mild traumatic brain injury: A randomized clinical trial. Journal of Head Trauma Rehabilitation 2016;32(3):1–15.
9. Sohlberg MM, McLaughlin KA, Pavese A, et al. Evaluation of attention process training and brain injury education in persons with acquired brain injury. J Clin Exp Neuropsychol 2000;22(5):656–76.
10. Haskins EC, Cicerone K, Dams-O-Conner KD, et al. Cognitive rehabilitation manual: translating evidence-based recommendations into practice. Reston (VA): ACRM Publishing; 2012.
11. Ylvisaker M, Turkstra LS, Coelho C. Behavioral and social interventions for individuals with traumatic brain injury: a summary of the research with clinical implications. Semin Speech Lang 2005;26(4):256–67.
12. Twamley EW, Jak AJ, Delis DC, et al. Cognitive symptom management and rehabilitation therapy (CogSMART) for veterans with traumatic brain injury: Pilot randomized controlled trial. J Rehabil Res Dev 2014;51(1):59–70.
13. Waid-Ebbs JK, Daly J, Wu SS, et al. Response to goal management training in veterans with blast-related mild traumatic brain injury. J Rehabil Res Dev 2014; 51(10):1555–66.
14. Hawley L, Newman J. Social skills and traumatic brain injury: a workbook for group treatment. Authors; 2006. Available at: www.braininjurysocialcompetence.com.
15. O'Keeffe F, Dockree P, Moloney P, et al. Awareness of deficits in traumatic brain injury: a multidimensional approach to assessing metacognitive knowledge and online-awareness. J Int Neuropsychol Soc 2007;13(1):38–49.
16. Crosson B, Barco PP, Velozo CA, et al. Awareness and compensation in postacute head injury rehabilitation. J Head Trauma Rehabil 1989;4:46–54.
17. Fleming JM, Strong J. A longitudinal study of self-awareness: Functional deficits underestimated by persons with brain injury. Occup Ther J Res 1999;19:3–17.
18. Miller WR, Rollnick S. Motivational interviewing: helping people change. 3rd edition. New York: Guilford Press; 2013.

19. Kiresuk T, Smith A, Cardillo J. Goal attainment scaling: application, theory and measurement. New York: Lawrence Erlbaum Associates; 1994.

20. Brooks JC, Shavelle RM, Strauss DJ, et al. Long-term survival after traumatic brain injury part II: life expectancy. Arch Phys Med Rehabil 2015;96(6):1000–5.

21. Cuthbert JP, Pretz CR, Bushnik T, et al. Ten-year employment patterns of working age individuals after moderate to severe traumatic brain injury: a national institute on disability and rehabilitation research traumatic brain injury model systems study. Arch Phys Med Rehabil 2015;96(12):2128–36.

22. Ray MR, LeBlanc MM, Manning RK, et al. Study of Cognitive Rehabilitation Effectiveness Study Manual, Chapter 4: Traditional Cognitive Rehabilitation for Persistent Symptoms Following Mild Traumatic Brain Injury (SCORE Arm 3). Defense and Veterans Brain Injury Center; 1–72. Available at: Pulled from https://dvbic.dcoe.mil/study-manuals. Accessed February 22, 2018.

## APPENDIX 1: RESOURCES AND CLINICAL TOOLS

Note: These resources are affiliated with and/or developed by the VA/DoD community.

- Free manuals and toolkits:
  - Study of Cognitive Rehabilitation Effectiveness (SCORE) Manual (Chapters 4 and 5): http://dvbic.dcoe.mil/research/study-manuals
  - mTBI Rehabilitation Toolkit (Chapter 7 and Appendix B): http://www.cs.amedd.army.mil/borden/Portlet.aspx?ID=065de2f7-81c4-4f9d-9c85-75fe59dbae13
  - Clinician's Guide to Cognitive Rehabilitation in mild TBI: Application in Military Service Members and Veterans: http://www.asha.org/uploadedFiles/ASHA/Practice_Portal/Clinical_Topics/Traumatic_Brain_Injury_in_Adults/Clinicians-Guide-to-Cognitive-Rehabilitation-in-Mild-Traumatic-Brain-Injury.pdf
  - Compensatory Cognitive Training (CCT); Compensatory Cognitive Training Facilitator Manual https://s3.amazonaws.com/cogsmart/Compensatory+Cognitive+Training+facilitator+manual+June+2013.pdf; Compensatory Cognitive Training Participant Manual https://s3.amazonaws.com/cogsmart/Compensatory+Cognitive+Training+participant+manual+July+2016.pdf; Cognitive Symptom Management and Rehabilitation Therapy (CogSMART) http://www.cogsmart.com/
- Clinical Practice Guidelines and Clinical Recommendations:
  - http://www.healthquality.va.gov/guidelines/Rehab/mtbi/
  - http://dvbic.dcoe.mil/resources/clinical-tools—Clinical Recommendations on Cognitive Rehabilitation of Service Members and Veterans following mild-moderate TBI (anticipated release summer 2018)

# Department of Veterans Affairs Polytrauma Telerehabilitation
## Twenty-First Century Care

Joel Scholten, MD[a],*, Cindy Poorman, MSPT[a,1], Lesli Culver, LCSW[b],
Joseph B. Webster, MD[c,d]

## KEYWORDS

- Telerehabilitation • Telehealth • Polytrauma • Traumatic brain injury • Amputation

## KEY POINTS

- Telehealth provides a unique opportunity to connect clinical providers to patients for evaluation and follow-up purposes.
- Using telehealth with mobile devices allows the provider to see the patient in their home or work environment, allowing greater individualization of treatment delivery.
- Telerehabilitation improves access to the vast array of clinical specialists required for evaluation and management of polytrauma injuries.
- Telehealth does not eliminate the need for face-to-face clinical care but can enhance delivery, coordination, and access to care.

## INTRODUCTION

The use of telehealth for the management of polytrauma and traumatic brain injury (TBI) patients provides a unique opportunity to leverage technology to enhance care for a complex patient cohort. TBI is increasingly viewed in a chronic disease framework but acute inpatient rehabilitation following TBI is just the initial phase of the rehabilitation process.[1,2] Telehealth provides an opportunity to facilitate clinical care and enhance support for community reintegration for individuals with neurologic injury.

Disclosure Statement: The authors have nothing to disclose.
[a] Physical Medicine and Rehabilitation, US Department of Veterans Affairs, 810 Vermont Avenue Northwest, Office #667, Washington, DC 20420, USA; [b] Department of Physical Medicine and Rehabilitation, James A Haley Veterans' Hospital, 13000 Bruce B. Downs Boulevard, 673-111E, Tampa, FL 33612, USA; [c] Department of Physical Medicine and Rehabilitation, Virginia Commonwealth University School of Medicine, Richmond, VA, USA; [d] Physical Medicine and Rehabilitation, Hunter Holmes McGuire VA Medical Center, Building 514, 1201 Broad Rock Boulevard, Richmond, VA 23249, USA
[1] Present address: 4100 East Mississippi Avenue, Suite 825, Room 804, Glendale, CO 80246.
* Corresponding author.
E-mail address: joel.scholten@va.gov

In addition, telehealth provides an opportunity to connect experts to patients in more remote or underserved areas. For patients with complex and chronic rehabilitation needs in which the traditional rehabilitation team is expanded to meet the needs of the patient, telehealth can decrease health care disparity. This is especially true for veterans who have sustained combat and noncombat polytrauma injuries, defined as "two or more injuries, one of which may be life threatening, sustained in the same incident that affect multiple body parts or organ systems and result in physical, cognitive, psychological, or psychosocial impairments and functional disabilities. Traumatic Brain Injury (TBI) frequently occurs in polytrauma in combination with other disabling conditions, such as: traumatic amputations, open wounds, musculoskeletal injuries, burns, pain, auditory and visual impairments, post traumatic stress disorder (PTSD), and other mental health problems."[3] The use of telehealth can also assist in connecting various levels of expertise within health care systems, including the US Department of Veterans Affairs (VA) Polytrauma System of Care[4] and the VA Amputation System of Care (ASoC).[5] These were developed to provide a nationwide integrated system of rehabilitation services to ensure veterans and service members transition seamlessly between Department of Defense (DoD) and VA, and back to their home communities.[3] These specialty systems of care provide options for clinical rehabilitation, care management, patient and family education and training, psychosocial support, and advanced rehabilitation and prosthetic technologies.[3]

## HISTORY OF TELEHEALTH

The use of video conferencing in medicine had its beginnings in 1959 when clinicians at the University of Nebraska used a 2-way television technique to extend group therapy mental health services to remote areas. They connected to 3 VA hospitals in Omaha, Lincoln, and Grand Island, Nebraska. The results of these sessions were very positive. So much so that the clinicians commented that "two-way television group therapy may be the means for skilled mental health personnel to extend their services to persons in distant areas which have an insufficient number of therapists."[6]

The 1990s brought significant changes in the telehealth world with the introduction of electronic medical records, digital communications, and the rapid growth of the Internet.[7] Today, telehealth brings health care providers in primary and specialty care to areas devoid of these resources. Telehealth has been implemented in the US private health care sector but challenges with payment and state licensure have hindered the full utility of virtual care. The telerehabilitation efforts described in this section will highlight services that have been developed and are available in the VA.

The VA's Telehealth Services mission is to "provide the right care, at the right place and at the right time" through the effective and appropriate use of health information and telecommunications technologies.[8] Telerehabilitation also strives to meet this mission by improving access to rehabilitation specialty care services, particularly with patients in rural and highly rural areas.

## TELEREHABILITATION

Telerehabilitation provides a range of conventional rehabilitation services at a distance using communication technologies.[9] Telerehabilitation is relatively new to the area of telehealth, with most development coming in the last decade. The growth of telerehabilitation has been hindered by the hands-on requirements of some rehabilitation disciplines. Many clinicians have thought that it was not possible to evaluate or treat patients without being able to touch them. However, these challenges are slowly being extinguished through the use of telepresenters (TPs) and innovative technologies. TPs assist in telehealth encounters by serving as the provider's hands during the clinical encounter and also support the clinical, business, and technical areas needed to deploy, implement, and manage telehealth clinics.[10] The clinical background and training of the TP should match the requirements for the individual clinic. For example, a licensed practical nurse may be an appropriate TP for a TBI clinic follow-up visit to assess effectiveness of headache treatments but a physical or occupational therapist skilled in obtaining joint range of motion and other measurements may be required for a specialty wheelchair evaluation clinic. As a result of using TPs, telerehabilitation is now being seen as an exciting alternative model of care that can assist patients in gaining their ultimate functional outcome.[10]

Telerehabilitation can be used to diagnose, evaluate, and manage patients of all ages with physical and/or cognitive impairment and disability. Early experience with telerehabilitation has shown that it can provide continuity and coordination of care across a continuum to help patients in their transition back to their local communities. Telerehabilitation advantages include (1) expedited access to care, (2) improved clinical communication and transitions between locations of care, and (3) potential elimination of unnecessary travel for patients and their families.

Telerehabilitation can also be provided directly in the patient's home. This allows clinicians to observe how patients participate in activities of daily living, provide recommendations for assistive devices, and evaluate the home environment for modifications to facilitate greater independence. Telerehabilitation can be provided through the following modalities[11]:

- Clinical video telehealth

Clinical video telehealth is the use of real-time interactive video conferencing, sometimes with supportive peripheral technologies, to assess, treat, and provide care to a patient remotely.

- Store-and-forward telehealth

Store-and-forward telehealth is the use of technologies to asynchronously acquire and store clinical information (eg, data, image, sound, and video) that is forwarded to or retrieved by a provider at another location for clinical evaluation.

- Home telehealth

Home telehealth is a program into which patients are enrolled that applies care and case management principles to coordinate care using health informatics, disease management, and technologies, including in-home and mobile monitoring, messaging, and/or video technologies. This program allows patients with chronic disease to take control of the management of that disease through personalized at home care.

## IMPLEMENTATION OF TELEREHABILITATION IN VA

Telehealth has been implemented in VA through identification of potential applications based on a particular diagnosis. There have been significant advances in using telehealth to address symptoms of TBI; mental health conditions, including posttraumatic stress disorder PTSD[12]; and pain[13,14]; thus covering the polytrauma clinical triad.[15]

## TRAUMATIC BRAIN INJURY

The VA initiated telehealth in the setting of TBI polytrauma through the establishment of a dedicated Polytrauma Telehealth Network connecting Department of Defense acute care hospitals to the VA's inpatient TBI rehabilitation programs, also known as polytrauma rehabilitation centers. This network enhanced communication between health care teams from both agencies by connecting via video conference to review clinical care and treatment planning while transferring patients between systems. This enhanced communication helped minimize potential errors during the transition with review of medications and specific restrictions and treatment plans, and provided a better patient and caregiver experience. These video conference meetings were also used to connect VA treatment teams when patients were transferred from a poly-trauma rehabilitation center following rehabilitation to another VA facility closer to the patient's home.

As telehealth use throughout the VA increased, providers began using telehealth in other areas of TBI or polytrauma care. In 2007, the VA deployed a TBI screening and evaluation program to ensure that every veteran leaving active duty service after September 11, 2001, was screened for possible TBI and, if positive, referred for an evaluation by a TBI expert.[16] VA convened a group of TBI experts to review and approve a comprehensive TBI evaluation protocol that could be completed by tele-health. This protocol allowed a TBI expert located at a VA medical center to evaluate a veteran at a remote location with the assistance of a TP, usually a nurse or nursing assistant. This program was initially implemented at 17 VA medical centers in 2012 and later disseminated throughout the VA health care system. Both veterans and TBI providers have noted high satisfaction with this virtual protocol.[17]

As VA providers became more comfortable with using telehealth technology, addi-tional TBI applications have been implemented, including TBI or polytrauma clinic follow-up visits, cognitive therapy, mental health counseling, and family meetings with the interdisciplinary treatment team.[18]

## AMPUTATION

Amputation is often associated with polytrauma. Amputations have medical, phys-ical, social, and psychological ramifications for individuals and their family mem-bers. Optimal management of this condition requires a comprehensive, coordinated, interdisciplinary program of services throughout the continuum of care. This includes offering the latest practices in medical interventions, prosthetic limb technology, and rehabilitation strategies to restore function and optimize qual-ity of life.[11,19]

In 2008, the VA established the ASoC with the goal to enhance the quality and con-sistency of amputation rehabilitation services. The ASoC is an integrated, national health care delivery system that provides lifelong holistic care and care coordination for veterans who have undergone amputation. Within the ASoC, a telehealth program has been deployed to enhance the veteran experience and improve outcomes by providing specialized amputation clinic services closer to the veteran's home.[20] Since 2008 there has been steady growth in the VA's tele-amputation services.

Tele-amputation services improve access to comprehensive specialty amputation care for veterans through the VA's secure video conferencing network. The benefits that can be expected from telehealth include improved access to specialty care and improved continuity of care. Telehealth allows VA medical centers with limited special-ized amputation rehabilitation services to partner with other VA medical centers with the needed expertise to provide care locally and reduce the need for veterans to travel. The ability to reduce travel burden is especially important for many veterans with am-putations who have significant mobility issues. For other veterans who have realized the active lifestyle that prosthetics and rehabilitation services have made possible, requent travel can affect their employment and participation in family or recreational activities.

Different types of tele-amputation services are being provided by the VA (**Box 1**). The first and most common is the interdisciplinary team amputee clinic. At this clinic, there is a full amputee care team at the provider site, including a physician, physical or occupational therapist, and prosthetist. The TP at the patient site is generally a nurse, medical assistant, or physical therapist. Services include initial evaluations and follow-up visits, which may be conducted with the veteran in their home or other community location.

Prosthetist-support clinics include a prosthetist at the provider site and commonly include other members of the clinic team (physician and therapist) at the patient site. Services provided by this clinic include assisting in developing the prosthesis

---

**Box 1**
**Types of tele-amputation services**

*Interdisciplinary amputee clinic*

- Provider site: amputee care team (physician, physical therapist or occupational therapist, prosthetist)

- Patient site: patient and a TP

- Services provided:
  - Initial patient evaluations and follow-up visits
  - Artificial limb and rehabilitation prescription
  - Assessment of a new prosthesis after delivery
  - Follow-up for comorbidities and complications

*VA prosthetist amputee clinic*

- Provider site: VA prosthetist

- Patient site: patient, VA physician and therapist

- Services provided:
  - Assist team in developing prosthesis prescription
  - Assessment of a new prosthesis or changes in prescription

*Support groups*

- Multiple sites are connected via videoconferencing

- Patients are able to interact and establish peer supports

- Patients are provided counseling support and education

*Telehealth to community-based prosthetic providers*

- Provider site: VA prosthetist or entire amputee care team

- Patient site: patient and contracted community-based prosthetist

- Services provided:
  - Assessment of a new prosthesis or changes in prescription
  - Follow-up for comorbidities and complications

*Telehealth to the veterans' home*

- Provider site: amputee care team or individual provider

- Patient site: patient and caregiver, if needed

- Services provided:
  - Assessment of a new prosthesis or changes in prescription
  - Follow-up for comorbidities and complications

prescription and in verification of a new prosthesis or new prosthetic components that have been provided by a contracted prosthetist in the community. The VA can also use telehealth services to evaluate veterans while they are being seen at the office of a contracted prosthetist in the community at the time of delivery of the artificial limb.

Amputee support groups are also being conducted with the support of telehealth. For this service, multiple sites are connected via videoconferencing into a joint support group. Veterans have a chance to interact with each other and receive support and education. Telehealth services have also been used to connect individual peer supporters to peer mentees.

## TELEREHABILITATION ENTERPRISE-WIDE INITIATIVE

The VA Office of Rural Health (ORH) implements enterprise-wide initiatives to increase access to care for 3 million veterans living in rural communities who rely on the VA for health care.[21] VA implemented the Telerehabilitation Enterprise-Wide Initiative in 2017 to enhance access to specialized rehabilitation services for rural veterans through the development of a hub and spoke model. Hubs are located at 4 VA sites with rehabilitation expertise to provide care to spoke sites in rural areas with limited expertise.

Hub sites provide specialized rehabilitation services, clinical care, and consultation through telehealth via various telerehabilitation protocols. These protocols provide a standardized approach for the clinician to provide telehealth services based on traditional face-to-face rehabilitation practices in addition to administrative guidance to set up and run specific rehabilitation clinics. Protocols have been developed in a variety of areas, including but not limited to

- TBI: A TBI specialist or TBI team connects via secure video to a veteran patient at another VA site or in the veteran's home to complete an initial TBI evaluation, follow-up visit, or family conference. If the visit occurs in a VA facility, the extent of physical examination depends on the training of the TP.
- Amputation: An amputation specialist or amputation team connects via secure video to a veteran patient at another VA site, prosthetic vendor, or in the veteran's home to complete an initial amputation evaluation, follow-up visit, family conference, or prosthetic limb checkout visit. If the visit occurs in a VA facility, the extent of physical examination depends on the training of the TP.
- Home safety assessments: A TP, therapist, or team of therapists connect via secure video to the primary care or rehabilitation team at a VA medical center and the veteran's home environment is evaluated by the team via streaming video. Functional assessments, as well as physical modification recommendations, are completed during these visits with a goal of maximizing the safety of the home environment.
- Specialty seating and power mobility clinics: A seating and mobility specialist or team is connected to a veteran at another VA medical center or outpatient clinic to provide an evaluation and make recommendations for appropriate mobility devices. The TP assists the veteran in demonstration of the veteran's functional ability, as well as obtains appropriate measurements for prescribing the appropriate device. Follow-up video visits are used to provide additional education and training on the device, as well as to ensure that the device meets the veteran's needs.
- Cognitive therapy: Cognitive assessments and interventions are provided by speech language pathologists, occupational therapists, or psychologists to veterans at another VA site or in the veteran's home. Materials needed for cognitive

therapy sessions are sent to the veteran before the visit via secure e-mail. A TP may or may not be required for these sessions.

## POTENTIAL BENEFITS OF TELEHEALTH

As technology continues to improve and telehealth becomes integrated into all clinicians' standard practice, the authors anticipate that telerehabilitation will be used to provide greater support and services in the community to individuals with polytrauma. There are definite potential benefits to integrating telehealth into a rehabilitation practice. Early adoption of telerehabilitation in the area of polytrauma includes using telehealth to promote compliance with rehabilitation recommendations, provide ongoing education, update home exercise programs, and to support caregivers.

## LIMITATIONS

Use of telerehabilitation in clinical care can be limited buy the skill and expertise of the presenter assisting in the clinical evaluation. Another limitation is the acceptance of virtual care modalities by patients and providers. Patients may not fully embrace virtual care because some may see this as an intrusion into their private lives if a clinician is seeing them in their home; however, many other patients anecdotally report high satisfaction with this care delivery. Providers are typically trained in face-to-face clinical assessment and treatment, and transitioning to utilization of telehealth does require some additional training and time for providers to develop adequate comfort to successfully provide virtual care.

Telehealth has the ability to disseminate polytrauma expertise from specialized hubs to potentially underserved areas (see previous discussion). In addition to the clinical limitations previously listed, there are policy and regulatory limitations that will likely impede uptake of telehealth. Currently, there is significant variability between states on the restriction of providers practicing telehealth, especially when patients are not located in the same state where the provider is located. Federal agencies are likely better positioned to fully implement telehealth due to the ability of the federal government to impose federal supremacy and overrule various state licensure regulations. Currently, the VA is posing regulations to allow virtual care anywhere in the country using the Anywhere to Anywhere program for providers in the VA health care system.[22]

## FUTURE DIRECTIONS

Implementation of telehealth in the rehabilitation setting will likely offer significant benefits to patients with polytrauma by improving access to experts, and by improving support and connection with providers when patients are in their home setting. Individuals with polytrauma have complex symptomatology and will likely have ongoing medical, rehabilitation, and community reintegration concerns. Using telehealth can enable the vast array of necessary rehabilitation providers to connect and support patients in the home environment. The future of telerehabilitation remains to be seen and implementing virtual care into every rehabilitation provider's standard of practice will be impeded until state licensure and payment issues are resolved.

## REFERENCES

1. Malec JF, Hammond FM, Flanagan S, et al. Recommendations from the 2013 Galveston Brain Injury Conference for implementation of a chronic care model in brain injury. J Head Trauma Rehabil 2013;28:476–83.

2. Masel BE, DeWitt DS. Traumatic brain injury: a disease process, not an event. J Neurotrauma 2010;27:1529–40.
3. Department of Veterans Affairs, 2013. VA polytrauma system of care handbook. [WWW document]. Available at: https://www.va.gov/optometry/docs/VHA_Handbook_1172_01_Polytrauma_System_of_Care.pdf. Accessed September 24, 2018.
4. Department of Veterans Affairs, 2015. Polytrauma/TBI system of care. [WWW document]. Available at: https://www.polytrauma.va.gov/system-of-care/index.asp. Accessed September 24, 2018.
5. Department of Veterans Affairs, 2015. Rehabilitation and prosthetic services. [WWW document]. Available at: https://www.rehab.va.gov/asoc/. Accessed September 24, 2018.
6. Wittson CL, Affleck DC, Johnson V. Two-way television in group therapy. Ment Hosp 1961;12(11):22–3.
7. Brennan DM, Mawson S, Brownsell S. Telerehabilitation: enabling the remote delivery of healthcare, rehabilitation, and self management. Stud Health Technol Inform 2009;145:231–48.
8. Department of Veterans Affairs, 2018. Telehealth Serv. About telehealth services. [WWW document]. Available at: http://vaww.telehealth.va.gov/about/index.asp. Accessed September 24, 2018.
9. Russell TG. Telerehabilitation: a coming of age. Aust J Physiother 2009;55:5–6.
10. Department of Veterans Affairs, 2018. Telehealth Serv. Telerehabilitation resource center. [WWW document]. Available at: http://vaww.telehealth.va.gov/clinic/rehab/trehb/index.asp. Accessed September 24, 2018.
11. Dept of Veterans Affairs, 2017. VA telehealth services [WWW Document]. VA Telehealth Serv. Available at: https://www.telehealth.va.gov/. Accessed September 24, 2018.
12. Department of Veterans Affairs, 2016. PTSD: National Center for PTSD. PTSD and telemental health. [WWW document]. Available at: https://www.ptsd.va.gov/professional/treatment/overview/ptsd-telemental.asp. Accessed September 24, 2018.
13. Flynn DM, Eaton LH, McQuinn H, et al. TelePain: primary care chronic pain management through weekly didactic and case-based telementoring. Contemp Clin Trials Commun 2017;8:162–6.
14. Müller KI, Alstadhaug KB, Bekkelund SI. A randomized trial of telemedicine efficacy and safety for nonacute headaches. Neurology 2017;89:153–62.
15. Lew HL, Otis JD, Tun C, et al. Prevalence of chronic pain, posttraumatic stress disorder, and persistent postconcussive symptoms in OIF/OEF veterans: polytrauma clinical triad. J Rehabil Res Dev 2009;46:697–702.
16. Department of Veterans Affairs, 2015. Screening and evaluation of traumatic brain injury in Operation Enduring Freedom, Operation Iraqi Freedom, and Operation New Dawn Veterans. Screen. Eval. Trauma. Brain Inj. Oper. Endur. Freedom Oper. Iraqi Freedom Oper. New Dawn Veterans. [WWW document]. Available at: https://www.va.gov/vhapublications/ViewPublication.asp?pub_ID=5376. Accessed September 24, 2018.
17. Martinez RN, Hogan TP, Lones K, et al. Evaluation and treatment of mild traumatic brain injury through the implementation of clinical video telehealth: provider perspectives from the Veterans Health Administration. PM R 2017;9:231–40.
18. Hernandez H, Scholten J, Moore E. Home clinical video telehealth promotes education and communication with caregivers of veterans with TBI. Telemed J E Health 2015;21:761–6.

19. Dept of Veterans Affairs, D. of D., 2017. VA/DoD clinical practice guideline for rehabilitation of individuals with lower limb amputation [WWW Document]. VADoD Clin. Pract. Guidel. Rehabil. Individ. Low. Limb amputation. Available at: https://www.healthquality.va.gov/guidelines/Rehab/amp/VADoDLLACPG092817.pdf. Accessed September 24, 2018.

20. Webster J, Poorman C, Cifu D. Guest editorial: Department of Veterans Affairs amputations system of care: 5 years of accomplishments and outcomes. J Rehabil Res Dev 2014;51. vii–xvi.

21. Department of Veterans Affairs, 2018. Office of Rural Health enterprise-wide initiatives. [WWW document]. Available at: https://www.ruralhealth.va.gov/providers/Enterprise_Wide_Initiatives.asp. Accessed September 24, 2018.

22. Sweeney E. 2017. Fierce HealthCare. VA proposed rule would override state licensing restrictions to expand access to telehealth. [WWW document]. Available at: https://www.fiercehealthcare.com/regulatory/va-telehealth-practice-restrictions-state-law-proposed-rule. Accessed September 24, 2018.

# Assistive Technology in Polytrauma Rehabilitation

Melissa Oliver, MS, OTR/L

## KEYWORDS

- Assistive technology • 3D printing • Integration of technology • AAC • EADLS
- Electronic cognitive devices • Adaptive sports

## KEY POINTS

- Assistive technology provides opportunities for individuals to engage in daily activities and life roles.
- Individuals with polytrauma injuries will benefit from assistive technology in areas of communication, cognition, mobility, interaction with their environment, and participation in recreation activities.
- Customized assistive technology solutions through 3-dimensional (3D) printing, 3D scanning, and electronics is another tool that allows individuals increase function and independence.

The era of technology encompasses the daily lives of most Americans from answering cell phones through watches to reconnecting with high school friends to the house automatically turning on the security alarm, lowering the thermostat, and turning off lights when they leave home. The Pew Research Center studies the trends in the use of Internet and technology. Their findings display how much Americans rely on their technology; in 2015, 84% of American adults used the Internet,[1] 91% owned some type of mobile phone, 56% owned a smartphone,[2] and the purpose of using smartphones ranged from looking up heath information to online banking to applying for a job.[3] Therefore, when an individual has been injured or diagnosed with a life-changing disease, the use of technology can still have a significant role in their recovery and connection to their surroundings.

Assistive technology (AT) is a broad term that includes rehabilitation, modified and assistive devices for people with disabilities or illnesses, as well as the procedures used in selecting, locating, and using them. AT devices provide individuals the opportunity to participate in their life roles by increasing their level of function and independence, which in turn, decreases caregiver burden. AT also allows for

---

Disclosure Statement: The author has nothing to disclose.
Assistive Technology Program, Physical Medicine & Rehabilitation Service, McGuire VA Medical Center, 1201 Broad Rock Boulevard, Richmond, VA 23249, USA
E-mail address: melissaotr@gmail.com

increased involvement in community, vocational/avocational and social environ-ments. According to Public Law 108-364 The Assistive Technology Act of 1998, as amended (2004), AT is "any item, piece of equipment, or system, whether ac-quired commercially, modified or customized, that is, commonly used to increase, maintain, or improve functional capabilities of individuals with disabilities."[4] An AT interdisciplinary team determines through an evaluation process if a client with spe-cific polytrauma injuries may benefit from AT; however, not everyone requires or may benefit from AT. The types of AT devices range from wheeled mobility devices to communication devices to cognitive aids to electronic aids to daily living (**Table 1**).

This article focuses on AT devices that could assist individuals with polytrauma injuries. Within the Veterans Affairs (VA) Health Administration, there are Assistive Technology Centers of Excellence at the 5 VA medical centers that have poly-trauma rehabilitation centers. These centers have dedicated staff in AT. Although each center might run differently, they all have the same 2 missions: (1) to enhance the ability of Veterans and Active Duty Members with disabilities to fulfill life goals through the coordination and provision of appropriate interdisciplinary AT services and (2) to serve as an expert resource to support the application of AT

**Table 1**
**Examples of assistive technology**

| Assistive Technology Devices | Examples |
| --- | --- |
| Communication Aids | • White boards<br>• Speech and augmentative communication aids<br>• Speech generating devices<br>• Writing and typing aids |
| Computer Access Aids | • Accessibility features in operating systems<br>• Alternative input devices<br>• Alternative output devices<br>• Voice recognition software |
| Daily Living Aids | • Clothing and dressing aids<br>• Eating and cooking aids<br>• Toileting and bathing aids |
| Education and Learning Aids | • Cognitive aids<br>• Early intervention aids |
| Vision and Reading Aids | • Glasses<br>• Literacy and reading software<br>• Magnifiers |
| Environmental Aids | • Environmental controls and switches<br>• Home-workplace adaptations<br>• Ergonomic equipment<br>• Home assistant devices |
| Mobility and Transportation Aids | • Ambulation aids<br>• Scooter and power wheelchairs<br>• Manual wheelchairs<br>• Alternative access methods<br>• Vehicle conversions |
| Seating and Positioning Aids | • Wheelchair cushions<br>• Trunk control positioner |
| Recreation and Leisure Aids | • Sports aids<br>• Adaptive toys and games<br>• Travel aids |

within the VA health care system. The AT programs provide expertise for other VAs that may not have specialized AT services and/or rehabilitation engineering, which is provided through telehealth services and/or AT conferences and in-services.

The AT evaluation process takes into account several variables such as the client, their goals, and environments. The AT evaluation is an ongoing process with collaboration between clients, family, caregivers, and the interdisciplinary team. Engagement in life roles is the goal of AT intervention. Clients who are independent with a given activity when using equipment (as opposed to requiring assistance) have been noted to experience higher levels of autonomy and self-sufficiency.[5] AT devices can also maximize independence, increase efficiency, increase sense of control, decrease caregiver burden, support function in different environments, and provide a level of privacy and dignity; also the devices are more portable, therefore, more appealing. One of the main challenges of AT devices is that one size does not fit all; for example, one client with a traumatic brain injury may be able to successfully use a smart device to remember to take their medication, whereas another client who also has a traumatic brain injury may find accessing the smart device very challenging due to physical limitations. In addition, the use of AT devices has the potential to increase a client's level of frustration and anxiety due to technology overload; therefore, it is critical to monitor their tolerance level before, during, and after AT intervention because technology may be overwhelming. When learning new devices, training requires more than a one-time visit otherwise carryover may not occur; but it may not be covered by insurance. In addition, the potential repairs may be costly. The purpose of this article is to explore the AT evaluation process, selection and matching AT devices, and training strategies specifically for clients with polytrauma injuries who may need AT devices.

## EVALUATION

The AT evaluation focuses on the clients' and/or caregivers' goals in identifying their roles and daily functions affected by injury or illness. During the evaluation process, the AT therapist explores the client's past and current use of technology along with their motivation to use technology as part of their rehabilitation. Collaboration between client and their rehabilitation team members about the type of AT device that will best meet their needs is critical to the recovery process and inclusion of technology. As part of the evaluation process, trial and training of the AT devices will determine the effectiveness of the AT devices.

The Human Activity Assistive Technology (HAAT) model is the frame of reference that is used during the evaluation to guide the decision-making process. The HAAT was designed specifically for AT and consists of 4 components: human, activity, AT, and context (**Fig. 1**).

Human components review the abilities of the person specifically in physical, cognitive, and social areas. In addition, the human aspect reviews the skills and abilities of the client. Activity component reviews the client's self-maintenance (self-care activities, shopping, money management), productivity (school, volunteer, work), and recreation and leisure activities. The context, while not part of the title of the model but is vital to the decision-making process during the AT evaluation, sets the stage of where the AT device will and can be used to achieve the client's goals. The context component considers physical, social, temporal, and cultural contexts. AT component focuses on what the human technology interface is, the processor or device, environmental interface where there is a link between the device and the

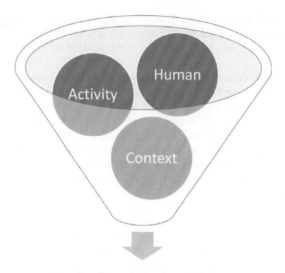

## Assistive Technology

**Fig. 1.** The Human Activity Assistive Technology model.

external environment, and the activity output.[4] Considering each element separately and interactively helps to select, design, and implement appropriate AT that fits the client and their lifestyle.

When selecting an AT device, a hierarchy approach of the AT evaluation and selection leads to the most effective AT decision. **Fig. 2** shows the hierarchical approach to the AT selection process.[6] During the evaluation process, the hierarchy approach to AT starts with changes to the task and then the environment. If both modifications do not affect the client's success, then move to the selection and trial of devices working through each moving to more complex options till a possible solution or combination of solutions is identified.

Commercially available products are broken down even further into no technology, low technology, and high technology. For example, a client who wants to remember to take their medications can use post-it notes as a no-technology solution, alarm on a clock as a low-technology solution, and a web-based calendar that interfaces with a smart watch, smart tablet, and home assistant devices to remind them to take their medications as a high-technology solution.[7]

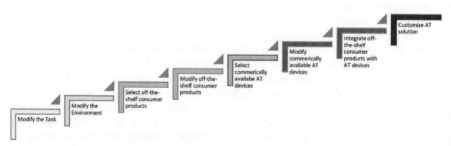

**Fig. 2.** The hierarchy of AT selection process.

In addition, the selection of AT device may be based on where the client is in their rehabilitation. The questions that should be asked include the following:

- Is this an acute need?
  - If so, the technology will change as the client is progressing through rehab.
- Is it a chronic need with a more permanent solution?
- Is it a progressive disease?
  - If so, the technology may change from low technology to high technology back to low technology solution as the disease changes.

Other important factors for the selection of AT devices include determining the least invasive device; environment where the device will be used; pros and cons of the AT devices; client's current knowledge; and usage of devices and their physical, mental, and cognitive strengths and challenges (**Fig. 3**).

The key to success during the AT evaluation is the collaboration with other services, co-treatment with treating clinicians in several different sessions, training of all staff involved in the client's care, and comprehensive training and education to caregiver

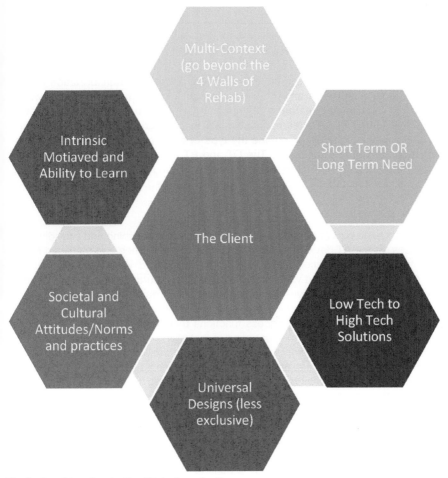

**Fig. 3.** Consideration in the AT device selection.

and/or family members. Also, it is important to remember that AT is creativity and that no 2 individuals are the same, meaning what works for one may not work for another. In addition, there is no wrong way to use AT tools because it may be designed for one purpose but work to accomplish something totally different.

## INTERDISCIPLINARY TEAM

The interdisciplinary team includes an AT specialist who is typically a rehabilitation therapist (occupational therapist [OT], physical therapist [PT] and/or speech language pathologist [SLP]). Their role in the team is not only to evaluate clients' needs, goals, and environments specific to AT but also to serve as experts in the various AT devices and services. Therefore, it is the responsibility of the AT specialist to learn new devices and become knowledgeable in the device functions and capabilities as well as understand the limitations. The AT specialist will collaborate with other team members through education, training, and, if possible, co-treating using the specific AT device in order to determine the best technology fit for the client. Physicians play a critical role because they evaluate the client's current medical and mental status as well as identify precautions before referring to AT. An AT interdisciplinary team approach works well when the team is made up of various disciplines because they provide diverse perspectives to a specific need. For example, wheeled mobility clinic will include an AT specialist (OT or PT), who is specialized in seating and mobility, a rehabilitation engineer, who is specialized in alternative access and integration of technology, and driver's rehabilitation therapist, who is knowledgeable in adaptive driving device and transportation needs. Another good example of an AT interdisciplinary team is adaptive sports where an OT, PT, and certified recreational therapist (CRTS) who specializes in adaptive sports evaluate a client's recreational goals in comparison with their strengths and challenges in order to determine the type of sport and adaptive sports equipment required to meet their goal. The OT and PT are trained in seating and positioning, whereas the CRTS is in the adaptation of sports and its equipment, resulting in an appropriate sports and/or leisure device.

## FUNDING

Funding is a large part of the evaluation process when prescribing and providing any AT devices. Some AT devices are covered by private insurance and Medicaid/Medicare with strong justification. However, the functions and various options built in most AT devices are limited when it comes to funding source approval; for example, Alternative and Augmentative Communication (AAC) device is "locked down" if Medicaid is paying for the device, meaning that the client is not able to use the environmental control or computer access functions that are built into the AAC device because it is not the primary medical need of that client. Medical justification should include the following: demographics, diagnosis, prognosis, limitations, abilities, activities unable to perform, goals, and equipment requirements instead of a specific device name. Funding sources require that the AT therapist have evaluated 2 or more AT devices that could meet the client's needs. A comparison chart of the trial devices in the documentation including why the device does or does not meet the clinical/medical needs demonstrates the due diligence required by most funding sources. Insurers typically will deny the request initially; therefore, clinicians need to be prepared and respond timely with answers to request for additional information or an appeal. Insurers, usually, will select the least expensive device. Most AT devices are not covered by traditional funding sources.[8] Examples include consumer devices used as an AT device (ie, tablet with medication reminder applications (APPs) or do it your-self (DIY) home automation to control lights within the home environment). Clinicians need to research the terminology used in the insurance policies to include it in the documentation to increase funding success. Funding sources approvingly take into consideration letters of support from the client's primary care providers, caregivers, family, and therapists that are included with the requested documentation.[9] **Box 1** shows funding sources that include, but not limited to, the following:

## ACCESS

Access is the interaction between the client and the AT device. The access methods vary depending on the type of AT devices but needs to be as simple as possible considering the capabilities of the client and their goals. Equipment abandonment is a significant consideration particularly given the expense of equipment. Direct, indi-rect, and combination selections are the access options. Direct selection is when the client has almost immediate cause and effect with the technology such as when they use their hands, styluses head pointing, eye gazing, or controlling the cursor with a mouse. This type of selection allows for quicker responses of the AT devices. For example, the client pushing the joystick forward and the power wheelchair starting to drive forward or a client pushing the "Volume Up" button on the TV remote turning the volume up in sound. Styluses provide a direct selection option if adaption is required due to a hand tremor or contracture (**Fig. 4**).

Direct selection method in some situation can be fatiguing depending on the task demand and role responsibilities such as using a mouth stick to type documents within their job responsibilities and using it to control their TV through their Electronic Aids to Daily Living (EADL) device. Clients with hand limitations due to hemiparesis or contractures could still use direct selection by using a head or mouth stick. If a client has more physical mobility limitations but good head control, then head pointing is an option where it tracks movements of a reflective dot on a hat, glasses, or head. The cameras for head pointing can be internal or external to the AT device such as on a computer. Eye gaze tracks eye movements using infrared light reflected off the client's retina. Eye gaze is most effective if the client is limited to no head movement. The eye gaze technology will work even with clients who wear glasses

---

**Box 1**
**Funding sources**

Individual with Disabilities Education Act (IDEA) (1997), school districts are required to provide AT devices for students in order to participate in school activities (ie, AAC device)

Medicare and Medicaid (government health insurance), with some limitations

Private insurance companies typically take the lead of Medicare and Medicaid

Worker's compensation

State Departments of Rehabilitation Services for clients who have vocational or educational goals

Private funding

Charity Organizations

Support groups

Low-interest loans specifically for AT devices through state AT programs

# Styluses

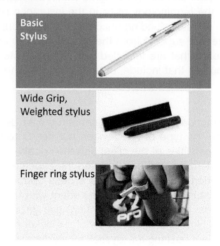

| Basic Stylus | |
| Wide Grip, Weighted stylus | |
| Finger ring stylus | |

**Fig. 4.** Examples of stylus.

(bi- and trifocals) and/or only one functional eye but calibration is required for each client. A client's retina reflects onto the AAC device shown as a red dot to select a particular option (**Fig. 5**).

Indirect selection is used when the client does not have the ability to accomplish direct selection due to limited dexterity, fine motor control, strength, range of motion, and/or coordination. Scanning is the method that indirection selection uses where a device is programmed to highlight a selection in a particular pattern such as row/column, linear, or step as seen outlined in red on the AAC device in **Fig. 6**. Switches are used during the indirect selection process as the interface between the client and the AT device. Switch activation methods include depress and release, proximity, sip and puff, head grip and release, minimal muscle activation, voice, and hand moisture.[9] The selection of the type of switch will determine the success of the client's overall usage. **Table 2** provides examples of different switch options.[9]

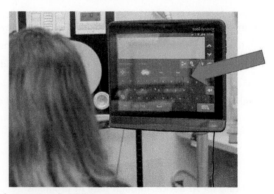

**Fig. 5.** Example of eye gaze for AAC access.

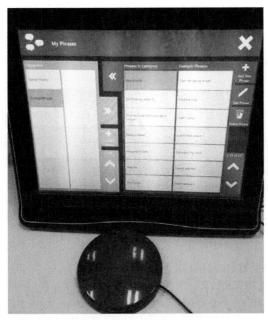

**Fig. 6.** Example of scanning on AAC device.

## MOUNTING

Mounting of AT devices and access methods manages the placement and interaction between the client and AT device. The following items should be considered when determining the mounting options:

- What environment will the AT device be used?
- Mobility: manual or power wheelchair?

**Table 2**
**Examples of types of switches (Webster & Murphy, 2018)**

| Type of Switch | Outcome | Example |
|---|---|---|
| Button switch | Body movement activates the device | Jelly Button |
| Light touch switch | Minimal movement activates the device | Microlight switch |
| Pneumatic switch | Provides stability when used | Sip-and-puff switch |
| Electromyelogram (EMG) switch | Senses muscle movement and provides switch closure to activate a device | Tinkertron EMG switch |
| Proximity switch | Detects the presence of a body part/movement to activate the switch | Candy Corn switch |
| Eye blink | Aims a sensor at the eye, blinking breaks the beam, which then activates the device | Eye blink AT switch |
| Breath control | Breath to activate the device | Sip-and-puff switch |
| Bite switch | Electromechanical to activate a device | Bite ability switch |

- Hospital bed usage?
- Other seating options?
- Access methods?
- Need to access while using transportation?
- How many devices?
- Does the client need to move the device on and off the mount?

Client's position in relation to the access method and AT device will determine the effectiveness and successfulness of the AT device. For example, a client who uses direct selection may be in a hospital bed but need to use their computer for work and be placed directly in front of them otherwise they will not be able to be independently access their computer (**Fig. 7**).

A client who uses a sip-and-puff switch to activate the call bell for nursing staff requires the switch to be mounted to the right side of their hospital bed for easier access because they are unable to use their left side due to a stroke (**Fig. 8**).

Other examples of mounting can be seen in **Fig. 9**.

## AREAS OF ASSISTIVE TECHNOLOGY
### Augmentative and Alternative Communication

AAC is the word used to describe extra ways of helping people who find it hard to communicate by speech or writing. The American Speech Language and Hearing Association defines augmentative communication as "An area of clinical practice that attempts to compensate (either temporarily or permanently) for the impairment and disability patterns of individuals with severe expressive communication disorders."[10] It includes any method of communicating beyond speech that may include a combination of gesture, eye gaze, writing, picture selection, or computer use. Clients who can benefit from AAC devices include those with cerebral palsy, intellectual disabilities, laryngectomy, autism, cardiovascular accident, traumatic brain injury, amyotrophic lateral sclerosis, Parkinson disease, and multiple sclerosis.

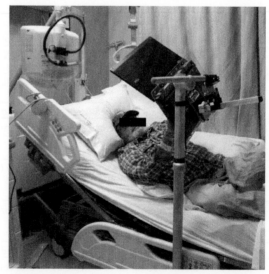

**Fig. 7.** Rolling floor mount for computer access while in a hospital bed.

# Less is More

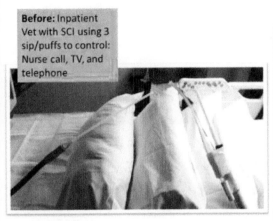

Before: Inpatient Vet with SCI using 3 sip/puffs to control: Nurse call, TV, and telephone

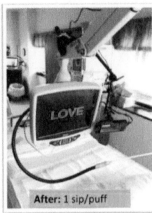

After: 1 sip/puff

**Fig. 8.** Bedside access mounting.

An AAC evaluation primarily involves the SLP and OT although other interdisciplinary team members can participate. The SLP gathers a history of the client's communication before the need for an alternative method is assessed, including their education level, living environment, and social supports and in addition, the client's receptive/expressive language skills (word knowledge, symbol knowledge), cognition (awareness, memory, executive functioning), and literacy skills (word recognition and reading comprehension). The OT evaluates visual skills (visual acuity, visual fields, blind spots) and motor abilities (fine motor, gross motor, positioning and seating needs) to assist with possible access methods.

### Nonspeaking Systems Versus Low Technology Versus High Technology

AAC systems include nonspeaking systems, low-tech devices, and high-tech devices. Nonspeaking systems require the individual to use their body to express needs and wants; therefore, there is no cost and requires minimal training. Examples include communication boards such as flip charts, E-Tran board, or dry-erase board. Low-tech AAC devices typically are inexpensive, low maintenance, time consuming, and provide communication through either text or symbols. Low-tech AAC examples are communication boards with a laser pointer, boogie board, and GoTalk. High-tech AAC devices are expensive and require training for both the client and their caregiver, troubleshooting training, maintenance requirements, positioning, multiple access modes, individualization, and some offer wireless connections and environmental control options. Examples include text to speech device such as a LightWriter SL-40 or a tablet with AAC text to speech APP. Other examples for dynamic screen communication devices are TobiiDynavox I-Series, Talk to Me Technologies, Zuvo, or Prentke Romich Accent. Depending on the client's specific needs, modification requirements, and access methods, the AT team will individualize the solution (**Table 3**). Clients who may not have access to an AT provider can review the sample resource list for ideas and contacts (**Box 2**).

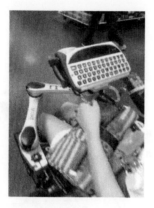

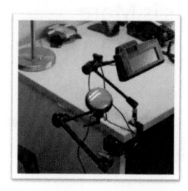

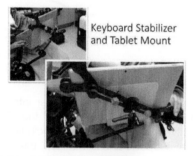

Keyboard Stabilizer
and Tablet Mount

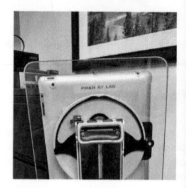

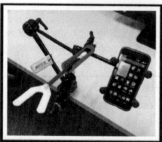

**Fig. 9.** Additional examples of mounting.

| Table 3 | |
|---|---|
| Examples of AAC solutions for different diagnosis | |
| **Who Can Benefit from AAC?** | |
| **Diagnosis** | **Potential Assistive Technology Solution** |
| CVA with fine motor and visual deficits | iPAD with Communication APP |
| Parkinson's Disease with tremors in head, voice and hands | Lightwriter |
| ALS | iPAD with communication APP, AAC device with eyegaze system; EMG switch for AAC device |

| Box 2 |
| --- |
| **Resource list** |

Abledata
  www.abledata.com
  800-227-0216

Ablenet
  www.ablenetinc.com
  800-322-0956

Adaptivation
  www.adaptivation.com
  605-335-4445

Alliance for Technology Access
  http://ataccess.org/

Association of AT Act Programs
  http://ataporg.org
  217-522-7985

Assistive Technology Industry Association
  http://atia.org
  877-687-2842

Brain Actuated Technologies, Inc.
  http://brainfingers.com
  937-767-2674

BrainLine
  www.brainline.org

Broadened Horizons
  www.broadenedhorizons.com
  612-851-1040

Clarity Products
  http://Shop.clarityproducts.com
  800-426-3738

Closing the Gap
  http://closingthegap.com
  507-248-3294

CSUN Technology and Persons with Disabilities Conference
  http://csun.edu/cod/conf/
  818-677-1200

Daedalus Technologies, Inc.
  www.daessy.com
  604-270-4605

DO-IT Technology and Universal Design
  http://uw.edu/doit/resources/technology.html

Infogrip, Inc.
  www.infogrip.com
  800-397-0921

Making Cognitive Connections
  http://id4theweb.com/

Mount'n Mover
  www.mountnmover.com
  888-724-7002

Prentke Romich Company
  www.prentrom.com
  800-262-1933

RESNA (Rehabilitation Engineering and Assistive Technology Society in North America)
http://resna.org
703-524-6686

Smarthome
www.smarthome.com
800-762-7846

Talk to Me Technologies
www.talktometechnologies
877-392-2299

Tash
http://tash.org
202-540-9020

Tobii Dynavox
www.tobiidynavox.com
800-344-1778

X10
www.x10.com
888-384-0969

In addition, high-tech AAC devices have infrared (IR) control ability, which allows the device to learn other IR devices such as TV remotes, stereo system remotes, and cable or streaming system remotes where the client is able to control his environment, email, and power wheelchair functions.

### Wheeled Mobility

Wheeled mobility facilitates a client getting from one point to another when they have an impairment of lower limb function (amputation), impairment of balance or gait (Multiple Sclerosis), impairment of endurance (congestive heart failure), morbid obesity, or cognitive impairment (dementia) providing opportunities to access more environments and increasing level of independence. Complex Rehab Technology refers to medically necessary, individually configured devices that require evaluation, configuration, fitting, adjustment, or programming to meet the specific medical and functional needs of an individual.[11] Wheeled mobility technology continues to evolve where the types and quality of materials are lighter, more durable, and functional (ie, lighter weight frame for easier and safer transfers and ability to lift in and out of a vehicle), improvement in the user-technology physical interface (ie, driver mechanisms, electronics, and seat functions), and sharing of control between the user and the technology. Types of manual wheelchairs include basic folding wheelchair, custom lightweight wheelchair, and rigid frame wheelchair. The types of motorized wheeled mobility devices include the following (**Fig. 10**, **Table 4**):

- Scooter—that has 3 or 4 wheels guided by a tiller with a limited seat modification capability
- Power wheelchairs—driven by a joystick or alternative input device with a variety of seat options.
- Add-on power-assist device—device that is mounted to an existing manual wheelchair and provide propulsion assistance to reduce the amount of wheel turns and assist with higher resistance surfaces.
- Enhanced function power wheelchairs—has augmented capabilities such as elevate, tilt, recline, stand, and access various terrains.

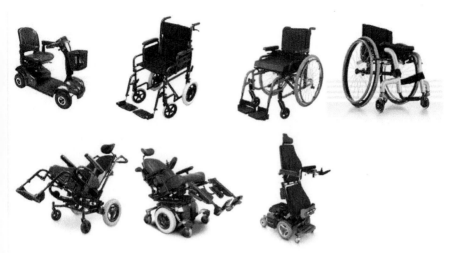

**Fig. 10.** Examples of types of wheeled mobility.

The wheeled mobility team includes the client, family and/or caregivers, physician, PT, OT, rehabilitation engineer, vendor/manufacturer, third party payer, if applicable, and/or teacher/vocational rehab counselor/employer. Full spectrum of services includes referral, assessment (more than measurements and specs), equipment recommendation and selection, funding and procurement, product preparation, fitting/training/delivery (ensure equipment can be used safely and effectively and provide maintenance and troubleshooting information), follow-up maintenance and repair, and outcome measures (**Fig. 11**). During the assessment process, the following aspects of the client are included:

- Past medical history
- Functional cognition
- Visual perceptual function
- Cardiopulmonary function
- Range of motion and strength
- Spasticity/tone/coordination
- Postural evaluation
- Self-care, activities of daily living (ADL), instrumental activities of daily living (IADL) tasks

| Table 4 Types of wheeled mobility | |
|---|---|
| **Types** | **Examples** |
| Dependent mobility systems | Transport wheelchairs Tilt-n-recline wheelchairs |
| Independent manual systems | Lightweight manual wheelchair One arm drive wheelchair |
| Independent powered mobility systems | Scooter Push-rim activated power-assist wheelchair Add on power-assist wheelchair |
| Powered mobility systems | Enhanced function power wheelchairs (ie, elevate) |

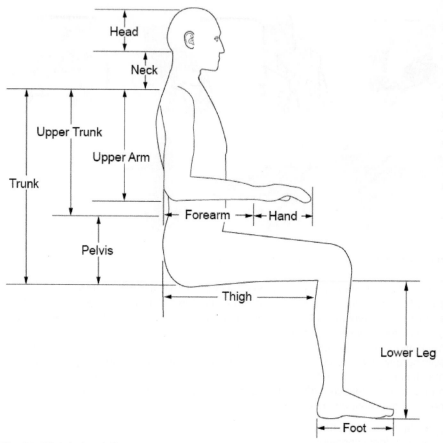

**Fig. 11.** Wheeled mobility measurement diagram.

- Home accessibility
- Community reintegration
- Vocational needs
- Transportation
- Goals and expectations
- Pressure management
- Functional mobility (environment)
- Transfers

The overall goal for seating and positioning is to achieve stability with seating posture but still allow dynamic control of movement. Other features of a wheelchair include type of frame (rigid or folding), functions (tilt, recline, standing), weight, seat type, back type, arm supports, leg and foot supports, wheel locks, head support, driving options, electronics, and accessories (ie, ventilator tray, attendant control). Seating and positioning evaluation considers other interaction needs such as with an alternative driving method and access to AAC device, if applicable. Part of the selection is trailing of the equipment including safety training on how to maneuver on/off curves and different terrains. **Fig. 12** demonstrates safety training for wheeled mobility.

Seating goals for clients with brain injury include accommodating changes in functions, managing abnormal tone, maximizing mobility, minimizing development of de-
formities, and upper extremity support. Skin integrity is crucial in the selection and
maintenance of a wheeled mobility device and cushions. Risk factors for skin breakdown and/or wounds include local pressure, sustained pressure, friction and shearing,
poor nutrition, infections, age, heat and moisture, and age. Therefore, pressure mapping can help determine the type of seating surface that would optimize health skin
integrity and needs to be reevaluated on a regular basis especially if the client does
not have sensation or awareness of seating position. Once a wheeled device is
selected then measurements are completed and environmental access is identified.
Recommendations for measurements and features are seen in **Table 5**.[12–16]

**Fig. 13** demonstrates wheeled mobility device providing support and stability for an
above-the-knee amputation patient.

Power wheelchair electronics now have the ability to offer Bluetooth control from the
power wheelchair allowing for computer and smart device access. The electronics
provide IR control and input-output module for X-10 control and in addition, foot rests,
access to joystick or alternative drive access in all positions (**Fig. 14**), arm rest positioning, dependence on setting, level of expertise, and vendor and/or manufacturer.

Once the wheeled mobility device is procured and received, additional adjustments
may be needed to ensure optional stability and safety. During the fitting, the AT
specialist will review all the functions of the wheeled mobility device including safety
features.

## Electronic Cognitive Devices

Electronic cognitive devices (ECDs) are a product or system that is used by a client to
compensate for cognitive impairments and support their ability to participate in ADL
skills or IADL skills (**Table 6**). Typical cognitive problems that would benefit from
ECDs include attention, memory, task sequencing, multitasking, organization, time
management, and adapting to transitions and changes in routines. Therefore, ECDs
can assist with scheduling, reminders, time management, behavioral cues, directions,
engagement in daily tasks, and engagement in work tasks. ECDs range from re-
corders to smartphones to tablets to wearable technology.

Neuropsychological testing or cognitive testing completed by SLP and/or OT identifies the client's cognitive strengths and deficits, which helps to guide the direction of
selecting an ECD. In addition, other aspects to take into consideration when selecting
an ECD include the client's balance, vision, hearing, speech, behavioral changes, and

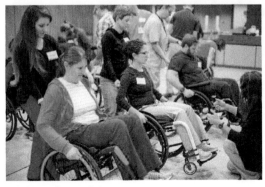

**Fig. 12.** Wheeled mobility safety training.

**Table 5**
Recommendations for wheeled mobility measurements and features

| Front Seat Height | Rear Seat Height |
|---|---|
| Seat angle | Seat frame width |
| Seat frame depth | Back frame height |
| Seat to back angle | Leg rest length |
| Leg rest angle | Horizontal and vertical axle position |
| Wheel camber | Caster type and size |
| Wheel type and size | Rolling resistance |
| Downhill turning tendency | Y axis control (ie, ease of turning) |
| Pitch axis control (ie, wheelies) | Static stability |
| Transportability | Footprint |
| Propulsion efficiency | Postural support and stability |

safety awareness. When approaching the ECD decision processing, the AT specialist starts with technology the client already has and is comfortable using because it is more likely to be used as a compensatory device.

The benefits of AT for cognitive deficits provide supports for attention, memory, and executive functioning.[17,18] According to Sohlberg and Turkstra, "the increasing use of

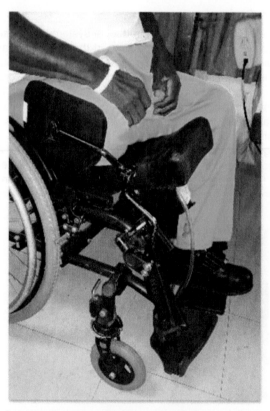

**Fig. 13.** Example of amputation above the knee and wheeled mobility seating and support.

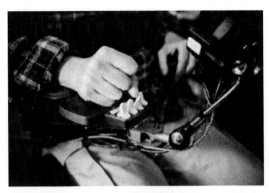

**Fig. 14.** Access to seat functions on power wheelchair.

technology to help individuals compensate for cognitive impairments is one of the most notable advances in neuropsychological rehabilitation in recent years."[19] Clients with a mild traumatic brain injury (mTBI) wanting to return to school having difficulty with recall and thought processing would benefit from a digital recorder or smartpen. Also, a client who is unable to remember to take medications may benefit from a medication reminder pillbox system plus a medication reminder APP on their smart device (**Fig. 15**).

When considering the use of mobile APPs as an AT strategy, the following should be considered: (1) what is the purpose?, (2) what features of the APP are required to achieve the goal?, and (3) are there other aspects that the identified APP will provide for the client?[20] Other considerations include APP overload, type of mobile devices (iOS, Android, or Windows), mounting needs, accessories, and access methods. Once an APP has been selected, the AT provider begins the training that will include identifying the benefits of smart devices as a memory aid, developing basic skills around the functions of the smart device itself (ie, power button, home button, settings), and training on the cognitive skills the APP will be using (ie, setting reminders in calendar appointment to assist with recall). Following a brain injury, clients may need continued support with problem-solving and decision-making; therefore,

| Table 6 Electronic cognitive devices | |
| --- | --- |
| No Tech Cognitive Aids | Wall calendar Day planner Sticky notes Stop sign |
| Low-Tech Cognitive Aids | Digital recorder Recording pens Simple flip cellphone Computer calendar Medication reminder watch Pillbox with alarm Bluetooth object tracker |
| High-Tech Cognitive Aids | Smart phones/tablets Various APPS Home assistant devices Wearable technology |

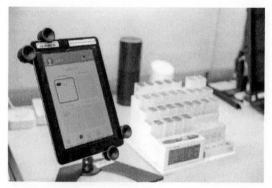

**Fig. 15.** Example of medication reminder system.

multiple APPs can assist with those deficits but may also require additional supports depending on the severity of the brain injury from caregivers and/or family (**Box 3** Case Study #1).

Wearable technology also has evolved from tracking steps to monitoring vital signs and sleep to appointment reminders to responding to text messages and phone calls. Wearable technology is effective because the device is physically attached to the person; therefore, they are less likely to lose or misplace it, increasing the effectiveness of its purpose as an AT device. Wearable technologies may require the smartphone be within close proximity to operate and not all APPs are effective on the wearable device.

---

**Box 3**
**Case study #1**

Sarah is a 56-year-old woman who received a traumatic brain injury from blunt trauma in the 1980s, which resulted in communication difficulties, visual deficits, and difficulty with reading and writing. In 2012, she was diagnosed with end-stage renal disease (ESRD) in 2012 and left above knee amputation. She also was being considered for a transplant. Her personal goals were to manage her own schedule and medications. Her husband was supportive in the use of AT and will provide support after discharge. Sarah was referred to AT to explore devices to assist with her goals. She already has an iPAD with a communication APP. Because she already had an AT device (iPAD), the AT specialist started with it as it was being used daily. Therefore, various picture-based iOS APPs were trialed to address schedule and medication management.

*APPS trialed:*

• Calendar Management by Voice

• Electronic Calendar that syncs to Cloud-based system

• Cloud-based notes

• Visual Medication Management

*AT Solution:*

Sarah is using a Calendar management app that is set by voice recording with several reminders. This app will sync with her husband's Google calendar, which he can monitor and add any changes. She is now independent with the management of her calendar. She also uses Evernote app where she can record any notes she wants to keep about medical appointments or therapy sessions that are also Cloud based; therefore, her husband can also monitor. She has also become independent with medication management using a visual medication app (at the time it was Pillboxie).

Home assistant devices such as Google Home and Amazon Echo provide the opportunity to be used as an ECD because they can provide auditory reminders for To Do lists, shopping lists, medication reminders, and calendar events. Voice quality depends on its effectiveness. Multiple devices may be needed throughout the home if using in multiple locations for cognitive supports. In addition, Amazon Show can provide step by step visual instructions for the sequencing of daily tasks (ie, cooking, laundry, dressing) as well as the ability to visually see a person during phone calls.

## Adaptive Computer Access

Adaptive computer access is a specialized group of hardware and software designed to enable individuals with a wide range of disabilities to use a personal computer. Over the past several years, both Microsoft and Apple have improved the accessibility features and functions within the operating systems. Bill Gates, Chairman of Microsoft Corporation stated, "Our vision is to create innovative technology that is, accessible to everyone and that adapts to each person's needs. Accessible technology eliminates barriers for people with disabilities and it enables individuals to take full advantage of their capabilities."[21] Computer's operating systems can compensate for upper extremity limitations, sensory impairments, and cognitive impairments.

The client's goal for accessing a computer becomes the focus of the evaluation as well as the environment in which the computer will be used. As part of the evaluation process, whether the computer task itself and/or the environment where the computer is located can be modified will be reviewed, which would be easier for the client. The AT specialist needs to also understand the client's current computer technology and skills. For example, ask about the following:

- Have you ever used a computer?
- Do you own a computer?
- What type of computer (desktop or laptop)?
- Mac or PC?
- What type of operating system?
- How old is the computer?
- How do you use a computer?
- Why do you use a computer?
- What do you want to use the computer for now?
- What computer accessories do you currently have (ie, keyboard, mouse)?
- What computer software do you have and use?
- Do you use any alternative computer devices?

Other factors that need to be considered during the adaptive computer access evaluation include the client's current seating and positioning, lighting, workstation, and access to the computer itself.

There are 2 areas of computer usage to address mouse operations and text entry. Mouse operations are pointing, clicking, and dragging. Mouse (or cursor) functions can be adjusted within the operating systems including, but not limited to, button configuration, pointer sizes, speed of the pointer, and the function of the wheel on the mouse. If these accessibility options do not work and/or other mouse options are needed, then there are commercially available products (**Fig. 16**). Text entry is inputting numbers and letters. Within the operating system's accessible setting, text entry can be adjusted to include, but not limited to, magnifier, on-screen keyboards, high contrast, narrator, and speech recognition. Examples of commercially available adaptive text entry options are in **Figs. 17** and **18**. In

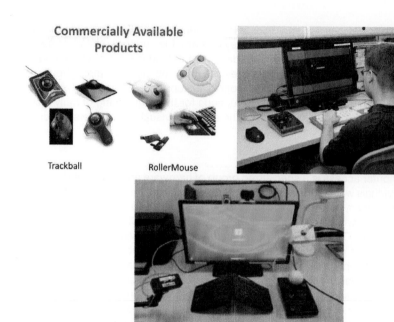

Fig. 16. Example of adaptive computer mice. Examples of adaptive computer access (both adaptive keyboard and mice). Examples of adaptive computer mice.

addition, power wheelchairs include the option of Bluetooth modules that allow the computer mouse to be controlled through the wheelchair's joystick or switches. **Table 7** shows computer access methods that can assist particular diagnoses (**Box 4** Case Study #2).

### Electronic Aids to Daily Living

EADL provide control of one's environment through alternative access, while increasing their level of function, typically within their home. EADL can also be used within a classroom and/or work setting depending on the client and their needs. A client with limited functional mobility and/or dexterity can benefit from the use of an EADL device to improve the interaction with their environment (**Fig. 19**). Most

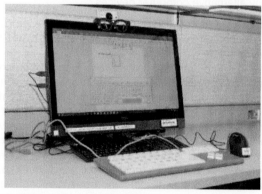

Fig. 17. Examples of adaptive computer access.

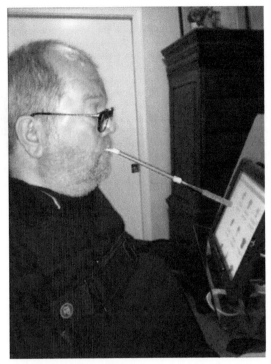

**Fig. 18.** Alternative computer access method.

electronic devices (lights, fans, air conditioning, TVs, and telephones) and many mechanical devices can be controlled (hospital beds, window blinds, and doors).

EADL are categorized into 2 types: (1) general-function EADL that controls a variety of devices and (2) specific-function EADL that controls only 1 identified device (ie, door openers, stand-alone adapted telephones, and page turners). General-function EADL are further divided into limited-output (also called basic) and multiple-output systems. An example of a limited-output EADL is a battery-operated device such as a toy and a simple electric device such as a table lamp. The alternative access method for limited-output EADL is through a switch (**Fig. 20**). If a client needs to control several items within their environment, such as audiovisual equipment (TVs, DVD players, cable, stereos), lights, simple appliances (eg, a fan), heating and air conditioning, electric beds, telephones, and power door openers, then the multiple-output system is required. Research has shown multiple benefits to clients who use EADL. Clients with limited physical mobility have demonstrated increase in overall independence and decreased

| Table 7 |  |
| --- | --- |
| **Examples of diagnosis that could benefit from adaptive computer access** | |
| **Who Can Benefit from Adaptive Computer Access** | |
| **Diagnosis** | **Potential Assistive Technology Solution** |
| CVA | Voice Recognition Software or Operating System |
| UE Amputation | Mini keyboard; finger mouse |
| Tremors | Vertical mouse; Sticky Keys; KEYS-U-SEE Keyboard |

**Box 4**
**Case study #2**

Erica is a 38-year-old Veteran who served for 8 years in the Army. She was working as an Admin-istrative Assistant at the local university, when in 2006 she was diagnosed with a brainstem me-ningioma. She underwent surgical resection and radiation therapy, which led to scarring, inflammation, and buildup of fluid on the brain where a shunt had to be placed. The brainstem meningioma resulted in right hemiplegia, mild visual impairment, and severe dysarthria. She was referred to AT for a full AT evaluation. Cognitive testing was completed and determined comprehension intact, memory intact, and attention span good. She already had AT devices, which were a power wheelchair and DynaWrite (text to speech communication device). Her goals were to finish her Master's Degree, communication through email, and shop on the internet. She was living in her parent's home and her laptop could be used in the bedroom or living room. Her main challenge was accessing the laptop due to right hemiparesis and dysarthria. AT specialist needed to evaluate both mouse and text access to assist her goal of computer access; therefore, the following AT devices were trialed:

*Mouse Access*

• Trackball

• Sticky keys

• Joystick mouse

• Enlarge cursor and pointer

*Text Access*

• Mini keyboard

• BIG KEYS yellow keyboard

• Word Q

• ZoomText magnification software

Through several AT treatment sessions for trials and training, the AT solutions included a joystick mouse with stick keys to increase speed and efficiency since the she is not able to push two or more keyboard commands (ie, Ctrl, Alt, Delete) and enlarge cursor and pointer to improve visual accuracy for mouse access. Text access solutions were BIG KEYS yellow keyboard for visual accuracy and touch access, Word Q to increase typing speed and Zoomtext for magnifier on the monitor.

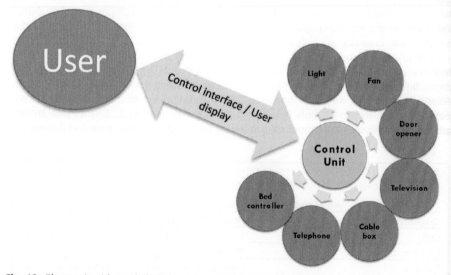

**Fig. 19.** Electronic aids to daily living—interaction process.

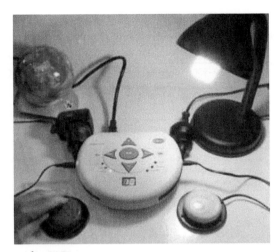

**Fig. 20.** Switch access for EADL.

frustration if they successfully used their EADL device.[22] In addition, this study found that these clients had significant and positive impact on the psychosocial well-being.[22] In addition, another study found nursing home staff have also reported a decrease in their frustration following introduction of the EADL.[23]

EADL have different transmission methods including IR, radio frequency, and home automation system. IR EADL devices are portable and require line-of-sight communication such as TV or universal remotes. Radio frequency EADL device is a device such as a garage door opener that does not require line-of-sight communication. Home automation systems use power line, which is existing AC house wiring; therefore, it is inexpensive but sensitive to the effectiveness of the current wiring. These systems use X-10 and Insteon modules to allow for communication between the device being controlled (ie, table lamp) and the wiring of the house. Another type of home automation system is home networks that use wireless radio frequency networks and wired local area network, which is more expensive and complex. Examples include Z-wave and Wi-Fi Bluetooth.[9]

DIY options for home environment control have increased significantly over the past few years such as Amazon Echo, Google Home, and Smart Things known as home assistant devices. Access to the option includes voice and/or APP on a smart device. Alternative access methods to the smart device may be required due to a client's upper extremity limitation; however, not all smart devices have accessibility features. Examples of access methods include the following:

- Functional fine or gross motor control, capacitive stylus or mouth stick, stylus holder, screen size, iOS: Assistive Touch, or Android: Easy Touch.
- Switch scanning on some smart devices include both wired (ie, RSL Steeper Pererro, Zygo ZyBox, Ablenet Hook) and wireless (Tecla Shield Uno/Dos, Ablenet Blue 2, RJ Cooper BSI) switches.
- Mouse control—Bluetooth mouse, USB wired
- Voice-controlled APPS

**Table 8** shows factors that need to be considered when deciding between DIY home assistant devices and professional home automation.

**Table 8**
**DIY versus professional home automation installation for environmental control units**

| | DIY ECU Options | Professional Home Automation |
|---|---|---|
| Cost | Range $59–$300 (depends on options) plus monthly monitoring (optional) | Range $1500–$4500 plus monthly monitoring (optional) |
| Installation | DIY | Professional installation |
| Access Options | Touch screen, voice control, mobile APP control | Touch screen, voice control, mobile APP control |
| APPs | Variable and limited control options; however, APPs can be controlled through some switch options built into the device | Well developed with variety of control options; however, APPs can be controlled through some switch options built into the device |
| Training | DIY | Professional training at time of installation |
| Technical Support | Minimal | Included in the professional installation |

EADL evaluations review the human and activity components to determine the most effective device by reviewing the client's goals, strengths, and limitations. An interdisciplinary team approach provides value during this process. For example, the OT and/or rehabilitation engineer will then provide a more in-depth evaluation of determining the most effective access method as well as education about different EADL, which include home automation systems and DIY options. In addition, EADL evaluations include specific aspects of the client's environment such as the following:

- What is the current environment access method?
- What does the client want to control?
- What does the client need to control (ie, in cases of emergency)?
- Where does the client want to control these items?
  - More than one room?
  - What environments?
- Does the client have Wi-Fi access?
- Does the client have a mobile device?
  - Type?
  - Current usage?
  - Motivation?
- What type of family/caregiver support does the client have in cases of troubleshooting the technology?

As discussed earlier in the article, access options include direct selection, indirect selection, or a combination of the two. Direct access is touch selection or voice selection. Totally hands-free option is possible; however, it is very sensitive to voice changes such as when someone has a cold their voice may change or voice quality changes due to breath control affecting the ability of the EADL device to understand the voice commands. Indirect access options include scanning, which is inefficient access method, but can use one or multiple switches to activate scanning; directed scanning is more effective but more complex than normal scanning and coded access such as Morse code. **Fig. 21** provide a sample of EADL device examples noting that as

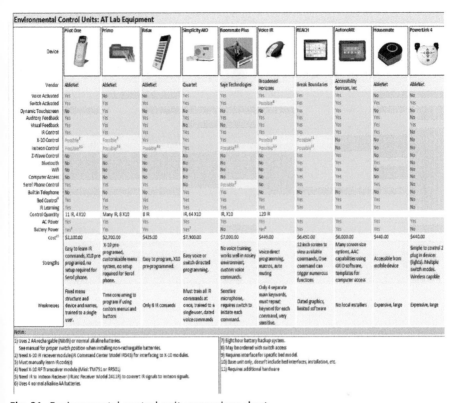

**Environmental Control Units: AT Lab Equipment**

| | Pilot One | Primo | Relax | Simplicity AIO | Roommate Plus | Voice IR | REACH | AutonoME | Housemate | PowerLink 4 |
|---|---|---|---|---|---|---|---|---|---|---|
| Vendor | AbleNet | AbleNet | AbleNet | Quartet | Saje Technologies | Broadened Horizons | Break Boundaries | Accessibility Services, Inc | AbleNet | AbleNet |
| Voice Activated | Yes | No | No | Yes | Yes | Yes | Yes | Yes | No | No |
| Switch Activated | Yes | Yes | Yes | Yes | Yes | Possible | Yes | Yes | Yes | Yes |
| Dynamic Touchscreen | No | Yes | No | No | No | No | Yes | Yes | No | No |
| Auditory Feedback | Yes | Yes | Yes | Yes | Yes | Yes | Yes | Yes | Yes | No |
| Visual Feedback | Yes | Yes | Yes | No | No | Yes | Yes | Yes | Yes | No |
| IR Control | Yes | Yes | Yes | Yes | Yes | Yes | Yes | Yes | Yes | No |
| X-10 Control | Possible | Possible | Yes | Yes | Yes | Yes | Possible | Possible | No | No |
| Insteon Control | Possible | Possible | Possible | Yes | Possible | Possible | Possible | No | No | No |
| Z-Wave Control | No | No | No | No | No | No | Yes | Yes | No | No |
| Bluetooth | No | No | No | No | No | No | Yes | Yes | No | No |
| Wifi | No | No | No | No | No | No | Yes | Yes | No | No |
| Computer Access | No | No | No | No | No | No | Yes | Yes | No | No |
| Serial Phone Control | Yes | Yes | Yes | No | Possible | Yes | Yes | Yes | Yes | No |
| Built in Telephone | No | No | No | Yes | Yes | No | No | No | No | No |
| Bed Control | Yes | Yes | Yes | Yes | Yes | Yes | Yes | Yes | Yes | No |
| IR Learning | Yes | Yes | Yes | Yes | Yes | Yes | Yes | Yes | Yes | No |
| Control Quantity | 11 IR, 4 X10 | Many IR, 8 X10 | 8 IR | IR, 64 X10 | IR, X10 | 120 IR | | | | |
| AC Power | Yes | Yes | Yes | Yes | Yes | Yes | Yes | Yes | Yes | Yes |
| Battery Power | Yes | Yes | Yes | No | Yes | Yes | Yes | Yes | Yes | No |
| Cost | $2,100.00 | $2,700.00 | $425.00 | $7,900.00 | $7,000.00 | $449.00 | $6,450.00 | $6,000.00 | $440.00 | $440.00 |
| Strengths | Easy to learn IR commands, X10 programmed, no setup required for Serol phone. | X-10 pre-programmed, customizable menu system, no setup required for Serol phone. | Easy to program, X10 pre-programmed | Easy voice or switch directed programming | No voice training, works well in noisy environment, custom voice commands | Voice direct programming, macros, auto muting | Only 4 separate main keywords, must repeat keyword for each command, very sensitive. | Many screen size capabilities using GIIO software, templates for computer access | Accessible from mobile device | Simple to control 2 plug in devices (lights). Multiple switch modes. Wireless capable |
| Weaknesses | Fixed menu structure and device and names, trained to a single user. | Time consuming to program if using custom menus and buttons | Only 8 IR commands | Must train all IR commands at once, trained to a single user, dated voice commands | Sensitive microphone, requires switch to initiate each command | 12 inch screen to view available commands, One command can trigger numerous functions | Dated graphics, limited software | No local installers | Expensive, large | Expensive, large |

Notes:

1) Uses 2 AA rechargeable (NiMH) or normal alkaline batteries. See manual for proper switch position when installing non-rechargeable batteries.
2) Need X-10 IR receiver module (X Command Center Model IR343) for interfacing to X-10 modules.
3) Must manually learn IR code(s)
4) Need X-10 RF Transceiver module (Mini: TM751 or RR501)
5) Need IR to Insteon Reciever (IRLinc Receiver Model 2411R) to convert IR signals to Insteon signals.
6) Uses 4 normal alkaline AA batteries.
7) Eight hour battery backup system.
8) May be ordered with switch access
9) Requires interface for specific bed model.
10) Base unit only, doesn't include bed interfaces, installation, etc.
11) Requires additional hardware

**Fig. 21.** Environmental control unit comparison chart.

technology changes some of the information in the chart (ie, price) may also change. This chart provides a comparison of the devices looking at specific device features and functions. Clients who may not have access to an AT provider can review the resource list for ideas and contacts (see **Box 2**).

Clients also want to control landline and/or cell phones, either via switch and/or via voice access. There are a variety of options for landline phone as seen in (**Fig. 22**). Photo Dialer connected to a landline phone identify important individuals that the client with a brain injury may only recognize by picture rather than trying to remember a number or name (**Fig. 23**).

The Sero! Phone is not voice accessible but is switch controlled and provides visual and auditory feedback. This phone works in combination with other EADL devices such as the Primo! or AAC dynamic devices. Voice Dialer 6000 is voice activated and provides auditory feedback. This device connects to the landline jack and then the phone itself and walks the client through setup. It also can store up to 40 names (**Fig. 22**). Smartphones have some built-in accessibility features allowing for switch and voice access, meaning more control of built-in features of the device itself. For example, iPhones have the ability to use a switch such as a Teckla Shield to access iOS features if a client is unable to provide direct access due to contractures. Individual APPs vary regarding the inclusion of elements that allow for use of the accessibility features that limit ability to use the switch access method. In addition, home assistant devices such as Amazon Echo and Google Home offer the ability to call others within their identified Amazon or Google community. **Table 9** provides examples of AT solutions for EADL needs for clients with specific diagnosis.

## Telephones: AT Lab Equipment

| Device | Serol | Ablephone 7000VC | RC-200 Ameriphone | Voice Dialer 6000 (Infinity III) |
|---|---|---|---|---|
| Vendor | AbleNet | Ablephone | Clairty | Ablephone (EnableMart) |
| Voice Activated | No[1] | Yes | Yes[4] | Yes[2] |
| Switch Activated | Yes | No | Yes | No |
| On Screen Menu | Yes | No | No | No |
| Auditory Feedback | Yes | Yes | Yes | Yes |
| Visual Feedback | Yes | Yes | Yes | No |
| IR Controlled | Yes | No | No | No |
| Primol / Pilot Controlled | Yes | No | No | No |
| Voice IR Controlled | No | No | No | Yes |
| Stand Alone Telephone | Yes | Yes | Yes | No |
| Speaker Phone | Yes | Yes | Yes | - |
| Phone Number Storage | Yes | Yes | Yes | Yes |
| Cost | $1,195.00 | $579.00 | $399.00 | $219.00 |
| Strengths | Primol And Pilot control with default settings, has limited AAC features, operates as a normal phone. | Inexpensive, easy setup, fully voice controlled, voice prompted training and setup. | Loud, sturdy, simpe, comes with remote switch, can plug in any ability switch, has sip/puff option. | Inexpensive, works with any phone, easy setup, voice prompted training and setup. |
| Weaknesses | Expensive, needs Pilot, Primol, or other ECU / AAC for voice control. | Commands trained to a single user, not as "refined" mechanically as the Serol. | Scanning interface, voice command is very simplistic. | Must use additional phone to operate tottaly hands free or with switch, commands trained to a single user. |

Notes:
1) Voice activated if combined with a Pilot or Primol ECU.
2) Voice dailing, but must use Ameriphone RC200 for total hands-free operation.
3) Voice activated if combined with a voice activated ECU.
4) Very simple voive activation for anser / hangup function, requires Voice Dialer for full voice control.

**Fig. 22.** Examples of adaptive landline phones.

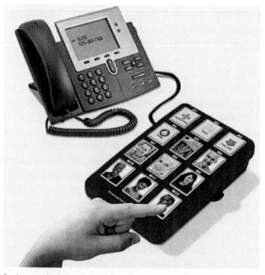

**Fig. 23.** Example of photo dialer.

**Table 9**
**Examples of EADL/environmental control unit recommends for different diagnosis**

| Who Can Benefit from ECU? | |
|---|---|
| Problem | Potential Assistive Technology Solution |
| Respiratory Failure; decrease strength and endurance | Voice and switch control Environmental Control Unit |
| Hemiparesis of dominant hand/Upper Extremity | Switch operated door opener and environmental control unit to control lights and TV; switch control bed controller |
| Deaf and Hard of Hearing | Clarity Alert Master |
| Mild Cognitive Deficit | Picture based phone (land line phone) |

## Safety, Alert, and Monitoring Systems

Safety in the home is also taken into consideration throughout the AT process. A safety plan gives clients, family, and/or caregivers a sense of control and security in emergency situations. Options for safety plans/devices include an alarm button on AAC device to alert a family member that they need help; another option is mounting a cellphone to a power wheelchair with alternative access to control to active "911." Monitoring systems also provide services that alert family and local emergency services if a button on a pendant is activated. Other monitoring systems offer fall detection. Monthly fee is typically required for the monitoring service.

Wandering behavior is another concern for some clients because they leave familiar environments, placing them in unsafe and unfamiliar ones. Wandering behavior can be diverted through low-tech solutions such as camouflaging doors and door knobs, red stop signs on the back of the door, or changing the type of door locks that will confuse the user.

There are devices that are added to the home environment to alert family/caregivers, such as motion detector placed on windows or doors as well as seat or bed alarms or vibrating alarm when the smoke detector is going off. In addition, tracking systems attached to the client such as on their shoes or wrist and a GPS tracking system locate them, which charges a monthly fee. A challenge with these systems is that clients may try to take them off. Some examples include, but not limited to, PAL (Protect and Locate) GPS, which is a watch with a band that locks (www.projectlifesaver.org), and GPS SmartShoe, where the technology is inserted into the shoe and tracked through GPS (www.gpssmartsole.com). In addition, there are GPS apps for tracking clients if they carry their phone or tiles/tags with them (ie, GPS tracker app, Find My iPhone, Tell MyGeo Android app).

Another area of safety and concern revolves around the use of the internet especially for vulnerable populations. Many news outlets report daily on Internet scams and identify theft and misuse of information. Clients who have frontal lobe damage have difficulty with self-awareness, problem-solving, safety/judgment, and inhibition. Therefore, this population can be a valuable group where others take advantage of them without any concern or warning to that person. AT team members provide training around safety when using the Internet. Topics typically discussed include the purpose of strong passwords (and how to remember them), identifying how a web page is secure, importance of virus protection on devices, phishing (practice of luring unsuspected Internet users to a fake Website), identify theft, and tips for using social media.

## Integration of Technology

Technology has evolved over the years that high-level devices have the capability to be used not only for the main medical purpose but also for alternative areas of need. For example, a power wheelchair is prescribed for mobility but also have the capability to have Bluetooth control on the computer and electronics to control IR receivers for environmental control. In addition, home assistant devices can not only control lights and TV but also set reminders for the client's day. In general, an AT specialist determines the best options for these kinds of cases especially because funding sources may only pay for the primary purpose of the AT device.

Learning technologies is another example of integration of technology needs. Clients with mTBI often want to return to school or work; however, because of cognitive deficits, specifically with executive function deficits, they struggle in the classroom, on-line classes, and/or on the job. However, through the use of educational software, APPS, and web-based sites, clients' success increases. Learning technologies is a broad range of communication, information, and related technologies that can be used to support learning, teaching, and assessment.[24] Learning technologies evolved from the education field for students who have learning disabilities. The types of deficits learning technologies assist with include word finding, word prediction, recall information, document accuracy, completion of assignments, and reading comprehension. Note-taking technology options are pen/paper, digital recorder, tablet, laptop, smartpens, and APPS. Literacy software includes Ginger, Kurzweil, Read and Write Gold, and SOLO. Text to speech books include Bookshare app, Learning Ally Website and APP, and Kindles. Word finding/prediction includes voice recognition software, Word Q/Speak Q. Most of this technology also opens an opportunity for adaptive computer access. For example, a client with a severe TBI resulting in hemiparesis could use word prediction software and/or voice recognition software to increase speed and accuracy (**Box 5** Case Study #3). Another client with a TBI and photosensitivity can use reading software program allowing them to listen to what is on the computer screen and not to have to try to read on their own or follow along.

## Adaptive Sports

Adaptive sports are sports played by persons with a disability, including physical and intellectual disabilities. As many disabled sports are based on existing able-bodied sports, modified to meet the needs of persons with a disability, they are sometimes referred to as adapted sports. However, not all disabled sports are adapted; several sports that have been specifically created for persons with a disability have no equivalent in nondisabled sports. Engagement in adaptive sports adds to the overall wellness and quality of life for the client.

Adaptive sports evaluation identifies a client's sport, recreational, and/or leisure goals, which include exercise, development of sports skills, engagement in leisure activities with family, and participation in team sports. The assessment takes into account the client's overall physical, cognitive, and mental strengthens and challenges as well as the environments in which they will participate in these activities. The types of adaptive sports range from bowling to fishing to skiing to cycling to softball to rugby and many in between. A few examples are discussed later.

Adaptive cycling includes hand cycles, recumbent cycles and wheelchair racers. When evaluating for the use of these devices, the AT team considers transfers, maneuverability (turning and backing up), shifting, braking, and safety issues when determining the most functional device.

---

**Box 5**
**Case study #3**

John is a 56-year-old Army Veteran who suffered a traumatic brain injury and stroke due to an assault. These events lead to right side hemiparesis, inability to ambulate, pain in both ears, visual deficits, and receptive and expressive aphasia. The patient was referred to occupational therapy for mobility needs, speech therapy for communication, and assistive technology for accessing his living environment. As an interdisciplinary team, they discussed the need for full evaluation including comfort level and motivation to using technology to meet his goals of communication, mobility, and accessing his living environments, which at the time was mainly the VA hospital's community living center. Speech therapy completed full cognitive testing, which indicated functional cognition. Occupational therapy completed neuromusculoskeletal and movement-related functional assessments and sensory deficits, finding that his dominant side was affected, right neglect, and right visual field cut. Overall, Veteran's frustration with staff and himself increased due to the lack of being able to successfully communicate with others.

Incorporating the HAAT frame of reference, John (Human Component) faced several challenges around communication, mobility, vision, and neuromuscular coordination. His goals (Activity Component) were to communicate, getting from one point to another independently, and accessing his surroundings (Context Component), which was the long-term care unit of the hospital because he did not have a discharge placement. Based on these components, the last HAAT component, Assistive Technology, was trialed.

*AT Equipment Trials:*

- Communication: low-tech picture device (Go Talk) and text to speech device (LightWriter)
- Mobility: 2 types of power wheelchairs (one front wheel drive and another mid-wheel drive) with left hand joystick for driving the wheelchair
- Mounting: REHAdapt and Mount'n Mover to add to wheelchair
- Environmental Control: access to TV remote, fan, and CD player

*Through various trials and trainings, the final AT solutions include the following:*

- Communication: LightWriter (text to speech device)
- Mobility: Permobil power wheelchair (mid-wheel drive) with left hand joystick
- Access: Mounting LightWriter to Permobil power wheelchair
- EADLS: Powerlink with Red Buddy Button to control fan and CD player and Large-Button Remote for TV access

---

Court Sport wheelchairs include sport-specific wheelchairs such as basketball wheelchair and a quad ruby wheelchair. The athlete's role on the team affects the decision on the design and configuration of the sports wheelchair, which then affects the athlete's performance.

Adaptive skiing offers many adaptive opportunities depending on the level of mobility and balance, sensory impairments, and/or upper body strength and coordination. Types of adaptive ski options include outriggers and monoski that uses short outriggers for balance.

Any of the seating sports requires further seating evaluation as the fit is critical for safety and performance as well as preserving skin integrity. Pressure mapping identifies any areas of concern and cushion requirements. Education about skin care is critical. **Fig. 24** shows examples of adaptive sports.

Adaptive shooting takes into account the fundamentals of rifle shooting, including aiming, breath control, hold control, trigger control, and follow through. In addition, the position of the athlete also affects the adaption required, such as offhand/

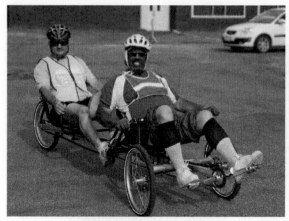
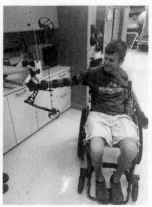
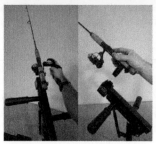
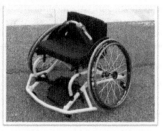

**Fig. 24.** Adaptive sports.

standing, unsupported, sitting, supported, kneeling, semi-supported, prone, and fully supported.

Adaptive fishing takes into account functional upper extremity coordination, strength and control as well as the position of the client while fishing—standing or sitting (wheelchair or no wheelchair). Additional considerations include type of fishing—salt water or fresh water—because that determines the fishing pole and weight.

### Training

Training plays a critical role in the success of the implementation of AT within the client's daily life roles and routines. Learning new everyday technology takes time but especially AT. Therefore, training is recommended to occur over multiple sessions and in different environments when possible to allow the client the opportunity to integrate the AT device into daily routines and functional activities. The benefits of multiple training sessions are that it allows the skills to become habitual, decreases the chances of equipment abundant, and increases successful usage.

Training occurs with not only the client but also the family and caregivers, teachers, and employers. Including all those involved with the client will also increase the chances that the AT device will be effectively used in the client's daily life. An effective way for the AT specialist to know if the client uses and understands the AT device is to have them train family and/or caregivers on how to use the device. This AT treatment session provides valuable information from how well the client knows the AT device to how effective they are in communicating its purpose to what other areas need to be worked on in future AT treatment sessions. Also, caregiver training increases compliance, ensures safety, develops skills if changes are needed, and increases awareness in maintenance requirements.

### Customized Assistive Technology Solutions

Over the years, the evaluation of AT devices traditionally required specialized professionals and/or companies to customize individual solutions OR the client, their family, or a very creative therapist, to develop a customized individualized solution. Rehabilitation professionals often have to use what is available to them (eg, duct tape, splinting materials, Velcro, and medical supplies) in order to assist the client to achieve their goal. The Assistive Technology Solutions in Minutes Book II offers solutions to every day challenges with limited resources for everything from mounting of devices to creating switches to creating a light for a cane.[25] However, over the past 5 years, other mediums that once were out of the reach of clients and rehabilitation specialists are now main stream and commercially available such as 3-dimensional (3D) printing and electronics. The Maker Movement has become a huge phenomenon where maker events are found in most cities, towns, universities, and health care systems. According to Mark Hatch, CEO, Techshop, "Making is a fundamental to what is meant to be human. We must make, create, and express ourselves to feel whole. There is something unique about making physical things. Things we make are like little pieces of us and seem to embody portions of our soul."[26] According to Susannah Fox, Former Chief Technology Officer at the US Department of Health and Human Services, "Healthcare is part of the innovation nation…we all need to be part of solving our problems in health care…need to prepare for the maker movement."[27] Students learn about 3D printing, designing, and simple electronics as early as elementary school. Clients are becoming their own problem solvers and not relying on health care professionals to find the solution as much anymore. Therefore, health care providers need to be skilled on making or at least be aware of the possibilities in order to meet the client's expectations.

Rehabilitation Engineering emphasizes engineering applications to meet the needs of and address the barriers confronted by individuals with disabilities.[4] Rehabilitation Engineering builds the bridge between rehabilitation and customized solutions. As part of the interdisciplinary team, rehabilitation engineers work closely with the client and rehabilitation therapists to assess the problem. They will design and develop a prototype to test, reassess, and redesign, if needed till an effective solution is created. Client involvement in the design allows for personal investment in the solution and increases the likelihood they will use the final solution. Rehabilitation engineers are also unbiased technical experts providing technical background to assist in identifying the customized solution to help achieve the client's goals.

The tools that rehabilitation engineers use to develop customized AT solutions include, but not limited to, computer-aided design (CAD) software, 3D printing, 3D scanning, and electronics. The design process starts with an idea designed first on paper and then transition to CAD software, which allows the user to turn a 2D idea into a 3D solution (**Fig. 25**).

CAD software capabilities range from a basic design to functional features and details. The cost ranges from free to thousands of dollars. Also, 3D designs are available through open source warehouses such as the NIH 3D Printing Exchange. The design process also takes into account the type of material needed for the end product. 3D printing material ranges from plastics, glass, metal, human tissue, wax, sand and glue mixes, polymers, and edible food. Within rehabilitation and specifically AT, the most used type of material is plastics, such as ABS plastics, nylon, and carbon fiber. Most manufacturing process can be divided into 3 basic types: (1) cutting item made by removing material from a solid block (ie, carving, chiseling cutting), (2) forming item

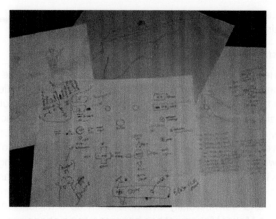

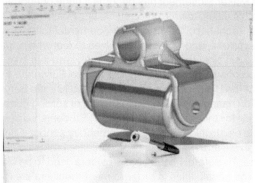

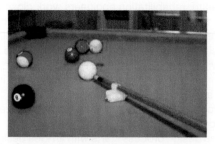

**Fig. 25.** 3D Printing from design to solutions.

made by shaping a material; material is neither added nor reduced (ie, molding, casting), and (3) joining item made by adding weight and volume (ie, welding, riveting, and 3D printing) (**Fig. 26**).

3D in health care includes medical modeling for presurgery and education, dental, medical instrument repair, orthotics, and assistive technologies. 3D scanning is another specific area of customized solutions where a laser light digitally captures the physical shape of an object without contact and creates a 3D representation that then can be manipulated to meet a specific purpose (ie, hand splints) (**Fig. 27**). Resources for some of these tools are in **Table 10**.

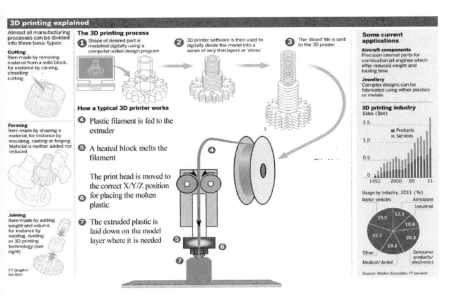

**3D printing explained**

Almost all manufacturing processes can be divided into three basic types:

**Cutting**
Item made by removing material from a solid block, for instance by carving, chiselling cutting

**Forming**
Item made by shaping a material, for instance by moulding, casting or forging. Material is neither added nor reduced

**Joining**
Item made by adding weight and volume, for instance by welding, riveting or 3D printing technology (see right)

FT Graphic
Ian Bott

**The 3D printing process**
1  Shape of desired part is modelled digitally using a computer-aided design program

2  3D printer software is then used to digitally divide the model into a series of very thin layers or 'slices'

3  The 'sliced' file is sent to the 3D printer

**How a typical 3D printer works**
4  Plastic filament is fed to the extruder

5  A heated block melts the filament

   The print head is moved to the correct X/Y/Z position
6  for placing the molten plastic

7  The extruded plastic is laid down on the model layer where it is needed

**Some current applications**

**Aircraft components**
Precision internal parts for combustion jet engines which offer reduced weight and tooling time

**Jewellery**
Complex designs can be fabricated using either plastics or metals

**3D printing industry**
Sales ($bn)

Usage by industry, 2011 (%)

Sources: Wohlers Associates; FT research

Fig. **26.** 3D process.

In the design process, the solution may require "brains" to the design, which is where adding of electronics come into play. The basic principles around electronics are inputs such as a client's action or sensor signal. Then based on the input, a decision is made from the "brains" of the device and appropriate result is outputted, which

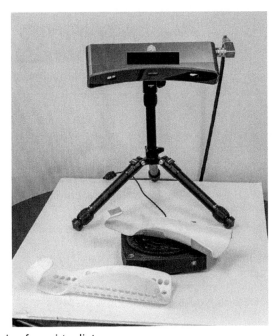

Fig. **27.** 3D Scanning for wrist splint.

**Table 10**
**Resources for 3D materials/tools**

| 3D Design Software | Free: |
| --- | --- |
| | • http://3dp4e.com/resources/free-3d-modeling-software |
| | • http://www.sketchup.com/products/sketchup-make |
| | • http://www.123dapp.com/sculptplus |
| | • http://www.123dapp.com/design |
| | • http://www.123dapp.com/catch |
| | • http://www.123dapp.com/meshmixer |
| | • https://www.tinkercad.com/ |
| | • http://pixologic.com/sculptris/ |
| | • http://www.3dtin.com |
| | • http://www.ptc.com/product/creo/elements/direct-modeling/express |
| | • http://www.freecadweb.org/ |
| | $50–$200 |
| | • http://fusion360.autodesk.com/ $25/mo |
| | • http://cubify.com/en/Products/Design $200 |
| | • http://cubify.com/en/Products/Invent $50 |
| | • http://cubify.com/en/Products/Sculpt $130 |
| 3D Scanning Options | Low Cost ($500–$1500) |
| | • Cubify iSense $500 (http://cubify.com/en/Products/iSense) |
| | • MakerBot Digitizer $800 (http://store.makerbot.com/digitizer) |
| | • Fuel3D $1500 (http://fuel-3d.com/) |
| 3D Printing Options | • 3D Printing |
| | • Contact a local university, high schools, library, or Makerspace/Hackerspace |
| | • Own a printer (Ultimaker, MakerBot, Afinia) |
| | • Make Magazine yearly review of consumer 3D printers |
| | • Use a printing service (Materialise, Shapeways, Sculpteo, Staples, Stratasys Direct) |
| 3D Printing/Making Options | • MakerHealth (www.makerhealth.co/) |
| | • Tech Garden (www.techgarden.org/) |
| | • Enable Community Foundation (www.enablecommunityfoundation.org) |
| | • FDA (www.fda.gov/MedicalDevices?productsandmedicalProcdures/3DprintingofMedicalDevices/) |
| | • NIH 3D Print Exchange (http://3dprint.nih.gov) |

may be a signal to the patient, physical action, or signal to another device. The tools when considering electronics include design software, hardware, firmware, fabrication, and development platforms. Basic electronic kits are available to provide simple electronic solutions; however, the more complex the solution the more likely a professional rehabilitation or an electronical engineer is required.

Customized AT solutions typically occur in one or more of the following situations:

1. When a client and their rehabilitation therapist have an immediate need to be met (**Fig. 28**)
2. Modifications to commercially available AT devices (**Fig. 29**)
3. Takes a design further in development to be more functional, durable, and reproducible (**Fig. 30**)
4. Customizing a solution that does not exist (**Figs. 31–34**).

Although 3D printing, 3D scanning, and adding electronics are new and exciting options in AT and rehabilitation in general, there are still challenges. First and

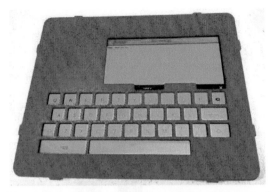

**Fig. 28.** Example of immediate need for 3D printing solution. This example is a keyguard for an iPAD for a specific communication APP. The patient had a stroke resulting in communication deficits and hand tremors making using a touchscreen challenging. Therefore, the keyguard provided accuracy. The keyguard could have been ordered but that would have taken weeks and the patient lived far away; therefore, one was made for him with the use of CAD software and 3D printing (ABS plastic).

foremost, a trained professional who understands design, the design tools, attention to details, and rehabilitation needs of clients is crucial to the success of the solutions and achieving the client's goals. The initial design is labor intensive taking hours upon hours to develop. It is not as simple as point, click, and print. The knowledge and awareness of types of materials and any safety concerns around that type of material determines the design and decision-making process. Attention to the final 10% of details makes or breaks the successful implementation. Depending on the design and type of material, the fabrication times vary in length. Finally, another challenge is that the tools and materials for the customized solutions are expensive. Although there are consumer 3D printers and electronics available, they have their limitations, including little to no technical support, limited materials, and limited print capacity.

## Simple Adapted Cellphone Access

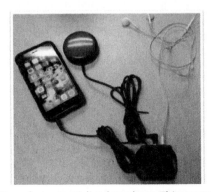

**Fig. 29.** Example of modification of commercialized products. This example is taking smartphone headphones switch adapted for individuals who cannot use the headset switches due to upper extremity limitations and not all smartphone functions can be controlled by voice.

# Custom Mouth Stick Holder

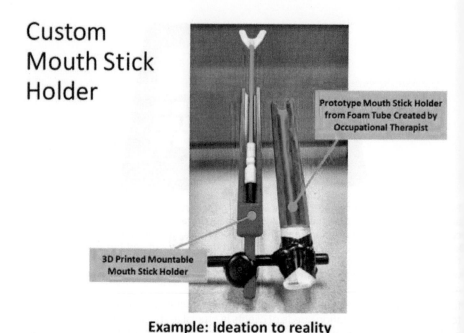

Prototype Mouth Stick Holder from Foam Tube Created by Occupational Therapist

3D Printed Mountable Mouth Stick Holder

## Example: Ideation to reality

**Fig. 30.** Customizing an idea. This example is of a mouth stick holder to increase independence with managing and accessing a mouth stick. An OT came up with the idea of using foam and duct tape. The AT Program took the idea, designed it, and 3D printed to make it more durable and reproducible.

### Assistive Technology Reevaluation

Reevaluation is an ongoing process and should be done throughout the AT treatment process and may change as the client improves. Another need for reevaluation includes if the client's needs are chronic or the disease is progressive. The AT team wants to ensure the AT device still meets their needs. As technology changes, there are newer and more effective ways for clients to achieve their goals. Additional reasons for changes in AT usage include the following: (1) clients find easier ways to achieve the goal; (2) perhaps simpler is better; (3) no longer meeting their needs; (4) no longer satisfied with the impact on the daily lives; (5) aging-related changes; and (6) the equipment is heavy, complicated, or required increase energy to use and therefore, equipment is abandoned.[28] Reevaluation of the AT equipment can take place during trial periods of the equipment. During that time, the client, family/caregivers, and other team members provide feedback about what worked and did not work as far as meeting their needs in their various contexts. Based on this information, a decision about permanent use is made. Key to success is the collaboration with other services and disciplines. Research has shown that a team approach with medical, functional, psychosocial, and technology components is the most effective.[29] Cotreatment with treating clinicians in several sessions, comprehensive training and education to caregiver and/or family members of the clients, and training to all staff involved in the client's care are other keys to successful implementation of AT devices in the client's life roles and environments. The efficiency and functionality of all the AT discussed here are expected to continue improving and playing valuable roles in allowing clients with a disability, injury, or illness to participate fully in society.

# Shake it Out

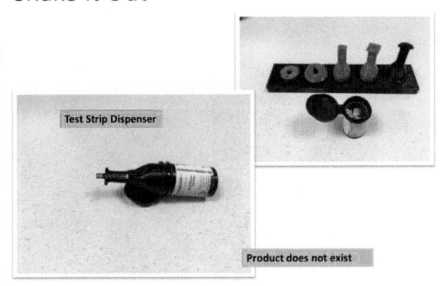

**Fig. 31.** 3D customized solution. This example is of a diabetes test strip dispenser. The client had had a stroke resulting in hemiparesis, sensory loss, and visual impairments due to the diabetes. His one goal was to test his own glucose. Through collaborations with the client, his wife, and the AT Program, a one-hand solution was designed and 3D printed. As seen here, there were multiple iterations as the design process is trial and error and attention to the final details before getting it right.

**FUTURE OF TECHNOLOGY**

AT devices have evolved over the past several decades. However, the speed of development of new devices and their capabilities has increase significantly over the last 5 years. For example, electronics on power wheelchairs over more than just functions and tablets are outdated as soon as they leave the store. So what is the Future of Technology specifically for AT?

## Utensil

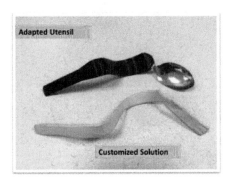

**Fig. 32.** 3D customized utensil. This example shows where an OT used splinting material to demonstrate the exact angles needed for an adaptive utensil and the 3D printed solution.

# Trumpet Valve Finger Guide

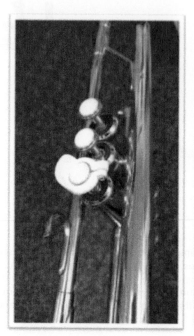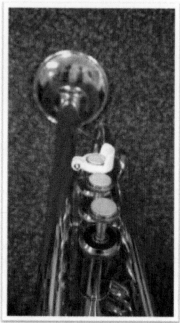

**Fig. 33.** 3D customized finger guide. This example shows where a 3D printed finger glide allowed for control of a tremor to continue to play a trumpet.

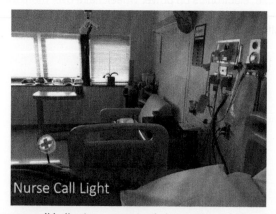

**Fig. 34.** Adaptive nurse call bell using customized electronics and 3D printing. This example is when a patient in a nursing home needed to call the nursing staff; however, due to hearing issues, he could not hear the chime on the nurse call bell to know that when he pushed it, it was activated. He therefore, continued to push the nurse call bell repeatedly. Through electronics and 3D printing they came up with a visual solution: when he pushed the nurse call bell, he would see the red crosslight up positioned at the end of his hospital bed.

Brain computer interfacing (BCI) uses electroencephalogram technology to allow for control of wheelchairs, keyboards, and video games. BCI has been researched for years testing out the possibilities and safety around its usage. Research is now focused on using BCI technology for connecting with AT devices specifically with communication, motor actions, and recovery.[30]

Assistive robotics is a growing field not only in industry but in health care as well. Robotics is being tested and research in meeting the needs of individuals with different daily needs. Personal robotics assists in providing caregiver tasks such as transfers and positioning in bed as well as a few household tasks. Canine service dog robotics provides guided serves to the blind and also, robotic features such as the exoskeleton assisting with mobility for someone with a spinal cord injury.

Virtual reality is a rapidly growing field. It is a computer technology that replicates an environment and simulates a user's physical presence to allow for the user to interact with that environment. Virtual reality creates sensory experiences (sight, touch, hearing, and smell), artificially, to allow for as much real world experience as possible. Virtual reality has been around in different forms for years especially in the form of simulators (ie, plane simulators). Within AT, driving simulators have been used to determine not only if someone can still drive but also what and if any adaptation is needed for their level of independence. Gaming then introduced interactive opportunities to engage the user with the activity on the screen. The Nintendo Wii and the Wii Fit open up the opportunity for interactive exercise and from a rehabilitation perspective, balance activities. Google Maps provides virtual tours of street views of different locations. Today, virtual reality products include a headset, where the individual is totally immersed into the virtual world. For example, someone in a wheelchair can hike over the mountain range or swim in the ocean or someone who has an amputated hand can play the piano. Research has shown benefits of virtual reality to include engagement in a range of activities that is free from limitations and allows them a sense of safety. In addition, the knowledge and skills acquired by individuals with an injury or disability using virtual reality devices transfers to the real world.[31] Virtual reality systems within rehabilitation provide another tool for clinicians to work with clients on skills within various environments, for example, a new wheelchair user learning how to navigate a busy interaction or grocery store. Research found that virtual reality training improved the gait speed and community walking time for individuals who had a stroke.[32] In another study, adults with TBI who used virtual reality to improve balance found greater improvements in quantitative measures and increased confidence with ambulation.[33] Other aspects of virtual reality provides experiences to individual who otherwise could not travel to locations around the world (ie, terminally ill WWII veterans visually visiting war memorials) or explore operating rooms to decrease anxiety before surgery or test out building designs for accessibility needs. However, although virtual reality is cutting edge, there are still challenges including possible motion sickness, disorientation leading to balance issues, technical issues with computer delays, and navigating nonvirtual surrounding, which can be dangerous without external sensory information. Nevertheless, the world of possibilities is wide open and research continues to explore and challenge those opportunities.

## ACKNOWLEDGMENTS

Tina Williams, MSW, for all of her love and support.

## REFERENCES

1. Perrin A, Duggan, M. American's internet access: 2000-2015. 2015. Available at: http://www.pewinternet.org/2015/06/26/americans-internet-access-2000-2015/. Accessed March 1, 2018.
2. Smith A. Smartphone ownership. 2013. Available at: http://www.pewinternet.org/2013/06/05/smartphone-ownership-2013/. Accessed March 1, 2018.
3. Smith, A. U.S. Smartphone use in 2015. 2015. Available at: http://www.pewinternet.org/2015/04/01/us-smartphone-use-in-2015/. Accessed March 1, 2018.
4. Cook AM, Polgar JM. Cook and hussey's assistive technologies: principles and practice. 3rd edition. St Louis (MO): Mosby; 2008.
5. Szymkowiak A, et al. A memory aid with remote communication: preliminary findings. Technol Disabil 2005;17:217–25.
6. Scherer M, Hart T, Kirsch N, et al. Assistive technologies for cognitive disabilities. Phys Rehabil Med 2005;17(3):195–215.
7. Lopresti EF, Milhailidis A, Kirsch N. Assistive technology for cognitive rehabilitation: state of the art. Neuropsychol Rehabil 2001;14(1/2):5–39.
8. Wallace J. Assistive technology funding in the United States. NeuroRehabilitation 2011;28(3):295–302.
9. Oliver M. Communication devices and electronic aids to activities of daily living. In: Webster JB, Murphy DP, editors. Atlas of orthoses and assistive devices. 5th edition. Philadelphia: Elsevier; 2018. p. 403–17.
10. American Speech-Language Hearing Association website. Augmentative and alternative Communication (AAC). 2016. Available at: http://www.asha.org/public/speech/disorders/AAC/. Accessed July 2, 2016.
11. National coalition for assistive and rehab technology website. Available at: www.ncart.us/. Accessed December 1, 2017.
12. Brubaker C. Ergonometric considerations. J Rehabil Res Dev Clin Suppl 1990;2:37–48.
13. Brubaker CE. Wheelchair prescription: an analysis of factors that affect mobility and performance. J Rehabil Res Dev Clin Suppl 1986;23(4):19–26.
14. McLaurin CA, Brubaker CE. Biomechanics and the wheelchair. Prosthet Orthot Int 1991;15(1):24–37.
15. Cooper RA. A perspective on the ultralight wheelchair revolution. Technol Disabil 1996;5:383–92.
16. Cooper RA. Rehabilitation engineering: applied to mobility and manipulation. Philadelphia: Institute of Physics Publishing; 1995.
17. Gillespie A, Best C, O'Neill B. Cognitive function and assistive technology for cognition: a systematic review. J Int Neuropsychol Soc 2012;18(1):1–19.
18. Gentry T, Wallace J, Kvarvfordt C, et al. Personal digital assistants as cognitive aids for individuals with severe traumatic brain injury: a community-based trial. Brain Inj 2008;22(1):19–24 (need more research and challenges are multifactorial).
19. Sohlberg MM, Turkstra LS. Optimizing cognitive rehabilitation. New York: The Guildford Press; 2011. p. 142.
20. Powell LE, Glang A, Pinkelman S. Systematic instruction of assistive technology for cognition (ATC) in an employment setting following acquired brain injury: a single case, experimental study. NeuroRehabilitation 2015;37(3):437–47.
21. Pratap A. Microsoft vision, mission and values. 2016. Available at: https://www.cheshnotes.com/2016/12/microsoft-vision-mission-and-values/. Accessed November 22, 2017.

22. Rigby P, Ryan S, Joos S. Impact of electronic aids to daily living on the lives of persons with cervical spinal cord injuries. Assist Technol 2005;17:89–97.
23. Croser R, Garrett R, Seeger B, et al. Effectiveness of electronic aids to daily living: Increased independence and decreased frustration. Aust Occup Ther J 2001;48: 35–44.
24. Association for learning technology website. Learning technology. 2015. Available at: https://www.alt.ac.uk/about-alt. Accessed July 1, 2017.
25. Willkomm T. Assistive technology solutions in minutes book II ordinary items extraordinary solutions. Durham (New Hampshire): University of New Hampshire Institute on Disability; 2013.
26. Hatch M. The maker movement manifesto. Columbus (Ohio): McGraw Hill; 2013.
27. Fox, S. StartUp health now. 2016. Available at: https://healthtransformer.co/the-maker-movement-in-healthcare-susannah-fox-hhs-content-f607d4c06380. Accessed December 1, 2016.
28. Hoge DR, Newsome CA. The source for augmentative alternative communication. East Moline (IL): LinguiSystems; 2002.
29. Culley C, Evans JJ. SMS text messaging as a means of increasing recall of therapy goals in brain injury rehabilitation: a single-blind within-subjects trail. Neuropsychol Rehabil 2010;20(1):103–19.
30. Millan JR, Rupp R, Muller-Putz GR, et al. Combining brain-computer interfaces and assistive technologies: state-of-the-art and challenges. Front Neurosci 2010. https://doi.org/10.3389/fnins.2010.00161.
31. Wilson PN, Foreman N, Stanton D. Virtual reality, disability and rehabilitation. Disabil Rehabil 1997;19(6):312–20.
32. Yang YR, Tsai MP, Chuang TY, et al. Virtual reality-based training improves community ambulation in individuals with stroke: a randomized controlled trial. Gait Posture 2008;28(2):201–6.
33. Thornton M, Marshall S, McComas J, et al. Benefits of activity and virtual-reality based balance exercise programmes for adults with traumatic brain injury: perceptions of participants and their caregivers. Brain Inj 2009. https://doi.org/10.1080/02699050500109944.

# Integrative Medicine and Health Coaching in Polytrauma Rehabilitation

Micaela Cornis-Pop, PhD[a,b], Kavitha P. Reddy, MD[c,d],*

## KEYWORDS

- Whole health • Health coaching • Complementary medicine • Polytrauma

## KEY POINTS

- Veterans Health Administration is transforming to a Whole Health System of care.
- Veterans Health Administration uses complementary and integrative health approaches.
- Health coaching is successfully implemented in polytrauma care and effects positive changes in patients' life satisfaction and well-being.

## INTRODUCTION

Over the last decade, there have been sizable changes in health care delivery models, with increased recognition that moving toward patient-centered and team-based care can result in improved patient outcomes and reduced financial burden to society. According to the 2009 Institute of Medicine summit on Integrative Medicine and the Health of the Public, "among Medicare recipients, 20% live with five or more chronic conditions (diabetes, heart disease, asthma, high blood pressure, and depression) and account for 2/3 of all Medicare expenditures, but only 55% of the most recommended clinical preventive services are actually delivered."[1] These findings continue to underscore the need to a shift from the disease and symptom–based care to patient-centered care, where patients and health care teams partner to promote health and well-being. The critical piece is empowering patients to make lifestyle and behavioral changes that support their long-term health and wellness.

Disclosure Statement: The pilot was supported jointly with internal funding by VHA's Offices of Patient Centered Care and Cultural Transformation and Rehabilitation and Prosthetic Services.
[a] Rehabilitation and Prosthetic Services, McGuire VA Medical Center, 1201 Broad Rock Boulevard, Richmond, VA 23249, USA; [b] Physical Medicine and Rehabilitation, Virginia Commonwealth University School of Medicine, Richmond, VA, USA; [c] Primary Care, VA St. Louis Health Care System, 3641 Olive Street, St Louis, MO 63108, USA; [d] Emergency Medicine, Washington University School of Medicine, St. Louis, MO, USA
* Corresponding author. 3641 Olive Street, St Louis, MO 63108.
E-mail address: Kavitha.reddy@va.gov

Culturally, there is a greater awareness among providers, health care teams, and patients that psychological, nutrition, environmental, and genetic influences contribute to disease progression, and impacting those factors can delay, and sometimes prevent, disease onset. There is also a much wider interest in education about healthy living. Concomitantly, health care educational institutions are putting greater focus on team-based care, patient-centered care, and the well-being of the providers they are training. The changes in public and institutional awareness of the value of a holistic approach to health issues affect the way medical care is delivered in both the private and public sectors nowadays.

The Veterans Health Administration (VHA) has been on the forefront of this journey, responding to the needs of our veterans, and incorporating Complementary and Integrative Health (CIH) approaches and health coaching into personalized health care plans.

## BACKGROUND

Several terms are frequently used to designate the new health care delivery model. For clarity, the authors provide the following definitions:

*Integrative Medicine and Health* reaffirms the importance of the relationship between practitioner and patient, focuses on the whole person, is informed by evidence, and makes use of all appropriate therapeutic and lifestyle approaches, health care professionals, and disciplines to achieve optimal health and healing.[2]

*Whole Health* is used within VHA to refer to patient-centered care that affirms the importance of the relationship and partnership between a patient and their community of providers. The focus is on empowering the self-healing mechanisms within the whole person while co-creating a personalized, proactive, patient-driven experience.

*Complementary and Integrative Health* approaches refer to group of diverse medical and health care systems, practices, and products that are not considered to be part of conventional or allopathic medicine. Most of these practices are used together with conventional therapies.[3]

## WHOLE HEALTH IN VETERANS HEALTH ADMINISTRATION

VHA's Whole Health system as a large-scale transformation in VHA care has been based on many years of lessons learned from grass-roots efforts at facilities across the nation exploring personalized health planning, health coaching, and integrating CIH into conventional care. From this emerged the vision of whole health. The key components of the Whole Health system include empowering patients, equipping them in self-care skills to support health and well-being, and a clinical approach that is based on high-quality evidence-based medicine and shared decision making around the patients' life goals (**Fig. 1**).

### *Empower: The Pathway*

In a partnership with their peers, veterans and their family explore their mission, aspiration, and purpose and begin their overarching personal health plan.

### *Equip: Well-Being Programs*

With a focus on self-care, skill building, and support, these programs are not diagnosis or disease based but support the personal health plan of everyone. Services include proactive, CIH approaches, such as stress reduction, yoga, tai chi, mindfulness, nutrition, acupuncture, and health coaching.

# The Whole Health System

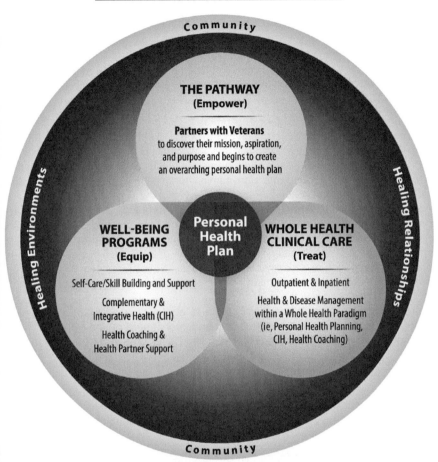

**Fig. 1.** Whole health system diagram. (*From* Available at: https://www.va.gov/PATIENTCENTEREDCARE/features/More_Than_Medicine.asp. Accessed September 24, 2018; with permission.)

## Treat: Whole Health Clinical Care

In the Veterans Administration (VA), community, or both, clinicians are trained in Whole Health and incorporate CIH approaches based on that veteran's personal health plan, grounded in the healing relationship.

To support this large-scale cultural transformation, VHA's Office of Patient-Centered Care and Cultural Transformation (OPCC&CT) has invested resources into educating and training VHA staff and volunteers in Whole Health curriculum over the last 5 years. Since fiscal year 2013, there have been about 6000 staff trained in whole health courses.

OPCC&CT partners with many VHA program offices to promote Whole Health care by having multidisciplinary advisory groups and representatives from multiple specialties working toward the common goal of impacting health care transformation.

To better understand the impact of the Whole Health model of care, OPCC&CT has developed multiple tracking strategies to evaluate patient-reported outcomes, utilization of hospital and pharmaceutical resources (including opioids), cost of delivering services, and the impact on the health of our veterans. Over the next several years, VHA will be monitoring these measures at several facilities that have committed to deploying the VHA Whole Health model of care.[4]

## COMPLEMENTARY AND INTEGRATIVE HEALTH IN VETERANS HEALTH ADMINISTRATION

Once relegated to backwaters of medical practice, CIH is increasingly recognized as a legitimate resource for health promotion by the public, the medical profession, and insurers. Data obtained from the National Health Information Survey at 3 points in time, 2002, 2007, and 2012, revealed growth in the use of CIH approaches (yoga, tai chi, and qi gong) for Americans, with nonvitamin, nonmineral supplements being the most commonly used approach.[5]

According to a recent 2015 Healthcare Analysis & Information Group survey on CIH services in VHA, administrative parent facilities report they provide at least one CIH service to veterans (93% 2015 vs 89% 2011). Although many facilities offer CIH services, the availability of these services is limited. As of 2015, facilities offering a CIH service, only acupuncture, chiropractic, mindfulness, Stress Management Relaxation Therapy, acupressure, and movement practices are offered at a rate equivalent to at least one-half day per week.[6]

In addition to this growing demand, there is also a growing body of evidence showing the potential health benefit of CIH as demonstrated by the evidence maps developed by VA's Health Services Research and Development:

- Acupuncture: https://www.hsrd.research.va.gov/publications/esp/acupuncture.pdf
- Yoga: https://www.hsrd.research.va.gov/publications/esp/yoga.pdf
- Tai chi: https://www.hsrd.research.va.gov/publications/esp/taichi-REPORT.pdf
- Mindfulness: https://www.hsrd.research.va.gov/publications/esp/cam_mindfulness-REPORT.pdf

Given the level of evidence for certain CIH approaches, in May 2017, VHA formally published Directive 1137, which outlined policy on the provision of these approaches in the medical benefits package for veterans.[7] Specifically, the directive stipulates that VHA must have a mechanism to make CIH available to veterans, either within the facility or through community partners. A multidisciplinary advisory panel approved 8 CIH approaches, which must be made available through VA resources, including acupuncture, yoga, tai chi, meditation, guided imagery, clinical hypnosis, biofeedback, and massage therapy. As standards for implementation are further developed and effectiveness is monitored, CIH approaches can have a significant impact as either monotherapy, such as acupuncture for low back pain, or adjunctive therapy, such as yoga[8] and mindfulness,[9] for anxiety/stress reduction.

## HEALTH COACHING

Health coaching has emerged as a valuable adjunct for the prevention and treatment of "lifestyle diseases," which are the greatest causes of morbidity and mortality in the developed world. By supporting beneficial lifestyle behavior changes, health coaching has been shown to help manage and treat diabetes, hypertension, hyperlipidemia, heart disease, cancer, and other chronic disorders. Health coaching is based on a working partnership between the patient and the clinician using tools such as motivational interviewing to raise awareness and engagement, tapping into a wellness vision that enables the patient to see new possibilities and a clear direction toward achieving the vision, goal setting, and accountability for sustainable change. The health coach is part motivational life coach, part counselor, and part clinician, who supports the patient to achieve personal goals of overall health and wellness.

The coaching literature has grown progressively over time. The Health and Wellness Coaching Compendium found 219 peer-reviewed articles in 2017 of which 150 are data based.[10] The Compendium results point to health coaching intervention as a treatment adjunct worthy of consideration for patients with cancer, diabetes, and heart disease. At the same time, the number of certified and practicing health coaches has soared, and a national standard board was launched in 2017.[11]

## HEALTH COACHING IN POLYTRAUMA: PILOT STUDY

The Polytrauma Integrative Medicine Initiative (PIMI) pilot, a 3-year study proposing to evaluate the feasibility of introducing Health Coaching in the care of veterans with complex symptoms related to traumatic brain injury (TBI) and polytrauma. PIMI was deployed at 3 VA Polytrauma Rehabilitation Centers in Palo Alto, Richmond, and San Antonio beginning in 2013.

The complex and often chronic medical and mental health problems of patients with TBI and polytrauma recommended this population for health coaching support to help personalize rehabilitation care and to create the conditions for patients and their caregivers to become competent in managing health care needs upon discharge from medical care and reintegration into community.

## METHODS

PIMI employed 9 health coaches certified through the Duke Integrative Health Coach Professional Training Program across the 3 sites of operation. The specific responsibilities of the health coaches included (1) providing individual and group health coaching services; (2) serving as resources, trainers, and mentors for Whole Health initiatives throughout the medical centers where they operated; (3) providing and facilitating access to CIH; and (4) collecting data for the PIMI evaluation. In addition to the polytrauma and Physical Medicine and Rehabilitation Clinics, the Health Coaches covered Primary Care, Pain Clinic, and Mental Health, as per clinical needs and referrals.

Clinical services provided by the PIMI health coaches included screening and evaluation for health coaching needs, individual and group interventions, and follow-up consultations. Service delivery pattern started with weekly appointments followed by bi-weekly and monthly visits, depending on the need. Most veterans favored a less intensive schedule of 2 times per month to once every 6 to 8 weeks. Initial visits tend to be longer, an average of 60 minutes, but as veterans make progress and moved into the maintenance phase, 30-minute visits became appropriate. Telephone and other virtual modalities were used for scheduling, maintenance, and follow-up care.

PIMI Health Coaches actively engaged with the local medical center leadership and clinicians to promote, to provide resources, and to partner in the development of patient-centered care models across the facilities where they operate. They either provide or facilitate provision of CIH services, including yoga, tai chi, massage therapy, and guided meditation. Health coaches participate in interdisciplinary team activities to discuss care plans for the veterans they serve and communicate information about the patient's adherence to treatment and progress toward health care goals.

The VA Center of Innovation on Disability and Rehabilitation Research in Gainesville, Florida, supported a 3-pronged approach to the PIMI program evaluation: (1) the formative evaluation considered whether health coaching is a valued intervention in the view of veterans and clinicians; (2) the prospective outcome study analyzed the effects of the health coaching intervention on participants' health and well-being; (3) a retrospective observational study explored the effects of health coaching on certain health variables. Findings from the pilot will drive further decisions regarding the role of health coaching in polytrauma care and options for expanding to other programs such as Primary Care and Pain Clinics.

## DATA COLLECTION
### Demographics

**Table 1** provides the abbreviated demographic summary of all veterans approached to participate in PIMI. Just more than a thousand veterans were asked whether they were interested in participating in the PIMI pilot (N = 1126). Data were captured on 749 veterans who agreed to participate and 377 veterans who declined. There are a few differences between the 2 groups:

### Service-Connected Injury

There is a significant association between PIMI participation and whether patient is service-connected (SC)-injured ($\chi^2$ (1) = 18.60, $P<.05$). The odds ratio of 1.8 indicated that if a veteran has a SC injury, the odds of their agreeing to participate is 1.8 times higher than if they do not have an SC injury.

### Employment

There is a significant association between PIMI participation and employment status ($\chi^2$ (1) = 19.248, $P<.05$). Of those who agreed to participate, 36.8% are employed, whereas only 29.3% of those who declined are employed. The odds ratio of 1.86 indicates that the odds of agreeing to participate were 1.86 times higher if the patient is employed than if the patient is not employed.

### School Attendance

There was a significant association between PIMI participation and school status ($\chi^2$ (1) = 26.95, $P<.05$). Of those who agreed to participate, 16.2% are in school, whereas only 5.3% of those who declined participation are in school. The odds ratio of 3.44 indicates that the odds of agreeing to participate are 3.44 times higher if the patient is in school than if the patient is not in school.
All other variables are not significant (see **Table 1**).

### Qualitative Evaluation

The following factors were used to measure PIMI implementation success: (1) PIMI health coaching being accepted by VA clinicians as a viable treatment option for veterans, referrals to health coaching were taken as clinician acceptance; (2) veterans accepted health coaching as a viable treatment option, veterans' verbal confirmation of health coaching as valuable was taken as acceptance; (3) health coaches' patient load was taken as a confirmation that health coaching was being regularly practiced at the VA implementation sites.
Data were collected from focus groups conducted at each site within 90 days of the start of PIMI (time #1), at 6 months after the initial round of focus groups (time #2), and at 1 year from the initial focus groups (time #3). Focus group sessions at each site were conducted with the following groups: health coaches (times 1, 2,

**Table 1**
**National Polytrauma Integrative Medicine Initiative demographic summary of all veterans, veterans agreeing to participate, and veterans who declined participation**

| Variable | Number of Veterans | Agreed to Participate | Declined Participation |
|---|---|---|---|
| Age (N = 1122) | Total N = 1126 | N = 749 | N = 377 |
| | 47.5 y (SD = 14.9) | 47.1 y (SD = 14.0) | 48.4 y (SD = 16.4) |
| | Range: 20–90 y | Range: 20–87 y | Range: 22–90 y |
| Marital status | N = 1081 | N = 745 | N = 336 |
|   Never married | 137 (12.7%) | 100 (13.4%) | 37 (11.0%) |
|   Living with significant other | 17 (1.6%) | 13 (1.7%) | 4 (1.2%) |
|   Married | 587 (54.3%) | 399 (53.6%) | 188 (56.0%) |
|   Separated | 49 (4.5%) | 35 (4.7%) | 14 (4.2%) |
|   Divorced | 267 (24.7%) | 183 (24.6%) | 84 (25.0%) |
|   Widowed | 24 (2.2%) | 15 (2.0%) | 9 (2.7%) |
| Race | N = 1026 | N = 693 | N = 333 |
|   American Indian/Pacific Islander | 11 (1.1%) | 8 (1.2%) | 3 (0.9%) |
|   Asian | 23 (2.2%) | 12 (1.7%) | 11 (3.3%) |
|   Black | 241 (23.5%) | 173 (25.0%) | 68 (20.4%) |
|   Hispanic | 279 (27.2%) | 190 (27.4%) | 89 (26.7%) |
|   White | 456 (44.4%) | 295 (42.6%) | 161 (48.3%) |
|   Mixed race | 16 (1.6%) | 15 (2.2%) | 1 (0.3%) |
| SC injured | | | |
|   No | 301 (26.7%) | 170 (22.7%) | 131 (34.7%) |
|   Yes | 825 (73.3%) | 579 (77.3%) | 246 (65.3%) |
|     %, 0%–30% | 13.9 | 15.1 | 11.0 |
|     %, 30% to 50% | 13.9 | 14.1 | 13.4 |
|     %, GT 50% | 72.2 | 70.8 | 75.6 |
| Employed | | | |
|   Yes (%) | 32.5 | 36.8 | 23.9 |
|   % Full-time | 63.4 | 63.8 | 62.2 |
| In school | | | |
|   Yes (%) | 12.5 | 16.2 | 5.3 |
|   Full-time | 56.7 | 60.3 | 35.0 |
| Top 3 diagnoses | N = 1067 | N = 715 | N = 352 |
|   1. Adjustment disorder (*ICD-9* 309–309.9) | 314 (29.4%) | 227 (31.7%) | 87 (24.7%) |
|   2. Diabetes (*ICD-9* 250–250.9) | 157 (14.7%) | 108 (15.1%) | 49 (13.9%) |
|   3. Spinal stenosis/lumbago, and similar (*ICD-9* 724–724.9) | 125 (11.7%) | 73 (10.2%) | 52 (14.8%) |
| Top 3 concerns/reason for referral | N = 1027 | N = 705 | N = 322 |
|   1. Overall wellness | 324 (31.5%) | 196 (27.8%) | 128 (39.8%) |
|   2. Diabetes | 130 (12.7%) | 92 (13.0%) | 38 (11.8%) |
|   3. Weight | 111 (10.8%) | 86 (12.2%) | 25 (7.8%) |
| Top 3 referral sources | N = 915 | N = 585 | N = 330 |
|   1. Primary care/PCP | 457 (49.9%) | 288 (49.2%) | 169 (51.2%) |
|   2. Polytrauma/PNS | 208 (22.7%) | 135 (23.1%) | 73 (22.1%) |
|   3. PM&R | 111 (12.1%) | 81 (13.8%) | 30 (9.1%) |

*Abbreviations:* PCP, primary care provider; PMR, physical medicine and rehabilitation; PNS, polytrauma network sites.

and 3); polytrauma and other VA clinicians and support personnel (times 1, 2, and 3); veterans enrolled in PIMI (times 2 and 3); and caregivers/partners of the veterans enrolled in PIMI (times 2 and 3). Focus group participants were drawn from a convenience sample of volunteers. Focus group sessions focused on the facilitators and barriers of implementing the PIMI pilot. Raw data from a total of 34 focus group sessions were audio-recorded and analyzed for key themes and subthemes.

### Personal Health Inventory

This instrument, developed by the OPCC&CT, offers a structured framework for exploring information, from the veterans' perspective, about their physical and mental health currently and in a "desired" state. Data for the PIMI pilot were collected using the September 18, 2012 version of the Personal Health Inventory (PHI). The first section of the PHI asks very broad questions about: (1) What really matters to you in your life? (2) What brings you a sense of joy and happiness? (3) What brings you a sense of sadness or sorrow? (4) What is your vision of your best possible health? The next section uses requires responses in 3 general areas using a visual analog scale from 1 (poorest) to 10 (best): (1) Physical Scale; (2) Mental/Emotional Scale; and (3) Life Scale. Ratings from the current state and desired state ("Where would you like to be"?) are recorded. Domains of interest include: Working the Body; Rest and Sleep or "Recharge"; Food and Drink; Personal Development; Family, Friends, and Coworkers; Spirit and Soul; Surroundings; Power of the Mind; Medical Prevention; and Medical Care Intervention.

At the end of the PHI, 3 additional open-ended questions ask the veteran to reflect on (1) what stands out about where you currently are and where you'd like to be? (2) If noting changes in your health and well-being choices, what do you think your health will look like 5 years from now? What might the worst case be? and (3) If you make changes in your health habits, what is your likely health 5 years from now? What might the best-case scenario be?

### Three-Month Follow-up

The PHI was readministered at 3 months following the initiation of the health coaching as a "temperature check" to gauge progress toward personal goal achievement. Scores from baseline to 3 months were analyzed using paired $t$ tests. Some health coaches continued to document their clients every 3 months, if the veterans remained in health coaching longer than 3 months. However, the number of cases that exceeded one 3-month follow-up was too small to provide meaningful longitudinal analysis.

### Observational Studies

Two observational studies were conducted at the request of specific PIMI sites to determine the effect of health coaching on health factors that were targeted through these interventions. Weight and hemoglobin A1C data from the veteran's medical record were compared at time points before and after health coaching was initiated.

### RESULTS
#### Qualitative Evaluation: Themes

##### Clinicians: health coaching reduces patient load burden
A theme that emerged over all time points with clinicians is that PIMI health coaching reduced the clinician's Patient Load Burden. Clinicians appreciated having "someone who can check up on the veteran," felt assured they could refer the veteran to "someone who cares" about their health, and noted that "Health Coaches can take the time we don't have" to provide necessary health counseling.

As Health Coaches reduce clinician psychological strain, they may also improve clinician self-efficacy. A new primary care physician stated that the positive changes brought by Health Coaching efforts remind him "of why I became a primary care doc [tor]." PIMI enabled him to feel as if he is positively impacting his patient's lives.

### Veterans: health coaching works

What makes the program worthy in the eyes of clinicians and veterans alike is that it works. Veterans and their caregivers said that health coaching has led to the following health improvements: weight loss, smoking cessation, improved relaxation techniques, overall mood improvement, an improved ability to sleep through the night, the ability to minimize focus on pain, an improvement in the ability to handle stress, and more positive family relationships.

Overall improvements provided some veterans with hope for the future for the first time in years. "They should call them life-coaches, not health coaches. It's my life that has been changed, not just my health." This hopefulness was directly related to the sense that veterans were in control of their own future and that they are developing the tools to successfully navigate that future. "Give us the tools. We'll take advantage of them." A guarded sense of optimism was evident.

### Veterans: improved self-efficacy

Veterans felt that health coaching enabled them to have more control over their health care and gave them a central voice in determining the health issues that most important to them. The PIMI health coaching program represented an opportunity for motivated veterans to take an active hand in shaping their medical care experience. Said one veteran, "I finally have a voice in my health care as [the] result [of health coaching]. I like that. A lot." Others said that "it makes me feel like I have some control" and "I'm doing this for me." Setting personal goals and achieving them left other veterans with a sense of pride. "I learned how to do things I didn't know I could do. It's unbelievable." Participation in the health coaching program appeared to remind veterans of the core strengths that enabled them to endure military training and military missions. One veteran said, "If you're made responsible to do it yourself, then you do."

### Veterans: shifting from an illness narrative to one of health

Part of the success of PIMI Health Coaching among veterans is how it restructures the illness narrative to one of health. Veterans move from a narrative where they are passive patients being treated for disease and injury ("Here, take this. You don't have to do anything.") toward one in which they are people who have the internal strength to accomplish any goal. "[The Health Coach] was the first one who told me not to accept my limitations, keep pushing." Veterans made statements like "It has helped me in actualizing goals," and "My pain is behind me. I can focus on my future now," or "It all starts with our minds." Phrases indicate an internalization (and implicit acceptance) of Health Coaching messaging.

### Veterans: continuity of care

Health Coaches support continuity of care within and outside VA. They serve veterans as patient advocates, informal mental health counselors, and rehabilitation consultants. They worked with veterans weekly to ensure they stayed on task with health goals. They also connected veterans to other VA and community resources. Said one veteran, "You can talk to [Health Coach] about anything, anytime" and "she knows what I need at the VA and gets it for me." Health coaching went well beyond the traditional boundaries of the hospital or clinic, and veterans and clinicians alike saw great value in this approach to care.

### Veterans: improved family relationships

Veterans discussed how Health Coaching improved their family relationships. Several veterans spoke of strained or nonexistent relationships resulting from their mental health issues. One veteran commented tongue-in-cheek that she "wanted to kill my daughters," but after several health coaching sessions focused on anger management and relaxation techniques, she finds that she "can handle them now." A male veteran explained that his "wife says I'm more present now." Asked to clarify, he said "I'm not just going through the motions. I'm present." Health coaching mindfulness techniques have helped him learn to root himself "in the moment," paying attention to others and his reaction to them. "It helped me with my family. I didn't really know how to deal with them. In this program, I found it. It helps me relax. ... I really enjoy being around my family now."

### Caregivers: reduction in caregiver burden

The authors did not speak with many caregivers of veterans during the evaluation of PIMI, but those they did speak to provide insight into the success of program. Caregivers told the authors in various ways that the Health Coach represented an additional caregiver, someone who provided additional caregiving support. One caregiver described the Health Coach as "a Godsend." Psychological strain resulting from being the primary caregiver has been well documented in the literature on caregiving and was no different for these caregivers. Health Coaches appear to lessen that strain for caregivers. They did this by providing caregiver support in the form of health education and a sympathetic ear. Said one caregiver, "I don't feel like I'm doing this alone." Another commented that the Health Coach "threw me a lifeline."

Health Coaches also reduced the caregivers need to navigate the VA system alone. The Caregiver could contact the Health Coach about treatment concerns possible medical needs and the Health Coach would then do the legwork of securing those services for the veteran. The Caregiver estimated her time burden was reduced by 10 hours a week or more.

**Patient health inventory: baseline Table 2** gives the initial scores PIMI clients assigned to the Physical Scale, Mental/Emotion Scale, Life Scale, and each of the

**Table 2**
**Baseline personal health inventory scores across domains (N = 547)**

| Variable | Current Score (Mean) | Desired Score (Mean) |
|---|---|---|
| Physical scale | 4.38 (SD = 2.04) | NA |
| Mental/emotional scale | 5.04 (SD = 2.39) | NA |
| Life scale | 5.26 (SD = 2.38) | NA |
| Working the body | 4.30 (SD = 2.11) | 8.43 (SD = 1.55) |
| Recharge | 4.70 (SD = 2.46) | 8.56 (SD = 1.54) |
| Food and drink | 5.31 (SD = 2.16) | 8.63 (SD = 1.36) |
| Personal development | 5.51 (SD = 2.39) | 8.56 (SD = 1.60) |
| Family, friends, and coworkers | 6.11 (SD = 2.76) | 8.51 (SD = 1.72) |
| Spirit and soul | 6.22 (SD = 3.18) | 8.65 (SD = 1.72) |
| Surroundings | 6.70 (SD = 2.42) | 8.86 (SD = 1.27) |
| Power of the mind | 5.65 (SD = 2.60) | 8.66 (SD = 1.39) |
| Professional care, prevention | 7.63 (SD = 2.13) | 9.32 (SD = 4.26) |
| Professional care, intervention | 7.69 (SD = 2.29) | 9.03 (SD = 1.30) |

Abbreviation: NA, not applicable.

**Table 3**
**Baseline to 3-mo changes in domain scores (N = 267)**

| Variable | Baseline Score Mean (S.D.) | Desired Score Mean (S.D.) | Follow-Up Score Mean (S.D.)* |
|---|---|---|---|
| Physical scale | 4.4 (2.0) | NA | 6.4 (1.9)* |
| Mental/emotional scale | 5.1 (2.2) | NA | 6.9 (1.9)* |
| Life scale | 5.3 (2.5) | NA | 7.1 (1.8)* |
| Working the body | 4.4 (2.1) | 8.5 (1.4) | 6.2 (2.0)* |
| Recharge | 4.8 (2.5) | 8.6 (1.4) | 6.1 (2.3)* |
| Food and drink | 5.5 (2.1) | 8.7 (1.4) | 6.9 (1.9)* |
| Personal development | 6.0 (2.4) | 8.6 (1.4) | 7.7 (1.9)* |
| Family, friends, and coworkers | 6.4 (2.8) | 8.6 (1.7) | 7.6 (2.1)* |
| Spirit and soul | 6.7 (2.5) | 8.9 (1.5) | 7.8 (2.0)* |
| Surroundings | 6.9 (2.5) | 9.0 (1.2) | 8.0 (2.1)* |
| Power of the mind | 5.9 (2.6) | 8.8 (1.3) | 7.4 (2.0)* |
| Professional care, prevention | 7.8 (2.1) | 9.5 (6.0) | 8.8 (1.6)* |
| Professional care, intervention | 7.9 (2.0) | 9.2 (1.2) | 8.7 (1.5)* |

* Indicates statistically significant positive gain in scores.

12 subdomains when veterans begin to work with the Health Coaches. These numbers represent the mean score of the 547 PIMI participants who completed the PHI questionnaire at baseline. The scores range from 1 (worst) to 10 (best). In general, the initial scores are in the 4 to 6 range. Participants have the lowest rating on the Physical Scale (mean = 4.38) and the highest rating on the Life Scale (5.26). Of the subdomains, Working the Body (which includes movement and physical activities like walking, dancing, gardening, sports, lifting weights, yoga, cycling, swimming, and working out in a gym) received the lowest score (mean = 4.30). Another relatively low mean score is in getting enough rest and sleep and participating in activities that help to make one feel recharged (mean = 4.70). Prevention and Intervention have the highest scores at 7.63 and 7.69, respectively. Not surprising, the participants' desired scores in all domains are in the 8s and 9s (see **Table 2**).

**Personal health inventory: 3-month follow-up** To gain a "temperature check" on the PIMI participants, Health Coaches collected data on the quantitative scores of the physical, mental/emotional, and life scales, as well as the wellness domains at the 3-month mark. **Table 3** shows the differences between baseline and follow-up scores for 267 individuals where data are available. Using paired $t$ tests, statistically significant ($P<.05$) changes are evident for all variables and all show a positive gain in scores. These results indicate that health coaching has a positive impact on patient-centered outcomes (see **Table 3**).

**Table 4**
**Post–polytrauma Integrative Medicine Initiative HA1c and weight results**

| Health Outcomes | No. of Patients | After 3 mo in PIMI | | |
|---|---|---|---|---|
| | | Mean Change | Range | Statistical Significance |
| HA1c | 41 | −0.5171 | −2.2 to +0.9 | P<.0001 |
| Weight | 75 | −3.56 kg | −99.3 to +14.3 | P<.0001 |

Table 5
Pre–polytrauma Integrative Medicine Initiative and post–polytrauma Integrative Medicine Initiative HA1c and weight results

| Health Outcomes | No. of Patients | Pre-PIMI | | After 3 mo in PIMI | |
|---|---|---|---|---|---|
| | | Mean Change | Range | Mean Change | Range |
| HA1c | 22 | +0.56 | −50 to +1.7 | −0.48 | −1.9 to +0.9 |
| Weight | 48 | +2 kg | −10 to + 28.4 | −3.59 kg | −99.3 to +14.3 |

**Observational studies** Ad hoc analyses were provided by the evaluation team as requested from the pilot sites. Health Coaches and referral sources were eager to discover whether the health coaching process affected specific patient health outcomes. In one of the analyses, Health Coaches extracted health factor data to examine differences on HA1c (blood sugar) and weight between the time when health coaching was initiated and at 3 months into the process (**Table 4**).

A statistically significant decrease in both weight and hemoglobin A1C was achieved at 3 months after health coaching was initiated.

In the second analysis, the comparison was conducted for comparable time periods before and after health coaching was initiated (**Table 5**).

Patients did better on both their HA1c and weight during the health coaching period than in a comparable time before they started receiving health coaching interventions. In the pre-PIMI, the patients had an average gain of 0.56 in HA1c and 2kg. After working with the Health Coach, patients dropped an average of 0.48 in HA1c and lost 7.91 pounds. Although the number of veterans included in this analysis is small, the differences in mean change scores are statistically significant.

## SUMMARY

The PIMI pilot met its indicators of implementation success with the program evaluation showing uniformly high satisfaction of veterans with the health coaching services received, a high level of interest in availability of these services by providers, and fully successful integration of the PIMI services into the medical teams where health coaching is regularly practiced. In addition, an analysis of the health coaching outcomes yielded statistically significant positive changes in participants over domains of life satisfaction and well-being. Two further observational inquiries demonstrated significant improvements in health outcomes for the patients enrolled in PIMI, including reductions in both weight and blood sugar levels. The current observational studies of health coaching are some of the largest in the literature and have the additional advantage of using health coaches with standardized training and clinical practices.

## LOOKING FORWARD

By 2018, approximately 1750 VHA clinicians will have completed Whole Health coaching training. Findings from a survey conducted with participants in these trainings suggest positive changes in clinical skills with the addition of patient-centered perspective in their practice as well as organizational changes demonstrating a more engaged and active workforce.[12] In addition, the VHA Whole Health Coaching course is an approved transitional course, allowing participants to sit for the national certification examination through the International Consortium for Health and Well-Being coaches.

Recent congressional legislation, the Comprehensive Addiction and Recovery Act of 2016, requires that VHA rapidly increase the education, delivery, and research of

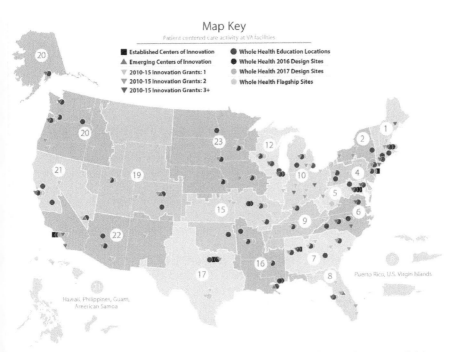

**Fig. 2.** Flagship sites including of the Whole Health model of care. (*From* Available at: https://www.va.gov/PATIENTCENTEREDCARE/features/Expanding_the_VA_Whole_Health_System.asp. Accessed September 24, 2018; with permission.)

Whole Health and CIH approaches targeting veterans with chronic pain, opioid use disorder, and chronic mental health disorders. In line with this commitment, VHA funded 18 flagship sites, including 2 polytrauma centers, to fully deploy the Whole Health model of care (**Fig. 2**). This large-scale endeavor will provide an opportunity to serve thousands of veterans through a whole health approach, evaluate outcomes related to patient engagement and quality of life, estimate costs of such a system, and assess utilization and cost avoidance associated with full deployment.

## REFERENCES

1. Institute of Medicine. Integrative medicine and the health of the public: a summary of the February 2009 summit. Washington (DC): The National Academies Press; 2009. Available at: https://doi.org/10.17226/12668. Accessed April 2, 2018.
2. Academic Consortium of Integrative Medicine and Health. Available at: https://www.imconsortium.org/about/about-us.cfm. Accessed April 2, 2018.
3. National Center for Complementary and Integrative Health, 2016 Strategic Plan. Available at: https://nccih.nih.gov/sites/nccam.nih.gov/files/NCCIH_2016_Strategic_Plan.pdf. Accessed April 2, 2018.
4. VA Patient Centered Care. Available at: https://www.va.gov/patientcenteredcare/. Accessed April 2, 2018.
5. Clarke TC, Black LI, Stussman BJ, et al. Trends in the use of complementary health approaches among adults: United States, 2002–2012. National health statistics reports; no 79. Hyattsville (MD): National Center for Health Statistics; 2015.

6. Healthcare Analysis & Information Group (HAIG). A field unit of the office of strategic planning & analysis within the office of the ADUSH for policy and planning. Available at: http://scienceblogs.com/insolence/files/2016/07/FY2015_VHA_CIH_signedReport.pdf. Accessed March 1, 2017.

7. VHA Directive 1137. Provision of complementary and integrative health. Available at: https://www.va.gov/vhapublications/ViewPublication.asp?pub_ID=5401. Accessed April 2, 2018.

8. Field T. Yoga clinical research review. Complement Ther Clin Pract 2011;17(1):1–8.

9. Marchand WR. Mindfulness-based stress reduction, mindfulness-based cognitive therapy, and Zen meditation for depression, anxiety, pain, and psychological distress. J Psychiatr Pract 2012;18(4):233–52.

10. Sforzo GA, Kaye MP, Todorova I, et al. Compendium of the health and wellness coaching literature. Am J Lifestyle Med 2017;20(10):1–12. Available at: http://journals.sagepub.com/doi/full/10.1177/1559827617708562. Accessed March 27, 2018.

11. Jordan M, Wolever RQ, Lawson K, et al. National training and education standards for health and wellness coaching: the path to national certification. Glob Adv Health Med 2015;4:46–56.

12. Collins DA, Thompson K, Arwood KA, et al. Integration of health coaching concepts and skills into clinical practice among VHA providers: a qualitative study. Glob Adv Health Med 2018;(7):1–8.

# Reintegrating Veterans with Polytrauma into the Community and Workplace

Paul Wehman, PhD[a],*, Lauren Avellone, PhD, BCBA[b],
Frederick Pecharka, MA, CRC, LPC-S[c], Katti Sorboro, MEd, CRC, PHR[d],
Joseph B. Webster, MD[e], Cynthia Young, MS, CRC[f],
Sharon Barton, MS, CRC, CRP[f], William A. Robbins, MD[g],
Samuel T. Clanton, MD, PhD[h]

## KEYWORDS

- Polytrauma • Employment • Vocational rehabilitation • Community integration

## KEY POINTS

- An intertwined model of medical and vocational support is critical to effective community reintegration for polytrauma patients.
- Transition to paid work for polytrauma patients should be rapid and facilitated by evidenced-based employment models.
- Interdisciplinary polytrauma teams should use advancements in technology to promote independence on-the-job and in the community.

Disclosure Statement: The authors have nothing to disclose.
[a] Division of Rehabilitation Research, Virginia Commonwealth University School of Medicine, 1314 West Main Street, PO Box 842011, Richmond, VA 23284, USA; [b] Rehabilitation Research and Training Center, Virginia Commonwealth University, 1314 West Main Street, PO Box 842011, Richmond, VA 23284, USA; [c] Louis Stokes Cleveland VA Medical Center, 1620 East 105th Street, Cleveland, OH 44106, USA; [d] Louis Stokes Cleveland VA Medical Center, 10701 East Boulevard, Cleveland, OH 44106, USA; [e] Department of Physical Medicine and Rehabilitation, School of Medicine at Virginia Commonwealth University, Hunter Holmes McGuire VA Medical Center, 1201 Broad Rock Boulevard, Richmond, VA 23249, USA; [f] Service Member Transitional Advanced Rehabilitation (STAR) Program, Hunter Holmes McGuire VA Medical Center, 1201 Broad Rock Boulevard, Building 514, Richmond, VA 23249, USA; [g] Polytrauma Transitional Rehabilitation Program (PTRP), Servicemember Transitional Advanced Rehabilitation (STAR) Program, Hunter Holmes McGuire VA Medical Center, 1201 Broad Rock Boulevard, Building 514, Richmond, VA 23249, USA; [h] Traumatic Brain Injury/Polytrauma Fellow, Hunter Holmes McGuire VA Medical Center, Virginia Commonwealth University, 1223 East Marshall Street, PO Box 980677, Richmond, VA 23284-0667, USA
* Corresponding author.
E-mail address: pwehman@vcu.org

Over the past 2 decades, the profile of patients entering polytrauma rehabilitation programs has changed. Due to medical advancements in trauma care, along with the changing methods of warfare stemming from a greater reliance on technology, survival rates have thankfully increased, but so has the number of service members returning with multifaceted injuries.[1,2] Veterans and service members face a variety of challenges while readjusting to community life after sustaining a polytrauma injury. Individualized and comprehensive treatment is necessary as each patient's symptoms will differ. Although traumatic brain injury (TBI) and posttraumatic stress disorder are commonly noted concerns linked to deployment, veterans and service members can also develop other comorbid postdeployment conditions including depression, anxiety, substance abuse, chronic pain, and sleep disorders.[1,3] Veterans also enter polytrauma rehabilitation programs following non–combat-related injuries sustained from car accidents or falls.[2]

Employment offers a number of quality-of-life benefits, including greater financial freedom, access to social circles, a sense of contribution to the community, and enhanced self-esteem. Additionally, veterans with TBI who achieve stable work have greater cognitive and motor independence and fewer self-report symptoms of anxiety, posttraumatic stress disorder, depression, and neurobehavioral symptoms than those reporting unstable work.[4] Successful return to work requires the collaborative efforts of numerous stakeholders, including the patient, family, health care providers, and vocational rehabilitation professionals. We address key themes that aid reentry to competitive employment for veterans and service members. Effective employment models and clinical strategies for implementation are presented. Two exemplar polytrauma programs in Veterans Affairs (VA) Hospitals located in Cleveland, Ohio, and Richmond, Virginia, are discussed. Finally, the integral role of technology in community reintegration is reviewed.

## VETERAN/SERVICE MEMBER EMPLOYMENT RATES

Current reports regarding unemployment rates among the veterans and service member population indicate continued cause for concern. In 2017, the US Bureau of Labor Statistics reported that approximately 4.9 million veterans (24%) had a documented service-related disability.[5] Of these individuals, 4.3% remained unemployed.[5] Higher rates of unemployment are also prevalent among specific subpopulations, affected by factors such as age and type of injury. For example, more than one-half of all unemployed veterans (59%) were age 25 to 54.[5] In a sample of 293 veterans and service members with TBI, very few (20.5%) were employed at a 1 year follow-up after injury and return to work was lengthy with a reported average of 6.5 months.[6] Ongoing vocational support services are clearly needed to meet the complex individualized needs of veteran populations.

## THEMES FOR SUCCESS

The themes presented are designed around the following question: What does it take for a patient to seamlessly transition back into the community following an injury? Each theme should be incorporated into the rehabilitation process to achieve successful employment outcomes and bolster community reintegration efforts.

### Listen to the Patient and Family

To assist in the most beneficial way, the team must have a deep understanding of the patient's personal goals surrounding employment and community life. A substantial discussion regarding the patient's ideas, expectations, and concerns for the future will help the team to devise the best plan of action and arrange the best support needed to achieve reintegration goals.

### Immediate Focus on Part-Time, Paid Work

Zeroing in on paid employment in integrated work environments as soon as possible is essential because it creates a positive ripple effect in other areas of life. During the reintegration process, participation in work allows the individual an opportunity to gain physical, emotional, and social competence.

### Integrated Medical and Vocational Rehabilitation Model

Using an intertwined approach that draws on the important strengths of both the physician and vocational rehabilitation specialist allows the patient to receive care that addresses symptom overlap across settings. Open dialogue and constant communication between the medical and vocational team is vital.

### Proactively Identify Threats to Success

One of the major advantages of a comprehensive team is the critical ability to detect deleterious factors that are likely to thwart success. It is important for teams to assess potential challenges (eg, mental health issues, a lack of motivation, or unrealistic goals) to obtain necessary intervention immediately.

## TRANSITION TO THE COMMUNITY AND HOME

Transitioning from polytrauma rehabilitation back into community and home life should be as seamless as possible. Carefully designing clear and measurable discharge goals for patients regarding both short- and long-term plans can enhance smooth transitioning. Tapping into long-distance technology, such as Telehealth, Zoom, and various mobile apps can help the individual to maintain access to supports during transfer of care. The fading of daily and weekly consults as the patient maintains targeted discharge goals in the community is necessary to promote autonomy and independence. Finally, connecting the patient with trained professionals who implement evidence-based models for securing employment can greatly enhance inclusion and reintegration into the community.

## EVIDENCED-BASED EMPLOYMENT MODELS

To achieve positive employment outcomes, a polytrauma team must help the patient to obtain employment and then proceed with putting any necessary supports in place to help the patient thrive. A current review of the literature supports the efficacy of the following employment models for individuals with disabilities.

### Supported Employment

Supported employment is a set of services aligned with personalized needs used to assist an individual with intensive disabilities obtain competitive employment. The supported employment approach maintains that all willing individuals are able to work, regardless of the severity of a disability. The implementation of supported employment involves a series of steps that include an employment specialist first learning about a job seeker before assisting them with job placement, on-the-job training, and job retention services.[7] There is a strong evidence base for supported employment, because it is associated with positive employment outcomes for a variety of disabilities including TBI,[8] psychiatric disabilities,[9] spinal cord injury,[10] autism,[7] and intellectual disability.[11]

## Customized Employment

Customized employment is an extension of supported employment that also facilitates competitive, integrated employment for individuals with the most significant disabilities.[12] The CE approach emphasizes the establishment of a mutually beneficial relationship between the job seeker and the business. To accomplish this goal, an employment specialist undergoes a discovery process with the individual, which allows for vocational themes to be identified based around the job seeker's strengths, needs, and interests. A job is then developed within a business that meets the specific abilities of the job seeker while also meeting the needs of the business in a tangible way, such as increased profits or efficiency. Job training and ongoing support are provided as the client becomes independent.

## Individual Placement and Support Model

The individual placement and support program is uniquely designed to meet the needs of individuals with psychiatric disabilities.[9] It integrates employment supports and mental health treatment to provide a comprehensive model for obtaining and sustaining competitive employment. A rapid job search is conducted to transition individuals to employment quickly while explicit attention is paid to personal preferences regarding work. Benefits counseling is incorporated to help individuals navigate how to keep receipt of government income, such as Supplemental Security Income or Social Security Disability Insurance, while working. Finally, ongoing supports are put into place for long-term employment success.[9,13]

## Spinal Cord Injury–Vocational Integration Program

Similar to other models mentioned, the spinal cord injury–vocational integration program integrates specialized treatment for patients with spinal cord injury with supported employment services. The objective is competitive employment regardless of the severity of the disability and involves a rapid job search, benefits counseling, and ongoing support. The results of a multisite, randomized research study examining the effect of a spinal cord injury–vocational integration program for veterans versus a treatment as usual condition indicated that those in the spinal cord injury–vocational integration program group were 2.5 times more likely to be competitively employed at the 1-year follow-up.[10]

In summary, veterans and service members can achieve successful employment outcomes when provided with an interdisciplinary team that collaboratively addresses both medical and vocational needs. Polytrauma centers across the United States have designed comprehensive programs for this specific purpose. The Cleveland Veterans Administration Medical Center and the Hunter Holmes McGuire VA Medical Center provide a description of model programs. In the following section, the article moves away from the didactic presentation to describe examples of currently operating polytrauma sites that have successfully incorporated vocational support within each program.

## POLYTRAUMA VOCATIONAL PROGRAMS
### Polytrauma at the Cleveland Veterans Administration Medical Center

The Louis Stokes Cleveland Veteran Affairs Medical Center (LSCVAMC) is a Polytrauma Network Site located in Northeast Ohio. The facility provides long-term rehabilitation services after injury to service members who incurred more than 1 injury at the organ level. The Polytrauma Specialty Vocational Program at LSCVAMC was developed to address the following challenges commonly reported by polytrauma patients: job loss, difficulty maintaining employment, failing formal training or academic courses of study, dissatisfaction with career outlook given the current skill set, a lack of ability to move forward vocationally during transition, and difficulty deciding on a vocational career. Therefore, the program was developed with the intention to provide customized vocational rehabilitation counseling plans that meet the individual profile of each veteran served. This customized approach is achieved by integrating the vocational rehabilitation counselor (VRC) into the polytrauma interdisciplinary treatment team. The VRC serves as a sort of a conduit between the polytrauma team and the veteran by providing necessary supports to ensure the veteran completes vocational goals and overcomes unique barriers to employment experienced by veterans (**Table 1**).

## Polytrauma Veteran Profile

Individual characteristics (eg, injury type, motivation to work, age, and inclination toward military culture) contribute to the type and intensity of support a veteran will need to transition to employment, as well as influence the type of vocational or educational goal the veteran desires to achieve. Data collected from chart reviews conducted between 2015 and 2017 involving 165 veterans referred by polytrauma providers to polytrauma vocational services at LSCVAMC offers a general profile of veterans receiving employment services.[14]

- The VRC receives consults primarily with veterans who have a mild TBI (93%) with an average age of 30 years.[14] Physical injuries are present 75% of the time and combine for either posttraumatic stress disorder and/or a general anxiety diagnosis 73% of the time.[14] Veterans seen by the VRC are primarily Operation Enduring Freedom/Operation Iraqi Freedom/Operation New Dawn Veterans (98%).[14] Case coordination can occur with the Operation Enduring Freedom/Operation Iraqi Freedom/Operation New Dawn case management program team while vocational services are being used.
- Service-connected veterans make up 79% of all consults received at the LSCVAMC.[14] A service-connected compensation can have both positive and negative impacts on the vocational planning process. One negative aspect includes an impact on motivation to participate in the vocational rehabilitation process. Of the veterans with service-connected disabilities, 74% hold a disability rating of 50% or greater.[14] This injury severity means they receive a higher stable monthly income, which potentially impacts the urgency of veterans participating in the vocational rehabilitation process.

## CONSULTATIONS AND INTERDISCIPLINARY TREATMENT TEAMS

Staffing for the LSCVAMC is illustrated in **Fig. 1**. Consults are received from treating providers on the interdisciplinary team, but primarily received from the polytrauma coordinator, as well as the medical director of the Polytrauma Center. The full-time VRC typically receives 4 consults per month and manages a caseload averaging 45 veterans.[14] Owing to the high demand for consults and caseload size, there are 1.25 full-time equivalent counselors associated with the polytrauma team.[14] The interdisciplinary treatment team meets on a weekly basis to discuss clinical updates, difficult cases, or new patients with mild or severe TBI. The dynamics of the injury requires cross-clinical communication on a consistent and available basis to address the vast needs of this population. Team members are readily available to provide feedback, support, updates, and outreach as vocational problems arise or support is needed by the VRC.

**Table 1**
Polytrauma barriers to employment for veterans reported at the Louis Stokes Cleveland Veteran Affairs Medical Center

| Barrier | Description |
|---|---|
| Difficulty accepting help | Gaining help can be perceived by veterans as a weakness. The veteran may refuse assistance from the Veterans Center or only take short-term assistance despite needing more substantial support. |
| Unfamiliarity with making decisions alone | Veterans tend to be more accustomed to following orders from leadership. Career planning can be difficult when making major decisions are left solely to the individual. |
| Lack of meaning and/or purpose in life | There is a sense of mission, fulfillment, and purpose while in the service. When veterans transition out of the military service, especially if forced to medically retire, there can be a void they look to fill. |
| Entitlement mentality | Some veterans may have a sense of power or right owed to them based on participation in the military. This can cause problems with communication and problem resolution on the job or during the job-seeking process. |
| Limited civilian work history | If veterans entered the military at the age of 18, time in civilian employment is usually limited. Generally, human resource professionals do not equate years of military service to that of civilian employment, so many veterans face difficulties transitioning to employment and competing against civilian peers. |
| Cultural fit | Veterans are frequently at a disadvantage with limited understanding of the cultural aspects of the civilian workforce, such as upward mobility, typical chain of command, "open door policies," employee supports, philanthropy efforts, and colleague relations. |
| Unrealistic salary expectations | Veterans who have years of military service with no formal education and/or who held military positions that do not exist readily in the civilian labor market can demonstrate unrealistic salary expectations because of their military pay. This factor can cause confusion, frustration, and a lack of motivation to work. |
| Lack of financial motivation | Stable service-connected compensation can lead to a lack of urgency or consistency in participating during the vocational counseling process, interfere with motivation to find work, and result in larger gaps in employment. |
| Adjustment issues | Issues faced by veterans can include acceptance of disabling conditions, stability with finances and housing, separation, loss, and reconnecting to the community. |
| Lack of knowledge regarding disability rights | Before entering the service veterans likely experienced few health barriers. Many veterans may not understand appropriate medication disclosure, how to access accommodations, and overall employee rights related to disabilities on the job. |

## POLYTRAUMA VETERAN STRATEGIES/PROGRAM PRINCIPALS

The primary strategies used within the Polytrauma vocational program align with recommendations made by BrainLine (Brainline.org). The 2 major strategies applied by the VRC to engage this veteran population are person-centered planning and resource

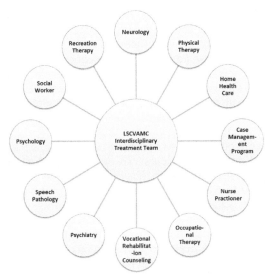

**Fig. 1.** Polytrauma interdisciplinary treatment team members at Louis Stokes Cleveland Veteran Affairs Medical Center (LSCVAMC).

facilitation. Person-centered planning is the foundation of Cleveland's polytrauma vocational program. Person-centered planning is the guiding principal during the entire process, meeting the veterans' needs vocationally without boundaries on the type of support that can be accessed. Supports accessed are customized to the individual person with respect to expectations, available resources, knowledge, skills, needs, abilities, and interests. Consults are received for veterans at different phases in the vocational planning process. The frequency and intensity of vocational preparation changes from veteran to veteran depending on many factors, such as stability with health and housing, support system, finances, benefits available, postmilitary transition, and motivation. The planning process is not static; it is a continuum type of service, changing as milestones are achieved, problems arise, or lifestyles change. Focus is maintained on meeting the veterans where they are and where they want to be, without limitation of available vocational services at the network site.

## DESCRIPTION OF SERVICES

The major driver in the type of services requested are due to the age of the population and benefits accessible. To reiterate, the average age of veterans consulted to the VRC is 30-year-old with a career mindset of potentially having decades left in the workforce.[14] The benefits accessible range from service-connected compensation providing a stable income, robust GI Bills, and potential academic funding with Vocational Rehabilitation and Employment. Many of the veterans accessing vocational support have held limited civilian opportunities in the workforce and have an inadequate understanding of careers outside of military-related occupations. Veterans tend to gravitate toward military-style professions despite the misfit with both physical and mental health.

The main service used but often not directly requested is vocational guidance and counseling. Assistance is frequently needed for career counseling and long-term planning owing to a lack of understanding about factors such as alternate military careers, labor market statistics, and action steps for moving forward with vocational planning. This type of vocational guidance and counseling has been the primary support needed for 37% of all consultations received.[14] Veterans who need assistance with career exploration and planning choose from customized support to fit comfort level, current phase in planning, available resources, and know-how in researching, The assistance available from the VRC often results in career counseling, referrals, informational interviewing, shadowing experiences, advocacy with associated programs, career assessments, and education on various topics pertinent to increasing vocational awareness of both internal and external factors.

The next most sought out support vocationally by Cleveland's Polytrauma Network Site is academic assistance, which occurs 35% of the time as being a primary need.[14] These consultations cover veterans who require assistance with transitioning to institutions, academic retention, and postacademic achievement. Academic support is often a continuum from guidance and counseling where the long-term plan identified turns into action steps. Academic supports range from career counseling, advocacy, coordination of on-campus supports, accessing mentors, technology training, addressing learning strategies, work experiences such as practicums or internships, communication skills, and general problem resolution.

There are many national and local resources targeted at helping wounded warriors secure employment. Polytrauma VRC harnesses local and national support as it aligns with the veteran's career field and long-term plan, leading to more advocacy on the veteran's behalf. This type of additional support can include resume development, military skill translation, interviewing skills, and education with job seeking for civilian employment. When gaps in employment occur, nonpaid work experiences have been coordinated with employers to help update the veteran's skills in meeting marketplace demand. Often these experiences are supported by agencies like Chapter 31 or Vocational Rehabilitation and Employment, who provide a stipend to the veteran (**Table 2**).

## POLYTRAUMA AT THE HUNTER HOLMES McGuire VA MEDICAL CENTER IN RICHMOND, VIRGINIA

In 2011, the Department of Veterans Affairs responded to a joint VA/Department of Defense Task Force's recommendation to address coordinated efforts on behalf of wounded warriors by launching the Service member Transitional Advanced Rehabilitation (STAR) program at the Hunter Holmes McGuire VA Medical Center in Richmond, Virginia. In January 2012, The STAR program was established as a pilot for injured service members and veterans who require comprehensive residential rehabilitation to successfully return to work and integrate into the community. After 1 year of achieving successful vocational and rehabilitation outcomes, the STAR Program was integrated into the VA Polytrauma System of Care. The STAR Program assists the service member with transitioning into various domains of community life (**Fig. 2**).

## DEMOGRAPHICS OF POLYTRAUMA PATIENTS

Since its inception, the STAR program has maintained high levels of success in terms of both patient satisfaction (93%) and program completion rates (93%).[15] The STAR program has served patients with varying severities of TBI as well as patients with other brain conditions such as stroke and anoxia. The program has also been able to successfully treat patients with a host of other neurologic, orthopedic, and mental health conditions. The population has been mostly male (82%), active duty service members (79%) from all branches of the military, with an average of 30 years of

**Table 2**
**Community supports and external stakeholders collaborating with the polytrauma specialty vocational program at the Louis Stokes Cleveland Veteran Affairs Medical Center**

| Community Support | Collaborating Capacity |
|---|---|
| Office of Workforce Development, Disabled Veterans Outreach Program (DVOP) | The primary objective of the DVOP is to decrease the rate of unemployment and underemployment among Ohio veterans. The program assists with resume development, resource identification, mock interviewing, employer education, veteran job fairs, among other areas. |
| Employment Collaborative of Cuyahoga County (ECCC) | This is a collaborative of 35 dedicated state, federal, private, and nonprofit entities who share resources and job leads, expanding job opportunities for veterans in the hidden labor market; holds 4 job or interview fairs a year for direct hire of attendees; and educates employers on inclusion of people with disabilities in the workforce, including veterans. |
| Northeast Ohio Military Employment Collaborative (NEOMEC) | The goal of this initiative is to assist veterans in the area with access to mentors and networking. Cleveland's VRC has begun working with the president on accessing mentors for polytrauma veterans along with facilitating employment workshops targeting transitional needs of veterans. |
| Cleveland's Society of Human Resource Managers (CSHRM) | CSHRM is a local chapter, affiliated with the international organization SHRM whose members are composed of human resource professionals. Cleveland's VRC is a member of this group and is on their Diversity & Inclusion committee. This collaboration enables interaction with a wide range of human resources professionals to build relationships with businesses. |
| Opportunities for Ohioans with Disabilities (OOD) | The OOD is a state vocational rehabilitation program. Veterans benefit from the OOD with access to costly services such as tools, interview clothing, work site assessments, retraining, and/or job coaching. |
| Vocational Rehabilitation & Employment (VR&E) or Chapter 31 | VR&E counselors work with eligible veterans in identifying career goals. Cleveland's Polytrauma VRC works closely with the veteran and VR&E counselor during this process to advocate, serve as a liaison with the medical center, conduct case management, complete documentation, and guide veterans on decision making. |
| Kent State University's Project Career Grant | This research project assists undergraduate 2 and 4-year college students who have a traumatic brain injury. The grant harnesses the use of technology and personal assistance to decrease academic deficits related to their disability. |

(*continued on next page*)

| Table 2 *(continued)* | |
|---|---|
| **Community Support** | **Collaborating Capacity** |
| Veterans Education Assistance Program (VEAP) | The VEAP is part of a larger national initiative that is, held locally at Cuyahoga Community College and targets first time veteran college students. The free program provides preparatory coursework, knowledge of on-campus supports, career counseling, and development of academic skills. Veterans going to any college can access this program. |

age.[16] The clinical volume served by the program averages 25 participants per year.[16] The program length of stay is based on the individual service member's treatment and employment goals with an average length of stay of 95 days or less.[16] STAR Program participants are referred by a variety of sources with the majority of referrals from military bases and VA medical facilities.

## VOCATIONAL REHABILITATION

The STAR Program uses an interdisciplinary team approach to provide high-quality medical care, rehabilitation services, and vocational rehabilitation services. A unique component of the STAR Program is the residential setting (patients are living at the program), which provides the opportunity for intensive, daily vocational and rehabilitation services. The patient's employment and community reintegration goals guide the direction of the patient's rehabilitation, and up to 40% of the patient's clinical schedule can include one-on-one therapy sessions with VRCs or work-related activities in the community.[15] VRCs are essential members of the core interdisciplinary team and the patient's vocational rehabilitation goals are directly integrated within the patient's medical and rehabilitation goals. VRCs working with the STAR Program focus on the following core areas: evaluation and job development, community-based support, and an education transition program.

### Evaluation and Job Development

Vocational rehabilitation services include a comprehensive intake, vocational evaluation, and assessment process to identify an employment plan that matches the skills,

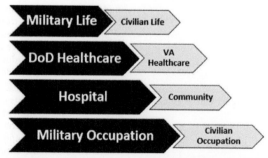

**Fig. 2.** The Service Member Transitional Advanced Rehabilitation (STAR) program facilitation of services. DoD, Department of Defense; VA, Veteran's Affairs.

abilities, aptitudes, interests, values, preferences, and personality traits of each service member. This process is followed by in-depth career exploration based on relevant labor market information and the development of up-to-date and accurate job search documentation, along with job search support, and an introduction to community, veteran, education, and employment resources.

### Community-Based Support

VRCs have established successful relationships with community-based employers and veterans organizations to provide veterans with a wide variety of vocational opportunities. STAR program service members also participate in workshops and trainings provided by employers and military veterans to facilitate transitioning to civilian employment.

### Education Transition Program

The STAR program created an educational transition and preparation component for participants who identify education and training as a necessary step to their vocational goals. The education program provides participants with preparation for college, including assisting with organizational skills, memory strategies, time management skills, and so on. The education transition services can also include arranging for the service member to sit in on a few class sessions at a local college to practice the strategies learned in a real college class environment.

Collaboration between the VRC and the STAR program team is key. The interdisciplinary team meets weekly to discuss patient goals and progress. **Table 3** provides a description of comprehensive polytrauma treatment services provided in the STAR program.

## MEASUREMENT AND EVALUATION

To monitor the individual success of patients, annual outcome measurement goals are developed by the STAR interdisciplinary team to assess the program. Preservice and postservice data are obtained by STAR Program therapists, and this information is added to the program database for analysis and reporting on a quarterly and annual basis. An informal survey conducted in fiscal 2016 of previous STAR patients indicated that of the previous participants that were contacted, most were still in active duty status, employed, or participating in an education program.[16]

In summary, the STAR program represents a novel model for the provision of vocational rehabilitation services within a comprehensive, residential rehabilitation setting for injured service members and veterans. As of September 30, 2017, 147 service members have participated in the STAR program.[16] Over time, the program has evolved to meet the changing needs of the populations being served. This evolution in primary population served includes a transition from combat-related injuries to non–combat-related injuries and illnesses. The program has also experienced a shift from injuries occurring overseas to more injuries occurring stateside. Despite this evolution, STAR has maintained high levels of success in terms of both patient satisfaction and program completion.[15]

## TECHNOLOGY OF POLYTRAUMA PATIENTS AND COMMUNITY REINTEGRATION

Using advanced technology can enhance vocational services provided to injured service members/veterans by meeting support needs on the job or helping to modify the vocational environment. Although there will always be a primary role for the experienced VRC, some aspects of existing vocational services inherently lend themselves

Table 3
Comprehensive polytrauma treatment services provided by the interdisciplinary team at Hunter Holmes McGuire VA Medical Center

| Service | Description |
|---|---|
| Therapeutic environment | Program participants reside in a homelike setting within the Polytrauma Transitional Rehabilitation Center. The floor plan includes individual living quarters, common living space, and facilities of daily living and recreation activities. |
| Medical care | Patients meet with a physician weekly and have access to emergency care or consultation when needed. Additionally, a nurse is available 24 h/d and 7 d/wk. The provision of medical care is comprehensive, covering general medical conditions in addition to disabling conditions. |
| Rehabilitation therapy | The individual needs of each patient are met via a multitude of available services including occupational therapy, speech therapy, exercise programs, and recreational therapy. Access to assistive technology or support for use of compensatory strategies is also provided. |
| Mental health | Psychologists, neuropsychologists, counselors, and psychiatrists perform various duties such as consultation, management of psychiatric medication, or neurologic testing. |
| Vocational rehabilitation | Certified vocational rehabilitation counselors meet weekly with patients to conduct services such as assessments, vocational exploration, vocational training, and job placement support. |
| Social work | Licensed clinical social workers meet weekly with patients to assist with plans for community reintegration. |
| Nurse case management | Case management is provided from date of admission through follow-up services to ensure sustained success with health and program goals. |

*Data from* Webster J, Kim J, Hawley C, et al. Development, implementation, and outcomes of a residential vocational rehabilitation program for injured service members and veterans. J Vocat Rehabil 2018;48(1):111–26.

to some degree of automation. For example, the development of common computer-based memory aids used in the general population (eg, phone apps that offer alerts or to-do list apps) can be specifically programmed and altered based on the needs of service members/veterans and the demands of the work setting. These applications can be used to automate the manual aspects of services currently performed by vocational counselors (eg, alerting the patient to ensure schedule adherence) to fade VRC support and foster independence on-the-job over time.

Technology can be used to help injured service members/veterans overcome both physical and cognitive barriers. Augmentative strategies for the physical functioning of injured veterans in the vocational environment include devices designed as cognitive and memory aids, for augmentative communication, and augmentation or functional replacement of limb movement. Patients with brain injuries may have intact or modestly impaired cognition, but still have sustained damage to the primary speech and language centers of the brain. Augmentative communication devices that use technological advancements of the manual communication board (common within existing Veterans Administration augmentative and alternative communication services), or more advanced devices using direct brain–computer interfaces, are possible strategies for improving the ability of patients to communicate and interact with their environment. Versions of these systems that are adapted for the work or educational environment may again integrate with the vocational context using schedule, location, and movement-based clues to establish the appropriate communication context to select among appropriate responses or to cue interactive behaviors that are appropriate for the situation in a controlled work environment.[17,18]

Injured veterans and service members with functional deficits related to physical impairments could benefit from engineering supports including advanced smart robotic orthoses and prostheses that have been developed to assist or replace nonfunctional limb movement in patients with spinal cord injury or brain injury. The concept of shared control, in which a functional device movement is produced using input from both the individual as well as a computer controller, could help to assist with vocational task completion. These devices could be placed in the context of work and specific work tasks and use a combination of environmental sensors (eg, computer vision to place user commands using personalized movement or advanced interfaces such as direct brain–computer interfaces into the context of the specific work-related task at hand).[19–21]

Taking advantage of the versatility of modern technology can help injured service members/veterans reintegrate into the community more efficiently and effectively. Often, devices already in the injured service members/veterans possession can be used, such as a personal cell phone or tablet to install immediate support on-the-job or in independent living settings. The use of commonplace devices for this purpose is also likely to provide comfort owing to familiarity and also alleviate concerns about stigma associated with using accommodations, because such devices are widely used by all members of a workforce for various purposes. As technology continues to rapidly advance, the benefits for injured service members/veterans are likely to continue to expand.

## SUMMARY

Employment is an important part of community reintegration for polytrauma patients and requires the knowledge and support of a well-defined interdisciplinary team. Collaborative communication between the patient, physician, other service providers and the VRC enables proper support to be put in place to achieve successful employment outcomes. A comprehensive team can work to effectively identify and eliminate barriers to employment, ensure the physical health and safety of the veteran on the job, install proper evidenced-based training or technological assistance to help the veteran thrive in employment, and assist with the continued development and refinement of long-term employment goals. Community reintegration and vocational success can be maximized when patients have access to a supportive and intertwined network of skilled professionals.

## REFERENCES

1. Phillips KM, Clark ME, Gironda RJ, et al. Pain and psychiatric comorbidities among two groups of Iraq-and Afghanistan-era veterans. J Rehabil Res Dev 2016;53:413–32.
2. Siddharthan K, Scott S, Bass E, et al. Rehabilitation outcomes for veterans with polytrauma treated at the Tampa VA. Rehabil Nurs 2008;33(5):221–5.
3. Pugh MJV, Finley EP, Copeland LA, et al. Complex comorbidity clusters in OEF/OIF veterans: the polytrauma clinical triad and beyond. Med Care 2014;52(2):172–81.

4. Dillahunt-Aspillaga C, Pugh M, Cotner B, et al. Employment stability in veterans and service members with traumatic brain injury: a Veteran's Administration traumatic brain injury model systems study. Arch Phys Med Rehabil 2018;99(2): S23–32.
5. Employment situation of veterans – 2017. U.S. Bureau of Labor Statistics Website. 2018. Available at: https://www.bls.gov/news.release/vet.nr0.htm. Accessed April 8, 2018.
6. Dillahunt-Aspillaga C, Nakase-Richardson R, Hart T, et al. Predictors of employment outcomes in veterans with traumatic brain injury: a VA traumatic brain injury model systems study. J Head Trauma Rehabil 2017;32(4):271–82.
7. Schall CM, Wehman P, Brooke V, et al. Employment interventions for individuals with ASD: the relative efficacy of supported employment with or without prior project search training. J Autism Dev Disord 2015;45(12):3990–4001.
8. Rumrill P, Wehman P, Cimera R, et al. Vocational rehabilitation services and outcomes for transition-age youth with traumatic brain injuries. J Head Trauma Rehabil 2016;31(4):288–95.
9. Modini M, Tan L, Brinchmann B, et al. Supported employment for people with severe mental illness: systematic review and meta-analysis of the international evidence. Br J Psychiatry 2016;209:14–22.
10. Ottomanelli L, Goetz LL, Suris A, et al. Effectiveness of supported employment for veterans with spinal cord injuries: results from a randomized multisite study. Arch Phys Med Rehabil 2012;93(5):740–7.
11. Wehman P, Chan F, Ditchman N, et al. Effect of supported employment on vocational rehabilitation outcomes of transition-age youth with intellectual and developmental disabilities: a case control study. Intellect Dev Disabil 2014;52(4): 296–310.
12. Wehman P, Brooke V, Brooke AM, et al. Employment for adults with autism spectrum disorders: a retrospective review of a customized employment approach. Res Dev Disabil 2016;53:61–72.
13. Drake RE, Bond GR. Introduction to the special issue on individual placement and support. Psychiatr Rehabil J 2014;37(2):76–8.
14. Sorboro K. Demographics of polytrauma specialty vocational program patients. 2017.
15. Webster J, Kim J, Hawley C, et al. Development, implementation, and outcomes of a residential vocational rehabilitation program for injured service members and Veterans. J Vocat Rehabil 2018;48(1):111–26.
16. Service Member Transitional Advanced Rehabilitation Program. FY17 annual outcomes report; 2017.
17. Beukelman DR, Fager S, Ball L, et al. AAC for adults with acquired neurological conditions: a review. Augment Altern Commun 2007;23(3):230–42.
18. Demmans Epp C, Djordjevic J, Wu S, et al. Towards providing just-in-time vocabulary support for assistive and augmentative communication. In: Proceedings of the 2012 ACM international conference on Intelligent User Interfaces; 2012. p. 33–6.
19. Ross RJ, Shi H, Vierhuff T, et al. Towards dialogue based shared control of navigating robots. In: International Conference on Spatial Cognition. Springer: Berlin (Heidelberg); 2004. p. 478–99.
20. Schirner G, Erdogmus D, Chowdhury K, et al. The future of human-in-the-loop cyber-physical systems. Computer (Long Beach Calif) 2013;46(1):36–45.
21. Collinger JL, Wodlinger B, Downey JE, et al. High-performance neuroprosthetic control by an individual with tetraplegia. Lancet 2012;381(9866):557–64.

# Adaptive Sports in the Rehabilitation of the Disabled Veterans

Check for updates

Kenneth K. Lee, MD[a,b,c,]*, Michael J. Uihlein, MD[d,e,f,g]

## KEYWORDS

• Adaptive sports • Disabled veterans • Sports medicine • Spinal cord injury

## KEY POINTS

• Adaptive sports, which contribute to the rehabilitation of military veterans, have deep roots, dating back to the 1700s.
• The expertise required to practice adaptive sports medicine is based on knowledge of the complexity of disability medicine and the uniqueness of the sports.
• Adaptive sports participants are challenged by the barriers of the disability, logistics, and complexity.
• In the long run, the upfront cost of sports equipment is a financially viable option for health care for individuals with disabilities.

## INTRODUCTION

At some point in our lives we all played catch, kicked a ball, ran a race, or played in an organized sport. Sports are ingrained in our society and are part of being a human. They bridge countries, cultures, and political divides. They teach individuals about goals, training, and the importance of a team. Members of the United States Armed Forces undergo training for physical fitness. The training also emphasizes the importance of teams and goals, such as completing a mission. When active duty members

Disclosure Statement: The authors have nothing to disclose.
[a] Spinal Cord Injury Division, Clement J Zablocki Veterans Affairs Medical Center, 5000 West National Avenue, SCI-128, Milwaukee, WI 53295, USA; [b] Department of Physical Medicine and Rehabilitation, Medical College of Wisconsin, Milwaukee, WI 53226, USA; [c] National Veterans Wheelchair Games, National Veterans Sports Programs and Special Events, US Department of Veterans Affairs, 810 Vermont Avenue, NW Washington, DC 20420, USA; [d] Emergency Medicine, Clement J Zablolcki Veterans Affairs Medical Center, 5000 West National Avenue, SCI-128, Milwaukee, WI 53295, USA; [e] Adaptive Sports Medicine Clinic, Spinal Cord Injury Division, Clement J Zablolcki Veterans Affairs Medical Center, 5000 West National Avenue, SCI-128, Milwaukee, WI 53295, USA; [f] Department of Emergency Medicine, Medical College of Wisconsin, Milwaukee, WI 53226, USA; [g] Men's U.S. National Sled Hockey Team, USA Hockey, Colorado Springs, CO, USA
* Corresponding author. 5000 West National Avenue, SCI-128, Milwaukee, WI 53295.
E-mail address: KENNETH.LEE8@VA.GOV

Phys Med Rehabil Clin N Am 30 (2019) 289–299
https://doi.org/10.1016/j.pmr.2018.08.001
1047-9651/19/Published by Elsevier Inc.
pmr.theclinics.com

of the United States Armed Forces or Veterans get inured, their previous training that emphasized perseverance, comradery, and team work make adaptive sports a perfect rehabilitation modality. Some will continue to play adaptive sports after completion of their rehabilitation for the continued health benefits and reintegration into the community. The introduction of adaptive sports to this unique population of disabled individuals helps with initial rehabilitation, and has lifelong physical, psychological, and social benefits.

There are many organizations throughout the world that promote adaptive sports. In addition, there are highly competitive venues for adaptive athletes, including the Warrior games for disabled Veterans from the US Armed Forces, and the Summer and Winter Paralympic Games. In 2013, Prince Harry of Wales helped create the Invictus Games for military veterans from around the world to "inspire recovery, support rehabilitation and generate a wider understanding and respect for those whose served their countries." (https://invictusgamesfoundation.org/)

Through the US Department of Veterans Affairs (VA) National Veterans Sports Programs and Special Events (NVSP&SE), veterans have additional opportunities in promoting health and healing through adaptive sports and recreation. One of the programs dates back to 1981.[1,2] The VA is a leader in rehabilitation sports programs and no other health care system offers the breadth of opportunities to empower and reinforce healthy activity and engagement following devastating injury or disease. Other programs sponsored by the Department of Defense or the community are the Endeavor and the Warrior Games.

## A BRIEF HISTORY OF ADAPTIVE SPORTS

Adaptive sports are played by individuals with varying disabilities and include a range of activities from simple maintenance of health and fitness to the elite sports of the Paralympic Games. Adaptive sports are defined by any modification of a given sport or recreational activity to accommodate an individual with a disability and their different ability levels. It is important to recognize that adaptive sports attempt to maintain the integrity of the original sport or game. For example, wheelchair basketball is a popular adaptive sport around the world. It is played on the same court with the same ball as able-body basketball. The athletes are in wheelchairs and play with minor modifications of certain rules that would apply to able bodies athletes. Adaptations of sport-specific equipment or special prosthetics led to competition in 22 different events in the 2016 Summer Paralympic Games and 6 events in the 2018 Winter Paralympic Games.[3] Today, the Paralympic Games are considered the pinnacle of adaptive sports. They showcase the athleticism and skill of disabled athletes from around the world. However, this was not always the case (**Fig. 1**).

In the late 1700s, in Sweden, adaptive sports began as medical gymnastics and underwent several revisions throughout the next century. Before that time, individuals with disabilities spent most of their lives on the margins of society or locked in institutions. The idea that physical activity and sport could aid in rehabilitation of the disabled eventually progressed to adaptive sport for recreation, and then to adaptive sport for competition.

Sir Ludwig Guttman (1899–1980) is considered to be the father of competitive adaptive sports.[4] Dr Guttman was a neurologist in Great Britain who introduced organized adaptive sports to his patients with spinal cord injuries (SCIs) as part of their rehabilitation program. He founded the National Spinal Injuries Center at the Stoke Mandeville Hospital, which hosted its First Annual Stoke Mandeville Games on July 28, 1948. This event was held on the same day as the opening ceremony of 1948 London

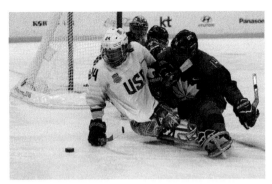

**Fig. 1.** United States Marine Corps Veteran, Josh Misiewicz, 2018 US Paralympic sled hockey team, PyungChang, South Korea. (*Courtesy of* Olympic Information Service/International Olympic Committee, Colorado Springs, CO, USA.)

Summer Olympics. It consisted of 16 paralyzed British military veterans and women engaged in an archery competition. This led to the establishment of International Stoke Mandeville Games in 1952. Then, in 1960, the Stoke Mandeville Games were held at the same time and location as the Olympic Games in Rome, Italy. This was considered the first Summer Paralympic Games, in which 400 athletes from 23 countries participated in 8 sports.

The history of adaptive sports in the United States is linked to military conflict, the civil rights movement, and the disabled rights movement. One of first laws addressed disabled military veterans from the Revolutionary War and was signed by President John Adams on July 16, 1798. The Military Disability Law provided an allotment for disabled veterans to help them reenter their communities.[5,6] Each military conflict has brought additional laws and support for disabled veterans. This has resulted in improved rehabilitation techniques, and the inclusion of adaptive sports and recreation therapy into treatment plans to help injured veterans recover from their wounds and return to society. The civil rights movement led to laws preventing all federal agencies from discriminating based on disability. Disability rights advocates pressed for passage of Architectural Barriers Act to ensure that there would be adequate access to public buildings for the disabled.

## ADAPTIVE SPORTS FOR MILITARY VETERANS

Whether veterans with disabilities use adaptive sports as a recreational pursuit or become an elite athlete, there is no denying the positive impact it has on the individual. Historically, it has been the combat wounded and returning service members who were the focus of adaptive sports programs through their rehabilitation, most notably those with SCIs and limb amputations.

One of the most visible programs in the United States is the VA's NVSP&SE, specifically the National Veteran Wheelchair Games (NVWG), which was founded by VA recreational therapists. The first NVWG was held in 1981 at the VA Medical Center (VAMC), Richmond, VA, hosting 74 veterans from 14 states. Since then, it has become the largest annual wheelchair and rehabilitation sports program in the world, hosting more than 550 disabled veterans from all 50 states.[2]

Other special VA adaptive sports programs include the National Disabled Veterans Winter Sports Clinic, National Disabled Veterans Summer Sports Clinic, and the National Disabled Veterans Training, Exposure, Experience (TEE) Tournament. These programs provide US military veterans a means to experience both summer and winter adaptive sports supported by VA physicians, clinical staff, physical therapists, recreational therapists, and prosthetists.[2] These programs expose disabled veterans to the VA's Rehabilitation Services and Prosthetic Services, Amputation System of Care, Automobile Adaptive Equipment, Blind Rehabilitation, Polytrauma–Traumatic Brain Injury System of Care, Recreation Therapy, and SCI System of Care and can provide the necessary equipment and expertise in adaptive sports (**Fig. 2**).

In addition, there is the annual Adaptive Sports Grant. This grant is a special program of the VA's NVSP&SE designated by Congress to support community organizations that provide adaptive sports and recreation services to veterans. This grant was initially authorized in 2013 as the US Paralympics Integrated Adaptive Sports Program. Now it provides 8 million dollars in annual funding to support more than 100 community adaptive sports programs that serve more than 10,000 disabled veterans.[2,7]

The VA is among the largest health care systems in the world, and it has been a pioneer in adaptive sports. US military veterans have access to equipment, services, and even training support to reach the elite level. Milwaukee VAMC is the first VA to set up an Adaptive Sports Medicine Clinic (ASMC) dedicated solely to adaptive sports with trained adaptive sports medicine physicians, physical therapists, and recreational therapists. This clinic provides medical evaluation and clearance for participation in VA-sponsored adaptive sport programs, treats injuries sustained during sporting events, and supports the medical justification for specialized equipment requisitions.

## ADAPTIVE SPORTS MEDICINE

Adaptive sports medicine combines the practice of disability medicine with sports medicine, incorporating knowledge of the specific sports and their patterns of injury and specialized equipment. In general, able-body sports medicine works with healthy individuals who succumb to a temporary illness and/or acute injury. The athletes tend to be in great physical condition with minimal underlying medical problems.

Adaptive sports medicine athletes have significant underlying medical or traumatic conditions, and complications related to the individual disability. There are also unique injuries related to the adaptive and assistive equipment used to compete.[8]

All adaptive sports athletes have baseline medical statuses that define their physical disability, such as SCI, amputation, polytrauma, and traumatic brain injury. Each condition is unique and must be understood by the individual athlete, as well as the health care provider. For example, an athlete with an SCI requires special attention to the care of the skin below the level of injury, especially when using tight-fitting adaptive

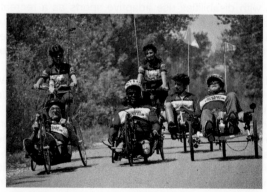

**Fig. 2.** Veterans handcycling group. (*Courtesy of* Badgerland Veterans Adaptive Sports Club, Milwaukee, WI, USA.)

equipment, and requires periodic pressure releases in endurance sports events. Understanding SCI and the potential for skin complications, along with equipment needs, can prevent devastating pressure injuries leading to potentially prolonged recovery.

A second example of the knowledge needed to understand the unique complications of an underlying disability is autonomic dysreflexia (AD). AD is a medical emergency that occurs in patients with SCI above thoracic nerve T6. It causes an imbalanced reflex sympathetic discharge and, if unrecognized or left untreated, can lead to potentially life-threatening hypertension, seizures, pulmonary edema, myocardial infarction, cerebral hemorrhage, and death.

Another example of the special medical needs when working with disabled athletes is knowledge of the proper care of a residual limb of an individual with an amputation. Many athletes with lower extremity amputations will push their limits and place their residual limbs at risk of damage and/or injury. Overuse of the residual limb in the socket of a prosthetic may result in a shift in hemodynamics that causes the limb to become edematous or ill-fitting, resulting in local trauma or skin breakdown. Specific knowledge of amputee care, including the use of stump shrinkers, skin protection, and evaluation of the socket fit, including gait, can mean the difference between the patient staying healthy and a medical complication that can affect the individual's activities of daily living.

Athletes involved in adaptive sports have many conditions that can affect their athletic performances and put them at higher risk than able-body athletes. One such injury is fracture. Many athletes with SCI have osteoporosis in their lower extremities. This places them at a higher risk for fractures. Fractures are not an uncommon condition seen in sports medicine. However, treatment of the fracture can be very different for an athlete with an SCI. Full-contact casts are not recommended unless there is compromise to a neurovascular structure due to impaired or absent sensation.

Another common condition that sports medicine providers commonly treat is overuse injuries. Overuse is common in able-body athletes because they push their limits during their training and competition. For athletes with disabilities, especially those who use wheelchairs as their main means of mobility, overuse injuries of the upper extremities can compromise mobility, independence, and the ability to perform basic activities of daily living. Many wheelchair users suffer from chronic tendinitis and bursitis of their shoulder, elbow, and wrist joints. As they add increased training load for competitions, their joints undergo superinflammation. Overuse can be a challenging problem to treat because it involves finding the right balance between performance and treatment, which often involves extended periods of rest.

In addition to these examples, many athletes with disabilities suffer from mental health conditions. These include depression, posttraumatic stress disorder (PTSD), and body image distortion. Athletes in this category can have exacerbation of these conditions during training or competition. Situational depression is a natural phenomenon for athletes when they lose an event but those who have depression due to their medical condition are at a higher risk for clinical depression; losing an event may trigger a relapse.

Many veterans suffer from PTSD. This is a major factor to consider while delivering care as an adaptive sports medicine provider in military veteran settings. During the opening and the closing ceremonies of the 2016 Invictus Games in Orlando, Florida, special plans were developed to identify and treat veterans experiencing PTSD. The ceremonies featured loud and extremely bright fireworks, as well as military helicopter flyovers, in the setting of a tightly packed crowd. These are all common triggers for military veterans suffering from PTSD. Athletes who have undergone a PTSD exacerbation during these events must have quick and safe access to treatment.

Adaptive sports medicine physicians who care for elite athletes or cover high-level adaptive sporting events may be exposed to athletes who are doping or boosting. As with any able-body sports, there are regulations that prohibit use of certain substances, methods, and medications in sport, including performance-enhancing drugs.[9] Athletes who have a medical need for medication that is banned in or out of competition in their sport can apply for a therapeutic use exemption (TUE) with the assistance of their sports medicine physician. The TUE will be reviewed by a committee associated with the individual sport, the US Anti-Doping Agency, or the International Paralympic Committee, depending on the sport and upcoming competition. One of the significant challenges for the TUE committee is the justifying of the medical necessity of a banned substance.

In addition to performance-enhancing drugs, there are natural physiologic conditions that are unique to SCI patients that can create an unfair advantage. One such tactic, termed boosting, is the use of AD in high-level athletes with SCIs.[10–12] The athlete would attempt purposefully cause AD to improve performance in endurance events. Typical ways to cause AD include increasing fluid intake before an event and then clamping a Foley catheter to cause bladder distention, or purposefully causing a noxious stimulus in an extremity. This is a high-risk, life-threatening practice and is considered as doping by the International Paralympic Committee. However, it is a very difficult scenario to monitor and prove.

Medical support for adaptive sports medicine must have all the able-body sports medical logistics but also must accommodate the various disabilities of adaptive sports athletes. To treat an individual with a PTSD exacerbation, a quiet room with a trained professional knowledgeable about PTSD is necessary. Examination tables must accommodate ease of transfer, as well as the lack of trunk control of many of the athletes. The medical clinic must be accessible to wheelchairs and to individuals with other movement disorders. Staff and volunteers involved in providing medical services must be educated on disability-specific medical emergencies and procedures, such as how to transfer in and out of the adaptive equipment. Another interesting and important aspect of adaptive sports medicine is the nonmedical logistical support that the medical staff provides during travels with an adaptive sports team. There are settings in which the medical provider is involved in fixing or modifying the adaptive sports equipment, driving a supply vehicle, and even helping find accessible restaurants for the team. As stated previously, it is important for an adaptive sports physician to know about the lives of the athletes with disabilities, including their equipment.

## THE BENEFITS OF ADAPTIVE SPORTS OR WHY DO WE NEED ADAPTIVE SPORTS?

A study by Lundberg and colleagues[13] found that the research participants felt stigmatized and stereotyped. Their adaptive sports and recreation participation provided them with opportunities to build social networks and experience freedom and success, positively compare themselves with others without disabilities, and feel a sense of normalcy. This brought them to the identity negotiating process. As potential athletes find themselves in this identity negotiating process through adaptive sports, understanding the exercise regimen becomes essential.

According to American College of Sports Medicine (ACSM) and the American Heart Association (AHA), individuals need moderate-intensity aerobic physical activity for a minimum of 30 minutes on 5 days each week or vigorous-intensity aerobic physical activity for a minimum of 20 minutes on 3 days each week to promote and maintain health.[14] In May of 2014, the Centers for Disease Control and Prevention recognized that individuals with physical disabilities have barriers that hinder physical activities.[15]

They reported that individuals with physical disabilities have the highest rate of inactivity of all the disability groups. The report also cited that 1 in 2 adults with disabilities get no aerobic physical activity compared with the 1 in 4 adults without disabilities. Finally, the report stated that adults with disabilities are 3 times more likely to have heart disease, stroke, diabetes, or cancer than adults without disabilities.

The barriers to physical activities can be divided into psychological, physiologic, and environmental factors. Psychological factors include low self-esteem and low confidence, decreased motivation, increased depression and pain, and higher stress. All these negatively affect quality-of-life (QOL) scores. Physiologic components include chronic health conditions, altered bowel and bladder function, irregular thermoregulation, and uncontrolled autonomic feedback. Environmental components include lack of accessible equipment and accessible exercise arenas, the prohibitive cost of adaptive equipment, and lack of experts in adaptive sports.

Benefits of adaptive sports come in 3 categories: psychological, physical, and social. Psychological benefits include increase in self-efficacy and confidence, higher motivation and optimism, and decreased depression and stress. These factors significantly improve QOL. The physical benefits include increased strength and coordination, higher balance and flexibility, improved independence performing activities of daily living, and decreased rate of chronic morbidities. Positive social implications include decreased discrimination, higher rate of employment and peer acceptance, improved communication skills, and friendship.

The literature supports how adaptive sports and recreation provide improvement in QOL, mental health improvement, and general health well-being.[16–19] Much of the evidence is anecdotal, generalized, and not prospectively researched.

A key outcome of adaptive sports and recreation is that it helps one attain employment after his or her disability. Most rehabilitation textbooks report 10% to 60% of individuals with an SCI return to employment, with most sources indicating 15% to 30%. One objective study showed that participating in the NVWG helped nearly 50% of veterans attain employment.[20] This is the first study that explored the perception of veterans on employment opportunities through participating in a NVSP&SE program.

## BREAKING DOWN THE BARRIERS

Adults with disabilities have inherent barriers due to physical and mental health impairments from chronic conditions such as SCI. There are many factors that can overcome some of the barriers, including increased opportunities (emergence of adaptive sport and recreation programs across the country), better education (more knowledge about techniques to accommodate for disability), and improved equipment (technological advances for overcoming limitations).

Many health care professionals lack the experience to provide guidance on adaptive sports. However, programs such as the Spaulding Adaptive Sports Medicine Clinic, Boston, Massachusetts, and the Milwaukee VAMC's ASMC are providing highly specialized care with staff trained in adaptive sports. When working with individuals with disabilities, it is important to know the background of adaptive sports and the chronic conditions of the individual receiving care. One must match and recommend aerobic physical activity options that match each person's specific disability and connect the individual with the appropriate adaptive programs.

The basics in getting individuals with disabilities involved in physical activities revolve around 5 factors[15]: (1) It is important to know the physical activity guidelines. Each individual should be educated on proper physical activity guidelines based on his or her disability and on the recommendation of the ACSM and AHA. (2) Ask about physical activity. Just because an individual has physical disability does not preclude them from the general inquiries about their current fitness schedule and goals or plan for increasing activities. It is important to look beyond the disability and put the person first. Proper disability etiquette is essential during this conversation. (3) Discuss the barriers to physical activity. This is a crucial step in adaptive sports consultation. Physical barriers are the reason many individuals with disabilities do not participate in adaptive sports. (4) Recommend physical activity options. It is important to address any barriers and physical limitations that effect participation in adaptive sports. Based on these findings, one can determine various options that are available for adaptive sports participation. Therefore, having the knowledge, or the resources, to refer the patient to appropriate adaptive sports programs is important. (5) Refer the patient to resources and programs. This last step is the beginning of the follow-through in adaptive sports. Referral to community programs that provide appropriate adaptive sports is the beginning of activities for an individual. It is vital that local programs have a relationship with the provider referring the person with disability so their progress can be followed.

## ADAPTIVE SPORTS LOGISTICS

Adaptive sports are resource-intensive and beginning athletes and programs are challenged by multiple barriers that must be overcome. Even the simple question of "Where do we play?" must be addressed. Many considerations should be taken into account when planning an adaptive sports program. For example, the accessibility of the event location must be considered and adapted as necessary. In addition, any adaptive equipment needed for the adaptive sport must be obtained. Wheelchair lacrosse is a new and emerging adaptive sport that is a good example of how to develop an adaptive sport program.

Wheelchair lacrosse founders stayed in the mainstream of not altering the sport of lacrosse but just adapting to it. However, there were barriers to overcome. Able-body lacrosse is played on grass but wheelchair lacrosse cannot be. So, the setting needed to be on a hard surface such as a de-iced hockey rink. Although it is easy to find large grass fields to host multiple lacrosse games, it is difficult to find enclosed rinks that are side-by-side or even in close proximity. Therefore, there are limits to the number of teams that can compete in a day. Typical locker rooms do not accommodate wheelchairs, so the teams must bring their own mobile storage. Protective gloves wear out within a weekend because wheelchair maneuvers shred them. The sports chairs endure wear and tear due to sport being used in a full-contact sport (**Fig. 3**).

Other adaptive sports have similar barriers and challenges, such as goalball for the visually impaired. It requires a quiet gymnasium, therefore the gym cannot be simultaneously used for other sports. Constant taping and retaping of the court wires (tactile

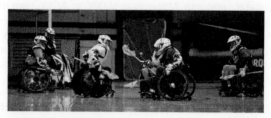

**Fig. 3.** Milwaukee Eagles wheelchair lacrosse team. (*Courtesy of* Wisconsin Adaptive Sports Association, Brookfield, WI, USA.)

court markings for the visually impaired athletes), as well as transportation of the athletes to venues, are important factors for a successful program.

Transportation is identified as a top barrier for persons with disability. Many adaptive sports require travel to different venues. Flights are challenging for many athletes with disabilities and hotels often have a limited number of accessible rooms. Many are unable to drive, so they depend on others. Renting a vehicle that has wheelchair accessibility and/or hand controls for driving is a major barrier. Usually, only 1 or 2 athletes can fit into a regular vehicle, considering the equipment they need to haul.

Sports that involve special equipment, such as the sports chairs, sledge hockey sleds, throwing stands for field events, racing chairs for track, and handcycles, are costly and require maintenance. Adaptive sports equipment is often custom-fitted, with cost ranging from $1200 to more than $10,000 each. Once procured, the toughest hurdle is storing and transporting the equipment to practices and events. Consider an individual with paraplegia who participates in paratriathlon. For this individual to travel to an event, she or he would need to travel with their own personal chair, a racing chair, and a handcycle. If she or he is competing in a court event, such as wheelchair basketball, then this must be added to the inventory such as commode and shower chairs. In addition, personal medical equipment, such as commode and shower chairs, must be included. This is just a single individual. If an entire team is traveling, the logistics and cost of transporting equipment is monumental.

These and other barriers to adaptive sports and recreation are described in a 2014 Summary Report from an Adaptive Sports and Recreation Expo held in Milwaukee, Wisconsin.[21] It showed that many participants of the Expo perceived the biggest barriers to participation in adaptive sport and recreation were transportation, lack of function, and caregiver availability. Many members of organizations supporting adaptive sports have a lower socioeconomic status, which limits their ability to purchase personalized adaptive sports equipment.

## ADAPTIVE SPORTS: IS IT WORTH IT?

Spending large amount of taxpayer's funds to purchase costly adaptive sports equipment can be questioned by those skeptical about the benefits of adaptive sports programs. A literature search provides 1 research study that showed a cost-benefit to providing physical activity to individuals with disability versus individuals without disability.[22] One of the best ways to demonstrate the cost-effectiveness of adaptive sports is through case studies.

Case 1. A 30-year-old veteran with T10 paraplegia and substance abuse postinjury had been in and out of rehabilitation for his substance abuse, as well as needing admission for medical reasons. Review of the cost for taking care of this veterans during the 5-year period of his substance abuse was more than 1 million dollars. This veteran was introduced to adaptive sports and was able to complete and sustain his substance abuse rehabilitation to stay in compliance with the various sports rules. A 3-year review of this veteran's care cost since his involvement in adaptive sports is $23,000. Most of this cost was in purchasing a specialty sports chair, a racing chair, and a handcycle. The veteran is now attending full-time school and seeking employment after graduation.

Case 2. A 44-year-old veteran with bilateral transtibial amputation from a roadside bomb during the Gulf War has been suffering from PTSD and various sequelae from the injury. This veteran initially had multiple visits to the VA due to adjustment issues. The VA spent $1800 during the initial phase of his rehabilitation for a basketball wheelchair. He is still using this chair after 20 years of playing wheelchair basketball and attributes his current and stable mental wellbeing to adaptive sports.

Case 3. A 72-year-old veteran with hereditary spastic paraplegia has not ventured out of the house for more than 6 years since decline in his neurologic condition. He has been visiting the outpatient clinic frequently with multiple admissions for various health reasons. Cost analysis for the veteran for the 6 years was more than $800,000. The veteran was introduced to adaptive sports and was tracked for 2 years on his hospital utilization and cost. The total cost was $4000 for 2 years, with half of it spent on an all-sports chair. Since his introduction to adaptive sports, the veteran had no hospital admissions, a significant decrease in utilization of the outpatient clinics, has bought a vehicle and a trailer, and has been participating in 5 different adaptive sports.

These cases exemplify how access to adaptive sports programs and equipment provided by the VA and local community programs can promote a healthy and active life style. This, in turn, has a positive impact on the individual and society by decreasing health care costs.

## SUMMARY

Adaptive sports and recreation can change the lives of those living with a disability. Individuals can be introduced to adaptive sports at any time during or after their initial rehabilitation. The many benefits, including physical fitness, psychological wellbeing, decreased health care costs, and reintegration into society, can last a lifetime. Physicians who treat adaptive athletes must have knowledge of the underlying disability, the specialized equipment, and the challenges adaptive athletes face on the field of play and in daily life. Adaptive sports are truly inspiring and will continue to amaze spectators and improve lives well into the future.

## REFERENCES

1. Annual report for FY2014: VA National Veterans Sports Programs & Special Events. U.S. Department of Veterans Affairs, Veterans Health Administration; 2014. Available at: https://www.va.gov/adaptivesports/docs/VA_Adaptive_Sport_Grant_Annual_Report.pdf. Accessed September 20, 2017.
2. Fact Sheet: VA National Veterans Sports Programs & Special Events. U.S. Department of Veterans Affairs, Veterans Health Administration; 2018. Available at: https://www.va.gov/adaptivesports/docs/Fact_Sheet_NVSPSE.pdf. Accessed September 20, 2017.
3. Paralympic movement, International Paralympic committee. Available at: https://www.paralympic.org/. Accessed September 20, 2017.
4. Dr. Guttman and the paralympic movement. The history press. Available at: https://www.thehistorypress.co.uk/articles/dr-guttman-and-the-paralympic-movement/. Accessed September 20, 2017.
5. A brief history of disability in the United States and Massachusetts. Massachusetts Office on Disability; 2016. Available at: https://blog.mass.gov/mod/tag/disability-history/. Accessed September 20, 2017.
6. De Luigi J. History of adaptive and disabled rights within society, thus creating the fertile soil to grow, adaptive sports. In: De Luigi J, editor. Adaptive sports medicine. Cham (Switzerland): Springer; 2018. p. 3–15.
7. Adaptive sports grant: VA National Veterans Sports Programs & Special Events. U.S. Department of Veterans Affairs, Veterans Health Administration; 2018.

Available at: https://www.va.gov/adaptivesports/va_grant_program.asp. Accessed September 20, 2017.

8. De Luigi J. Medical considerations in adaptive sports. In: De Luigi J, editor. Adaptive sports medicine. Cham (Switzerland): Springer; 2018. p. 59–69.
9. De Luigi J. Controversies in adaptive sports. In: De Luigi J, editor. Adaptive sports medicine. Cham (Switzerland): Springer; 2018. p. 385–92.
10. Webborn A. "Boosting" performance in disability sport. Br J Sports Med 1999; 33(2):74–5.
11. Blauwet C, Benjamin-Laing H, Stomphorst J, et al. Testing for boosting at the Paralympic games: policies, results and future directions. Br J Sports Med 2013;47(13):832–7.
12. Krassioukov A, West C. The role of autonomic function on sport performance in athletes with spinal cord injury. PM R 2014;6(8 Suppl):S58–65.
13. Lundberg N, Taniguchi S, McCormick B, et al. Identity negotiating: redefining stigmatized identities through adaptive sports and recreation participation among individuals with a disability. J Leis Res 2011;43(2):206.
14. Haskell W, Lee I, Pate R, et al. Physical activity and public health, updated recommendation for adults from the American College of Sports Medicine and the American Heart Association. Circulation 2007;116:1081–93.
15. Adults with disabilities, vital signs, center for disease control and prevention. 2014. Available at: https://www.cdc.gov/vitalsigns/disabilities/index.html. Accessed January 10, 2018.
16. Lundberg N, Bennett J, Smith S. Outcomes of adaptive sports and recreation participation among veterans returning from combat with acquired disability. Ther Recreational J 2011;45(2):105–20.
17. Prout B, Porter H. Psychosocial outcomes of participation in adaptive sports for adults with spinal cord injuries: a systematic review of the literature. Am J Recreat Ther 2017;16(1):39–47.
18. Hawkins B, Cory L, Crowe B. Effects of participation in a paralympic military sports camp on injured service members: implications for therapeutic recreation. Ther Recreation J 2011;45(4):309–25.
19. Scherer M, Gade D, Yancosek K. Efficacy of an adaptive kayaking intervention for improving health-related quality of life among wounded, ill, and injured service members. Am J Recreat Ther 2013;12(3):8–16.
20. Kim W, Lee L, Lans D, et al. Perception of employment by the veterans participating in the national veterans wheelchair games: a survey study. PM R 2018; 10(3):263–8.
21. Iverson M, Braza D, Lee K. 2014 summary report: EveryBODY plays! Adaptive sports and recreation expo. The Medical College of Wisconsin 2015. Available at: http://www1.mcw.edu/FileLibrary/Groups/PhysicalMedicineRehabilitation/Adaptive-sports-expo/SummaryReportEveryBODYPlays2014.pdf. Accessed January 10, 2018.
22. Xu X, Ozturk O, Turk M, et al. Physical activity and disability: an analysis on how activity might lower medical expenditures. J Phys Act Health 2018;15(8):564–71.

# Moving?

## Make sure your subscription moves with you!

To notify us of your new address, find your **Clinics Account Number** (located on your mailing label above your name), and contact customer service at:

Email: journalscustomerservice-usa@elsevier.com

800-654-2452 (subscribers in the U.S. & Canada)
314-447-8871 (subscribers outside of the U.S. & Canada)

Fax number: 314-447-8029

Elsevier Health Sciences Division
Subscription Customer Service
3251 Riverport Lane
Maryland Heights, MO 63043

*To ensure uninterrupted delivery of your subscription, please notify us at least 4 weeks in advance of move.

CPI Antony Rowe
Eastbourne, UK
March 22, 2019